Your Workout
PERFECTED

Nick Tumminello

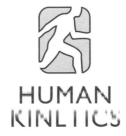

HUMAN KINETICS

Library of Congress Cataloging-in-Publication Data

Names: Tumminello, Nick, author.
Title: Your workout perfected / Nick Tumminello.
Description: Champaign, Ill. : Human Kinetics, 2019. | Includes
  bibliographical references.
Identifiers: LCCN 2018007762 (print) | LCCN 2017051930 (ebook) | ISBN
  9781492558149 (ebook) | ISBN 9781492558132 (print)
Subjects: LCSH: Physical fitness. | Exercise. | Weight training.
Classification: LCC GV481 (print) | LCC GV481 .T85 2019 (ebook) | DDC
  613.7--dc23
LC record available at https://lccn.loc.gov/2018007762

ISBN: 978-1-4925-5813-2 (print)

This publication is written and published to provide accurate and authoritative information relevant to the subject matter presented. It is published and sold with the understanding that the author and publisher are not engaged in rendering legal, medical, or other professional services by reason of their authorship or publication of this work. If medical or other expert assistance is required, the services of a competent professional person should be sought.

The web addresses cited in this text were current as of March 2018, unless otherwise noted.

Acquisitions Editor: Roger W. Earle
Developmental Editor: Laura Pulliam
Senior Managing Editor: Amy Stahl
Copyeditor: Michelle Horn
Senior Graphic Designer: Nancy Rasmus
Cover Designer: Keri Evans
Cover Design Associate: Susan Rothermel Allen
Photograph (front and back cover): © Human Kinetics
Photographs (interior): © Human Kinetics, unless otherwise noted
Photo Asset Manager: Laura Fitch
Photo Production Coordinator: Amy M. Rose
Photo Production Manager: Jason Allen
Senior Art Manager: Kelly Hendren
Printer: Sheridan Books

We thank The ZOO Health Club in Oakland Park, Florida, for assistance in providing the location for the photo shoot for this book.

Human Kinetics books are available at special discounts for bulk purchase. Special editions or book excerpts can also be created to specification. For details, contact the Special Sales Manager at Human Kinetics.

Printed in the United States of America   10 9 8 7 6 5 4 3 2 1

The paper in this book is certified under a sustainable forestry program. The paper in this book was manufactured using responsible forestry methods.

Human Kinetics
P.O. Box 5076
Champaign, IL 61825-5076
Website: www.HumanKinetics.com

In the United States, email info@hkusa.com or call 800-747-4457.

In Canada, email info@hkcanada.com.

In the United Kingdom/Europe, email hk@hkeurope.com.

For information about Human Kinetics' coverage in other areas of the world, please visit our website:
www.HumanKinetics.com

E7180

Your Workout
PERFECTED

Contents

PART I   Training Objectives

PART II   Exercises

PART III Programming

Exercise Finder

Chapter 5   Warm-Up and Mobility Exercises

Chapter 6   Upper-Body Exercises

Chapter 7   Lower-Body Exercises

Chapter 8   Core Exercises

Chapter 9   Conditioning Exercises

Acknowledgments

This book would not be possible if it weren't for several people. My good friend and business associate David Crump came up with the book's title. Eileen Escarda of Escarda Photo took all of the great exercise photos, along with the exercise models used in the photos: Jay Bozios, Serina Branch, Juli Lopez, and Korin Sutton. Gil Krohn and the staff at the ZOO Health Club in Oakland Park, Florida, allowed us to do the photo shoot at their facility. Jason Silvernail, DPT, coauthored chapter 15 with me. Many thanks to the Human Kinetics family—with special thanks to Justin Klug, Jeff Mathis, Roger Earle, and Laura Pulliam—for their involvement and hard work with me on this book. It's truly a privilege to work with these professionals in bringing this project to life, and I'm honored that they'll forever be a part of this book.

I'm so lucky that I get so much love and support from my mother, Faith Bevan; her husband, John Cavaliere; my father, Dominic Tumminello; my girlfriend, Romina Marinaro; and my close friends, Marc and Brenda Spataro, Kate and Daniel Blankenship, Ryan Huether, Rob Simonelli, Billy Beck, Deanna Avery, Paul Christopher, and Joe Drake from Gravity and Oxygen in Boca Raton, Florida.

As I think about all the people in the fitness and performance training field or related fields who have been a part of my life, I'm reminded that there's no such thing as a self-made person. I owe a debt of gratitude to the following colleagues for their friendship, continued support of my work, and help in my professional growth: John Rallo; Sivan Fagan; Nick Clayton; Brad Schoenfeld; Jim Kielbaso; Bert Sorin, Richard Sorin, and the Sorinex Equipment family; Matt Paulson, Ryan Ketchum, and the Fitness Revolution family; Nick Bromberg; Ethan and Liz Benda; Shelley Murray; Lindsay Vastola; Tim Arndt; Ben Cormack; Isa Olsson; Eric Helms; Karen Litzy; Bret Contreras; Alan Aragon; Lou Schuler; Luke Johnson; Chris Burgess; Mark Comerford; Bob Rossetti, Ron Rossetti, and the Northeast Seminars family; Dave Parise; Joel Seedman; Vince McConnell; Billy Beck; Jason Silvernail; Lars Avemarie; Bill Sonnemaker; James Fell; Tony Gentilcore; Marie Spano; David Jack; Tyler Christiansen; Quinn Sypniewski; Adrianne Ortiz; Bob Esquerre; Jeremy Boyd; Anastasis Charalambous; Jonathan Goodman; Andrew Vigotsky; Claudia Micco; Espen Arntzen; Steve Weatherford; Andrew Heffernan; John Spencer Ellis; Lee Boyce; Jonathan Mike; Robert Linkul; Nick Collias; Leah Lyons; Neil Pecker; Kennet Waale; Serkan Yimsel; Ian Houghton; Lara McGlashan; Chris Shugart; Matthew Sandstead; Rick Howard; and Elisabeth Fouts and the Power Systems family. I'm sure there are other people whose names deserve to be on this list. I owe those people a big handshake and a hug.

Finally, I thank all my clients—past, present, and future—for allowing me to continue to do what I love.

Introduction

If you're looking for a straightforward, realistic guide to working out that helps ensure that the work you're putting in is as smart, safe, efficient, and effective as possible, look no further!

There are four reasons most people work out: for fat loss, to build muscle, to improve function and performance, or for general fitness and health. This book simplifies the science and techniques behind each of these goals, clarifies misconceptions, and provides you with a variety of specific workout plans—gym workouts and bodyweight workouts—that you can use for each of the goals.

Chapter 1 focuses on fitness. If you always feel like you're failing when it comes to exercise because you're not interested in organizing your entire life around the gym, then chapter 1 is perfect for you! As discussed in chapter 1 and elsewhere in the book, exercising for general fitness and health purposes is a great goal to have. You don't always have to exercise for functional performance or a physique-related goal—the key is to understand who you are and what you want out of exercise.

Next, chapter 2 looks at function and performance. Chapter 3 is about fat loss. And chapter 4 is on the topic of physique. Each of the first four chapters identifies common myths that can create confusion and hold you back from improving in each of these four goals. These chapters also establish the scientific principles and methods you need to know in order to enjoy long-term success.

In chapter 5, Warm-Up and Mobility Exercises, you're provided with several warm-up sequences that get you ready for action so you can get more out of each workout. Chapters 6 through 9 detail a wide variety of exercises for the upper body (chapter 6), lower body (chapter 7), and the core (chapter 8) as well as exercises for conditioning (chapter 9). What makes these chapters unique is that in addition to providing easy-to-follow exercise descriptions, they also include a section on ways to perfect basic exercises, showing you how to do these exercises better than the way they are commonly performed.

Chapters 10 through 14 are the workout programming chapters, where everything you've learned in the previous chapters is put into action. Each of these chapters provides a multitude of workout programs for you to choose from depending on how many days per week you prefer to exercise based on your schedule. Chapter 10, General Beginner Programs, provides a workout plan for those who are just starting out or who haven't done any regular strength training in a while. Chapter 11, Fitness Programs, features workout plans for those who want to improve and maintain their overall health and fitness without necessarily focusing on a specific programming goal. Chapter 12, Function and Performance Programs, provides workout plans for those who aren't making a career in athletics but are interested in improving overall athleticism. Chapter 13, Fat Loss Programs, features workout plans for those who want to lose body fat while minimizing muscle loss. Chapter 14, Physique Programs, provides workout plans for those who are focused on aesthetics and are exercising to maximize muscle size.

All the workout programs provided in this book have been designed with the big-box gym member in mind. For instance, the programs combine exercises requiring immobile equipment (e.g., squat rack or machine) with exercises using mobile equipment (e.g., dumbbells, resistance bands). This mixture enables you to bring the mobile equipment to the immobile equipment and remain there without having to walk all over the gym and lose the equipment you're using to another member.

Since we're not always able to get to the gym and don't always have access to all the exercise equipment we'd like to use, chapters 10 through 14 also feature two alternative home gym workouts and two bodyweight workouts you can use to stay on track while training at home or on the road in a small hotel gym with limited equipment and space.

Although each of the programs provided in chapters 10, 11, 12, 13, and 14 is focused on a different training goal, the programs in each of these chapters involve many of the same exercises. This is because everyone should be doing upper-body exercises, lower-body exercises, and core exercises to ensure that their workouts are comprehensive. It's how those exercises are applied, organized, and priori- tized that makes the training programs in each chapter unique for each training goal. In other words, the programs in each of the programming chapters are set up differently because each emphasizes a different goal. This doesn't mean that you won't gain any muscle when doing the function and performance programs provided in chapter 12, or that you won't get stronger when using the fat loss training programs provided in chapter 13, for example. The benefits you'll get from doing the workouts in this book aren't mutually exclusive. But because the workout plans featured in chapters 10 through 14 each have a different emphasis, you will achieve the most in the area emphasized.

Regardless of the emphasis that you choose to focus on, the most import- ant factor is your ability to continue your workouts, and that means staying injury free. The final chapter of this book, chapter 15, Strategies for Minimizing Injury, identifies several potential risk factors for injury and provides simple and practical exercise recommendations you can use with any type of workout program to reduce your risk of suffering an injury.

If you're an inexperienced exerciser, you will appreciate the clear and user- friendly manner the information and workouts provided in this book are delivered in. If you're an advanced exerciser, fitness professional, or sport coach, you will certainly recognize the effectiveness of the training methods utilized here and will gain exciting new ideas, insights, and strategies for exercise programming.

Let's get to work!

PART I
Training Objectives

1 { Fitness

If you're like most people, you're not interested in being a gym rat who organizes your entire life around food and gyms. When it comes to diet, most people don't change their eating habits all that much, so they're mainly exercising to offset the foods they love to eat. And when it comes to exercising, most people aren't trying to win a contest for the best body on the beach. They're also not interested in chasing impressive lifting numbers. When people exercise, with or without the guidance of a personal trainer, they just want a great workout experience that challenges them but doesn't hurt them. They often gauge their success by how much they've enjoyed each workout, how they feel at the end of the workout, and how many workouts they've completed per week. If this sounds like you, then this chapter and the corresponding workout programs have your name on them!

Benefits of Resistance Training

Resistance training is most often associated with improvements in both aesthetics and athletics, since resistance training helps you develop muscle and strength. But what about the general fitness and health benefits of resistance training? Using resistance training as regular physical exercise has many benefits for your body and your mind.

Weight Management

In addition to its potential effectiveness in the prevention and treatment of metabolic syndrome, regular resistance training can help improve body composition (1,2).

You don't have to be a cardiologist to know that carrying extra body fat (i.e., being overweight) can place more stress on your heart and put you at a greater risk of dealing with health concerns, such as diabetes, increased blood pressure, high cholesterol, and an increased risk of heart attack.

Lower Risk of Disease, Death, and Functional Limitation

In addition to maintaining a healthier weight, creating higher levels of muscular strength by using a regular resistance training program is associated with a lower risk of all-cause mortality, fewer cardiovascular disease events, and a lower risk of developing functional limitations (3,4,5).

More Energy, Less Fatigue

Research indicates that regular resistance training may increase one's energy levels while decreasing feelings of fatigue (6). This comes as no surprise, since resistance training can help improve body composition. Put simply, carrying around more body fat makes you work harder both in life and in sport. Therefore, the more extra body fat you've got, the faster you'll get tired and feel fatigued. Following a regular resistance exercise plan can help you drop fat, especially when combined with good nutritional habits, and will help you to become more energy efficient and feel better throughout the day.

Bone Loss Prevention

In addition to promoting muscle strength and mass, resistance training also effectively increases bone mass (i.e., bone mineral density and content) and bone strength. It may reduce the chance of developing a musculoskeletal disorder (e.g., conditions of the bones, muscles, joints, and ligaments), such as osteoporosis (7,8). Additionally, resistance training may help slow or even reverse loss of bone mass in people with osteoporosis (9).

Reduced Anxiety and Depression

Research supports that resistance training, and physical exercise in general, may prevent and improve depression and anxiety. Studies dating back to 1981 have concluded that regular exercise, such as resistance training, can not only improve mood in people with mild to moderate depression but also may play a supporting role in treating severe depression. Other research has even found that exercise's effects lasted longer than those of antidepressants (10).

Research has also shown that physical exercise reduces anxiety by affecting the brain's response to stress. This evidence suggests that active people might be less susceptible to the undesirable aspects of stress and anxiety than sedentary people (11).

Improved Brain Function

Scientists once thought that our brains stopped producing new cells early in life, but more recently, it's been discovered that we continue to manufacture new brain cells throughout our lifetimes. The most potent stimulant for brain growth is physical exercise.

Research has shown that physical activity seems to stimulate the production of new brain cells and neurons and promotes their survival. This facilitates attention and concentration and helps lock in memories as they form. In later years, physical activity was associated with lower risks of cognitive impairment, Alzheimer's disease, and dementia in general (12). Another study concluded that, if exercise began by early middle age, it further reduced the risk of developing Alzheimer's (13).

Better Sleep

Sleep is the way our bodies rest and recover. Exercise elevates mood and reduces stress, and research has documented that exercise improves sleep patterns, which can help you become more alert in the daytime and helps promote better sleep habits at night (14).

Let's face it: If you're regularly exercising, especially with a challenging resistance training program, your body will need to rest and recover, making it likely that your sleep will improve.

Using resistance training to stay active and improve overall fitness and health while also enjoying the physical challenge it provides is a worthwhile goal. I just gave you seven scientifically founded reasons why.

Cardiovascular Exercise, HIIT, Muscle, and Beginners

Some say steady-state cardio interferes with muscle gains. But research indicates that in previously untrained men, adding low-impact aerobic exercise (like

Personal Trainers and Your General Health and Fitness

There are many obvious benefits of exercise, like building muscle and improved strength. There are also numerous, well-evidenced physical and mental health benefits that many trainers seem to be unaware of.

These include, as discussed earlier, disease prevention, preservation of bone mass, improved mood (even in those with depression), anxiety/stress reduction, improved sleep, an enhanced feeling of energy and well-being, the delay of all-cause mortality, and even brain growth.

Yet many personal trainers have this elitist idea that you're basically wasting your time working out unless you're training with a specific focus on physique or performance measures. This feeling is directed at recreational gym-goers who are working out for general fitness and health purposes but not focusing on a specific physique or lifting performance goals.

Many trainers look down on people who exercise for fitness and health, proclaiming that these people are "satisfied with being mediocre," as if those not interested in organizing their entire lives around gyms and food are somehow inferior humans.

These same trainers continue to be frustrated, wondering why some people "don't get it" or "don't care" as much as they do and ultimately end up not sticking around. But it's usually not that these people don't care; it's that they don't care about what the trainer wants them to care about. These trainers are the ones who just don't get it.

These personal trainers fail to realize that to most people, "getting results" from exercising isn't about achieving impressive deadlift numbers or building a wider back—those are gym rat goals. It simply means staying active, overcoming physical challenges, and enjoying each workout. Those are respectable and reasonable goals that personal trainers should encourage and be proud to facilitate.

cycling) doesn't jeopardize gains in strength or muscle size. In fact, it may even increase muscular gains (17).

Other evidence shows that aerobic exercise improves muscle size and aerobic capacity. These improvements are similar between younger and older men (18). It's likely that these results also apply to women because aerobic exercise alters protein metabolism and induces skeletal muscle hypertrophy. Ironically, it can also serve as an effective countermeasure for both women and men prone to muscle loss (19).

But keep these study results in perspective. They involve untrained people. As high-intensity interval training (HIIT) has grown in popularity, the standard 30-minute bout of steady-state aerobic training (the low-to-medium intensity exercise on a treadmill, elliptical, or bicycle) has become less popular. If you're just starting or restarting an exercise program, beginning with HIIT may increase your odds for injury.

It's a better idea to start with low-intensity aerobic exercise until you can run or use the elliptical or bike for about 30 consecutive minutes at a moderate intensity to increase your aerobic fitness. This gives you a better foundation for using high-intensity conditioning methods (16).

Steady-state cardio affects trained individuals. Look at bodybuilders: For years, they have been doing steady-state cardio while prepping for their shows and are able to maintain impressive amounts of muscle mass. This can't simply be chalked up to the influence of drugs, because there are plenty of natural bodybuilders who do this as well.

It's unrealistic to think that doing a reasonable amount of steady-state cardio will automatically cause you to lose hard-earned muscle, especially if you're emphasizing resistance training. For the intermediate or advanced exerciser who already has a solid training base, doing HIIT each workout is unnecessary. Too much in a week can be hard on the body and keep you from recovering sufficiently between workouts. A great method to use on recovery days is light to moderate cardio.

Resistance or Cardiovascular Training: Which One First?

Research has shown that performing aerobic exercise first in the workout may develop maximal *aerobic* power (20,21). Doing cardio first is best reserved for those who are training for an endurance event such as a marathon. The opposite is true for those training for general fitness and health purposes.

For example, one study demonstrated that fat oxidation and calorie burning were increased during the aerobic exercise component when it was done *after* resistance exercise (22). This increased metabolic effect was even more pronounced when the resistance exercise that preceded it was performed at a higher intensity. This is important to note; several other studies have shown that performing cardio first in the workout can compromise the performance of subsequent resistance training exercises due to residual fatigue, therefore reducing the mechanical tension—which will be discussed in more detail later—developed during the strength training portion of the sessions. This interferes with the strength and muscle gains (23,24,25).

How Personalized Is Your Training Program?

That many personal trainers have training biases is another problem. Some trainers follow a bodybuilding philosophy, others follow a powerlifting philosophy, others are more into Pilates, some do "3D functional training," others may be more into kettlebells, and the list goes on. Many personal trainers think that their chosen exercise method is the best, most complete method of training, and therefore advise everyone to exercise the same way. In other words, many trainers just end up giving their clients lessons on what that particular trainer likes to do instead of using the best modalities for *you*.

There are two types of personal trainers: *fitness professionals* and *fitness hobbyists*. Fitness hobbyists try to get other people excited about their pet exercise hobby, regardless of your individual goals, while the fitness professional fits the workout program to you, not you to the trainer's specialty or bias.

Improving your overall fitness and health is a goal with different parts. It's combination of fat loss, refining your physique, and performance training without specifically focusing on one over the other. Therefore, it requires several different exercise components. No single piece of equipment or type of training will be ever able to fully address all aspects of the goal when it has many parts. It makes sense to take a mixed approach to exercise programming, and that's exactly what all the workout programs in this book do!

You *Don't* Have to Be a Gym Rat or Do Extreme Workouts

It's commonly thought that to improve your overall fitness and health, you must either work out 24/7 or do extreme routines like the ones we see athletes and bodybuilders doing in magazines and on television. This is simply not true.

If you're trying to become a bodybuilder or a high-level athlete, you must exercise like one. However, if you're simply interested in getting into better shape, you certainly don't need to become a "health nut" who lives in the gym or does extreme workouts. For example, research has found that running even 5 to 10 minutes a day and at slow speeds (less than 6 miles per hour) is "associated with markedly reduced risks of death from all causes and cardiovascular disease." (15)

The fitness and health workout programs in this book involve resistance training, and they certainly keep you moving for longer than 10 minutes. These study results are not a workout recommendation. This research shows you don't need a long and complicated workout routine to reap all the benefits of exercise. You just need to get moving and keep improving.

Both Men and Women Need Intense Weight Training

Many men are comfortable with training to gain at least some muscle mass, so allow me to speak to women for a moment. When you talk about toning, enhancing, or shaping certain areas of your body, you mean building muscle and losing body fat. When it comes to developing your muscles, there is no such thing as exercises for "toning" muscle versus exercises for "bulking" it. Muscles only have one physiological way to grow, and that is called *hypertrophy*.

Muscle creates the shape of your body, and therefore more muscle equals more muscle tone. You can't build a perkier, rounder, or sexier anything without building muscle. To build (i.e., improve the shape of) that muscle, you need to stimulate muscle tissue. Those tiny pink dumbbells just aren't the tools for the job, because they don't challenge your body to become stronger and won't improve the shape of your body. But women will certainly benefit from the type of lifting just like men do.

Additionally, research has also found that doing resistance exercises first seems to increase the metabolic effects of the subsequent aerobic session (26), which is why all the workout programs in this book involve doing any cardio/conditioning activities after the resistance training portion of the workout.

It's important to understand that the studies about cardio compromising the performance of subsequent resistance training exercises refers to doing a full cardio workout (like a 30-minute run) in the same session as a full resistance training workout. This is not the same as placing small amounts of a cardio-based activity, like a 45-second bout of shadow boxing, for example, within a circuit along with the resistance training-based exercises. This type of circuit training can allow you to reap the metabolic benefits of both activities while making a fitness or fat loss-oriented workout more interesting and diverse.

Fitness trends come and go. And every new "best" workout claims to be better than the last "best" workout, demonstrating why what's popular is usually based more on marketing than on good science. You do not have to follow the latest workout trends to get into better shape (i.e., improve your fitness and health), and it's misguided to do so. Regardless of what's currently "in style," you should follow workout strategies that are based on scientifically backed exercise principles—described in the first four chapters of this book—that have repeatedly been shown to produce the results you're after. It's important to read the next three chapters as well as this one so that you can understand what these principles are.

2 { Function and Performance

This chapter is for those who want to improve performance, be able to perform a movement task faster or harder than previously (speed and power), lift progressively heavier weights (strength), lift the same amount of weight for more reps (muscular endurance), and reduce the recovery time needed to perform a series of exercise challenges (conditioning).

In this book, training for improved performance isn't about training for any specific sport; it's about training to improve the general physical qualities that determine overall athleticism—speed and power, strength, muscular endurance, and conditioning—that could be applied to any sport. Strength and conditioning workouts help you improve the physical qualities (i.e., more power or strength) that are not addressed by simply playing and practicing your sport. Focusing on improving overall strength and power can also help athletes decrease injury risk. Although much is often made about "sports specific" training, most athletes can benefit from adding overall strength, increasing explosive power, and improving conditioning levels. This can help you move faster, be stronger, and outlast the competition.

Just like when training for fat loss or building muscle, which are covered in the next two chapters, training to improve the power and strength that determine overall athleticism has its own set of myths and misunderstandings. This chapter identifies these myths and clarifies the misconceptions.

Training Principles and Methods for Function and Performance

Research shows that relative strength (i.e., how strong you are relative to your own bodyweight) is the greatest predictor of performance in sprint, vertical jump, and change of direction (1). Many trainers and coaches will assert that you can't become strong and powerful without focusing your training around the "big lifts," which are the traditional barbell bench press, squat, and deadlift. Saying that you can't get stronger and more powerful without emphasizing these exercises is an example of how people confuse training methods with training principles.

The *principle of specificity*, a universal training principle, dictates that adaptations to training will be specific to the demands the training puts on the body (2). Since the purpose of programming is to create the appropriate training stimulus to elicit specific adaptations, the first step in the programming process is to determine the desired training goals. The training goals ultimately determine the types of exercises and methodologies that need to be part of the workout program.

Specificity in training can be accomplished by targeting muscle groups, energy systems, speed of movement, movement patterns, or muscle action types (3). For example, if the goal is to become more explosive, the program should include explosive exercises (i.e., power exercises). If a someone has a multifaceted goal, such as improving overall health and fitness, it is basically training for a combination of fat loss, function, and physique without specifically focusing on one over the other. This program requires several training components because no single type of training will sufficiently address all the goals (4).

Another foundational training principle is the *principle of progressive overload*, which dictates that the training stress—based on frequency, intensity, and type of exercise as well as recovery processes—should exceed the training stress experienced during the previous workout (5). For example, if you're training to improve strength, you could gradually add heavier loads or perform more repetitions with the same load to ensure progress.

Now that you've got a general idea of training principles, we can discuss that when trainers and coaches talk about sticking to the basics, they've got a list of certain exercises (e.g., traditional barbell bench press, squat, and deadlift, etc.) they believe are foundational to improving human performance. But let's break that down.

The word *foundational* denotes an underlying basis or principle, something that's fundamental. When this definition is applied to exercise programs, it becomes clear that there aren't any fundamental exercises—often called the basics—that need to be used. There are only foundational or fundamental training principles, like specificity and overload, that need to be practiced. These principles dictate the exercises that should be included and how they're applied in a comprehensive training program. In other words, exercises are just methods that allow us to apply principles.

Many will judge a training program as either "good" or "bad" based on whether it uses a certain set of exercises deemed as the basics. This is putting methods before principles. When it comes to good program design, we don't go from the methods down; we go from the principles up. A good program isn't determined by the exercises it incorporates, but by how the training principles are utilized.

Some trainers and coaches will take things a step further when they assert that successful programming is all about *mastering* the basics, which translates to saying that good training involves mastering certain exercises. This isn't fully accurate either. First, if you're not trying to be a powerlifter or an Olympic lifter, there's no single exercise that you must do. When it comes to doing exercises like barbell deadlifts, you need to only use them in a way that's safe and helps you improve your overall strength or muscle growth. You need to possess basic competence in the lifts you're performing; however, you don't need to learn or practice the powerlifting specific skills required to be a master deadlifter.

As far as exercises go, there's no such thing as fundamental exercises. There are fundamental human actions, like pushing, pulling, rotation, locomotion, and level changes (6), and there are many conventional and unconventional exercise applications to choose from to express those (universal) human actions. For example, squats fall under the fundamental human action of "level changes." In other words, squatting is just one way of many for humans to perform the action of change levels.

The reason it's important to delineate fundamental human actions from traditional exercises is that when we think about squats, we usually think about how you move when you perform a barbell squat (front or back). And when we think that this type of squat represents a foundational human action that everyone should be able to do, we end up taking a one-size-fits-all approach and try to fit square pegs into round holes. Not everyone is built to squat that way.

However, when we realize that the traditional style of squatting is just one way to train the fundamental human action of level changes, we don't put it or any other exercise on a pedestal. We know that there are plenty of ways we can train level changes that better fit the individual based on their skeletal framework, body proportions, and injury history. This is why it's ridiculous when some trainers and coaches say, "You just don't know how to coach these lifts." People can't be coached out of their individual skeletal frameworks, body proportions, and injury histories. Trying to fit people to exercises instead of fitting exercises to people is one of the biggest training mistakes trainers and coaches make.

It comes down to this: Are you using the exercise, or is the exercise using you? Given the natural variations between our bodies, it doesn't make sense to tell someone that just because some lifters can do the traditional squat or deadlift that everyone should be able to do it the same way. Sure, you can force people to try, but it's a much smarter approach to select exercises based on individual needs.

When you have a grasp of training principles (i.e., movement specificity and overload), you understand that only those competing in weightlifting-oriented sports must do certain exercises. The big (barbell) lifts are a great way to create progressive overload because they provide a lot of value in your strength training, but they're not the only way. Resistance exercises are just a way to put force across joints and tissues to help them to grow stronger. That's it! Barbells, dumbbells, cables, machines, and bands are all just different tools that allow us to apply force across joints and tissues. And, unless you're in the gym to be a powerlifter, there's no reason your training should be overly focused on mainly improving your strength in the three big lifts. An athlete or gym-goer doesn't have to do a particular exercise to improve. The training program should adhere to training principles, and there's a wide variety of exercises that allow athletes and fitness enthusiasts to adhere to these principles and achieve their goals.

Research highlights that no form of exercise has magical properties. One study compared unilateral (single leg) versus bilateral (two legs) squat training for strength, sprints, and agility in rugby players. The results of this study found that Bulgarian split squats were just as effective as barbell back squats in improving measures of lower-body strength, 40-meter sprint speed, and change of direction (7). Another study also found that single-leg and double-leg training exercises increased strength and decreased fatigue in the lower body, with no differences between the single-leg and double-leg results (8).

Additionally, another study found that, although unilateral and bilateral training appear to affect muscle size adaptations similarly, and while both the unilateral and bilateral training groups had increases in both unilateral and bilateral strength, the unilateral training group had the greatest strength improvements in unilateral strength and the bilateral training group had the largest improvement in bilateral strength (9). In other words, although strength improved in both bilateral and unilateral training for the two groups, the magnitude of strength increases seems to be specific to the training type, which, again, is the principle of specificity at work. This highlights the importance of having a well-rounded strength training program that includes more than just traditional barbell exercises to strengthen your lower and upper body in a wide variety of stances, positions, and actions. That's exactly what the programs in chapter 12, Function and Performance Programs, will help you do.

Training Load for Function and Performance

Research indicates that although both high-load and lower-load training to failure can elicit significant increases in muscle hypertrophy (i.e., size) in well-trained individuals, high-load (heavy) training is superior for maximizing strength adaptations (10,11). That said, strength is your ability to produce force, and power is strength divided by time or how quickly you can produce force. Although lifting heavy weights can help improve your power, there's plenty of evidence to show that improvements in power are maximized (in both men and women) when you also regularly incorporate regularly low-load (lighter) exercises that require you to move fast (12,13).

This should come as no surprise because the principle of training specificity dictates that the adaptations you make to training will be specific to the demands the training puts on the body. As I also said earlier, if you want to maximize improvements in your overall strength, you must incorporate training with heavier loads (relative to your own strength level or 1RM). If you want to become more explosive, you've got to use explosive exercises. This is why the workout programs in the performance workout programs chapter emphasize both explosive exercises (exercises that involve lighter loads, sometimes just body weight) and heavy lifting.

When it comes to heavy lifting, it doesn't mean lifting a specific amount of weight that would impress the powerlifting community in barbell squat, deadlift, or bench press competition lifts. It simply means getting stronger than you were without sacrificing your overall health or physical capacity to participate in the other physical activities and sports you enjoy.

Sets and Reps for Function and Performance

Training for strength and power are similar when considering the number of sets and reps. The general rule for strength and power calls for doing more sets, around four to six or more sets, while keeping the reps low, in the one to five reps per set range (14). And, the general recommendations for rest between sets are similar for strength and power. A review of the research for rest intervals between sets for targeting specific training outcomes found that resting three to five minutes between sets produced greater increases in strength by allowing your body the optimal amount of time to recover, and higher levels of muscular power were demonstrated over multiple sets with three to five minutes of rest versus 1 minute of rest between sets (14). Resting longer than three to five minutes doesn't mean performance will increase further. Plus, you've only got so much time to work out anyway.

Training for Improved Conditioning

In addition to strength and power, you also need a high level of power endurance to perform optimally. The strength and power training methods in the workout programs in this book are great for improving your strength and power, but they're not so great for improving your *power endurance*, which is your ability to resist fatigue and be able produce the same level of power for a longer time—the length of competition. In other words, many of the low-rep, high-load training methods help you peak your power in short bursts, but they don't require you to call upon every ounce of strength you have and explode—even when you're tired.

Power endurance is only developed through exercise protocols that force you to be explosive while in a fatigued state. The conditioning protocols included at the end of many of the workout programs in the function and performance workout programs chapter increase your power endurance. They require you to expend a high amount of effort for extended periods of time, which is exactly what power endurance is, making them just what the doctor ordered for improving your ability to be explosive at the end of a competition when you're fatigued.

In short, if you don't train to outlast the competition, you won't outlast the competition. Using the conditioning methods in this book to complement your strength and power training will help you to be the last person standing when the smoke clears.

The major difference between training for strength and training for power is the weight load being used and the speed the movement is being performed. Strength training involves moving against higher loads (relative to one's strength level). Power training involves lighter loads (sometimes just body weight) and focuses on moving under control at high speeds.

Strength Training Myths

Many trainers, coaches, and exercise enthusiasts believe and continue to perpetuate common myths about strength training. To help you to make smarter choices in your training and to ensure that you're not running around your gym spreading misinformation, the following will address commonly held beliefs about strength training and separate the sense from the nonsense about them.

The Better the Lifter, the Better the Athlete!

Yes, strength matters for performance. However, there's a big difference between being a good athlete and simply being a good lifter in the gym. In other words, not every good athlete is a good lifter, and not every good lifter is a good athlete. For proof of this, look no further than the NFL combine results. Research has confirmed that there isn't a reliable link between combine performance and future NFL success. One such paper concluded that "the 40-yard dash, vertical jump, 20-yard shuttle, and 3-cone drill tests have limited validity in predicting future NFL performance." (15) Another paper found "no correlation of statistical relationship between combine tests and professional football performance." (16) The author also stated that "the results of the study should encourage NFL team personnel to reevaluate the usefulness of the combine's physical tests and exercises as predictors of player performance."

These athletes had "raw" physical ability, but what separated the NFL zeros from the heroes was the ability to use that talent as a platform to play the game well. This is important to understand; it's completely unrealistic to credit any workout program an athlete may use, much less a specific exercise like the bench press, for the success an athlete achieves. You've got to be careful trying to emulate what the world's best athletes are currently doing in their workouts; their success is caused by more than just what they do in a workout.

If any credit is given to a strength and conditioning program, it's mainly for improving your physical capacity (i.e., strength and power) to do what you already know how to do. Running faster doesn't help if you're running to the wrong spot on the field, and strength doesn't help if you miss a block or push your opponent in the wrong direction. But a strength and conditioning program can help an athlete have more gas in the tank (the conditioning) to express their skill and their will throughout the competition.

Always Do the Full Range of Motion

Partial reps are commonly thought to be just a way of "cheating." But they can be extremely beneficial for building strength. Incorporating them into your workouts helps develop strength better than just exclusively going with the full range of motion of many common pressing and lower-body exercises.

Chest presses and squats are both examples of exercises that are most difficult at the bottom of the range of motion. In presses, this is where the lever arm is the longest. The motion becomes easier as you get closer to the top of the range of motion, where the lever arm is shortening and giving you a mechanical advantage on the weight.

Research comparing the results from a group that trained with only a full range of motion squats (for 6 sets) twice a week to a group that trained with a combination of a full range of motion squats and partial range squats (for 3 sets each) twice a week found that although both groups improved their squat strength, the group that did the combination of full and partial range of motion had superior results (17). This was somewhat predictable. Using a weight that you can move during the most difficult part of the range of motion (where the lever arm is the longest) means that the load would be too light to create a sufficient overload stimulus in the less difficult ranges of motion (where the lever arm is shorter).

The point of this research is that a full range of motion doesn't necessarily elicit greater strength adaptations. The weight you're lifting isn't limited to how strong you are in the entire range of motion involved in the given exercise movement. It's limited to where the lever is the longest during that given movement, or practically speaking, when you are the weakest.

This is an excellent reason to incorporate partial reps into your training, so that you can provide the same relative overload to an area of the range of motion that involves a shorter lever arm. For example, in the case of doing a dumbbell press or bench press, mechanical partials involve moving the bar or dumbbells only through the top third of the range of motion. Since this is the part of the range of motion that involves a shorter lever arm, the weight used is heavier than what was used to perform the full range of motions. This is why the performance workouts in chapter 12 include some partial range of motion sets.

Add Plates Every Week

If this myth were true, then 30-year-olds who've been lifting consistently since they were teenagers should be hitting world record numbers. Since this clearly isn't the case, it's far more accurate to say, "You should get stronger every week, as long as you're changing your program every month or two."

Because the human body adapts, the principle of progressive overload will only take you so far. Everyone reaches a plateau at some point within a training program, and they're unable to keep progressively overloading the same exercises. This is where applying the principle of variation comes in.

Depending on how often you train each week, you should change your training program every three to five weeks or so depending on how many days per week you are training. This usually involves changing the exercises in the program, which is what the programs in chapter 12 will do. You can modify the order of the exercises, along with the sets, reps, and rest periods utilized. This gives the body enough time to adapt, but it usually isn't a long enough training period for the program to become boring, stale, or no longer beneficial. The lesson: Focus on using the same basic human movements—pushing, pulling, lower-body exercises, etc.—but in slightly different ways by using exercise variations.

Strength Training on Unstable Surfaces is More Functional

Does your trainer have you lifting weights while standing on unstable surfaces like wobble boards, a Bosu, or a fitness ball to improve your "functional strength" or "core stability"?

Here's the problem: The principle of overload is a universal training principle. Essentially, if you want to gain strength and improve your power, you must create sufficient overload on the body to stimulate such adaptations. However, research has shown the diminished force output suggests that the overload stresses required for strength training necessitates the inclusion of strength training on stable surfaces (18).

In short, lifting weights while standing or kneeling on a stability ball or on another type of unstable surface is a poor application of strength training because the environment created when doing so is not nearly as effective as being on a stable surface for stimulating gains in strength and power.

Now, some may claim that they're not using exercises that involve standing or kneeling on unstable surfaces to increase strength. Instead, they may say they're doing this to improve functional performance. However, research says otherwise: "Resistance exercise performed on unstable equipment may not be effective in developing the type of balance, proprioception, and core stability required for successful sports performance. Free-weight exercises performed while standing on a stable surface have been proven most effective for enhancing sports-related skills" (19).

If your goal is to improve (functional) performance, you need to consider where you are standing. Unless you're a circus performer whose act involves balancing on a big ball, the ground you're living, practicing, and playing on is stable. Also, don't confuse a slippery surface (like playing in the rain) with an unstable surface. Since functional training is about transfer, it's more functional for field, court, and combat athletes and those looking to improve their overall strength and power to train on the same stable surface they live, practice, and compete on.

Standing on unstable surfaces like a stability ball is a learned skill that's no different than learning to ride a bike. You get good at riding a bike by practice, and you'll get good at standing on a stability ball when you practice standing on it.

Let's consider another example involving balance. No one expects that being able to balance on a bike will offer much transfer into improved (functional) performance in activities other than riding a bike, so it doesn't make sense to think that standing on an unstable surface will be any different. Neither come close to replicating the force production and neuromuscular coordination patterns of running, jumping, punching, throwing, etc.

Isolation Exercises Are Nonfunctional for Improving Performance

Just because the performance workout emphasizes more strength and power training over the other workout programs in this book, it doesn't mean that isolation exercises are not also incorporated into the workouts.

Since isolation exercises do not necessarily reflect the specific movement patterns of many common actions in athletics, their positive benefits for improved performance potential is less obvious. This has led some personal trainers and coaches to mistakenly label isolation exercises as nonfunctional and therefore not valuable.

Performance improvements from exercise training aren't purely related to gains in strength and power. They can also be related to increased bodyweight from gaining muscle size (i.e., hypertrophy). Using some isolation and machine-based exercises to aid in getting *bigger* can help you improve your overall athletic performance in sports like football, basketball, baseball, tennis, golf, etc., where you're required to produce horizontal and diagonal forces when standing, such as when pushing an opponent or swinging a bat, racquet, or club. In that, one of the factors that determines our levels of stability and strength from our feet is our bodyweight.

A body's mass (or weight) contributes to stability because heavier bodies are harder to move and are more stable. Lighter bodies are the opposite: They're moved more easily and are less stable (20). Getting bigger (gaining muscle weight) can help you better use your strength by providing a greater platform from which to create and resist force.

Additionally, isolation exercises can also help reduce your risk of injury. For example, a research study about elite soccer players separated into two groups evaluated training in the groups. Although both groups used the same training programs, one group had additional, specific hamstring training using the lying leg hamstring curl machine and the other did not. The research showed that the addition of the lying curl increased sprint speed and decreased the risk of suffering a hamstring strain injury (21).

This agrees with other research, which showed that the lying leg curl exercise (where movement originates at the knee joint, such as when using leg curl machine) elicited significantly greater activation of the lower lateral and lower medial hamstrings compared to the stiff-legged deadlift (where movement originates at the hip joint, such as in a Romanian deadlift) (22).

The takeaway from this research is that a comprehensive hamstring exercise program should incorporate at least one exercise where movement is focused at the hip joint (such as the deadlift or other similar compound exercises) and one exercise where movement is focused at the knee joint (such as the leg curl machine or other similar isolation exercise) as each offers unique but complementary training benefits. Different regions of the hamstring complex can be regionally targeted through exercise selection. This is contrary to the common belief that just sticking to the "big" compound lifts provide a fully comprehensive training stimulus. It doesn't.

Training exercises for the hip adductors is another example of the importance of using isolation exercises for performance. A scientific review found that hip adductor strength was one of the most common risk factors for groin injury in sport (23). One study on professional ice hockey players found that they were 17 times more likely to sustain an adductor muscle strain (i.e., groin injury) if adductor strength was less than 80 percent of abductor strength (24).

It's not uncommon for personal trainers and strength coaches to claim that you don't need to do specific exercises to target your adductors, as compound exercises like squats and lunges do the job effectively. However, the research in this area shows this is false.

A review investigating the barbell squat found that a greater hip external rotation position (feet turned out) in a wide stance and increased load will increase hip adduction activation during this exercise (25). However, the highest values in muscle activity for the wide-stance squat (26), along with those found during a single-leg squat and a lunge, are relatively low compared to exercises that focus primarily on the hip adduction movement (27). To reach greater levels of muscle activation in the adductors, exercises targeted at training the hip adductors are superior to exercises like wide-stance squats, single-leg squats, and lunges.

These principles don't only apply to training the hamstring and adductor musculature. This research highlights the importance of including isolation exercises for overall development in addition to the other types of exercises when training for improved performance.

———

Since many people are not athletes trying to refine performance and are instead interested in focusing on fat loss, the next chapter clarifies many of the misconceptions about exercising for fat loss.

3 } Fat Loss

Many who exercise want to lose some extra body fat without losing muscle. But with the conflicting information (and just plain misinformation) out there, it's easy to fall prey to false beliefs about fat loss. Those false beliefs can hinder your long-term progress. Many people have lost fat, but most gained it back. People become confused and frustrated, thinking they've tried everything.

This chapter identifies several common mistakes so you don't make them and provides the simple-to-understand truth about how to eat and exercise for successful and safe fat loss without all the fads and diet dogmas.

Nutrition for Fat Loss: Made Simple

We can't talk about fat loss without talking about eating behaviors (a.k.a. diet). You won't find a more common question than, How should I eat for fat loss? For an answer you'll get lots of different opinions. The fact is, this issue, along with other issues like it, isn't about what this or that so-called expert says, and it's definitely not about what some athlete, trainer, or lean person at gym says. It's about what the body of scientific evidence—not just a single study—says when taken as a whole.

The International Society of Sports Nutrition (ISSN) has provided a list of conclusions and recommendations (for eating and exercising) in their position stand paper on diets and body composition. Here are a few of major takeaways from the ISSN's scientific paper (1):

- There are many diet types and eating styles. The various diet archetypes are wide-ranging in total energy and macronutrient distribution. Each type carries varying degrees of supporting data and unfounded claims.

- A wide range of dietary approaches (low-fat to low-carbohydrate/ketogenic, and all points between) can be similarly effective for improving body composition, and this allows flexibility with program design. To date, no controlled, inpatient isocaloric (i.e., calories matched) diet comparison, where protein is matched between groups, has reported a clinically meaningful fat loss or thermic (i.e., metabolic) advantage to the lower-carbohydrate or ketogenic diet.

- Common threads run through the diets in terms of the mechanism of action for weight loss and weight gain (i.e., sustained hypocaloric versus hypercaloric conditions), but there are also potentially unique means by which certain diets achieve their intended objectives (e.g., factors that facilitate greater satiety, ease of compliance, support of training demands).

- Diets focused primarily on fat loss (and weight loss beyond initial reductions in body water) operate under the fundamental mechanism of a sustained caloric deficit. This net hypocaloric (i.e., reduced calorie) balance can either be imposed daily or over the course of the week.

- The collective body of research about intermittent caloric restriction (i.e., intermittent fasting) demonstrates no significant advantage over daily caloric restriction for improving body composition. Increasing dietary protein to levels significantly beyond current recommendations for athletic populations may improve body composition. The ISSN's original 2007 position on protein intake (1.4-2.0 g/kg) has gained further support from subsequent investigations arriving at similar requirements in athletic populations. Higher protein intakes (2.3-3.1 g/kg Fat Free Mass) may be required to maximize muscle retention in lean, resistance-trained subjects in hypocaloric conditions. Emerging research on very high protein intakes (>3 g/kg) has demonstrated that the known thermic, satiating, and lean mass-preserving effects of dietary protein might be amplified in resistance training subjects.

- Most existing research showing *adaptive thermogenesis* (i.e., a slowing of metabolism) has involved diets that combine aggressive caloric restriction with low protein intakes and an absence of resistance training, essentially creating a perfect storm for slowing metabolism. Research that has mindfully included resistance training and adequate protein has circumvented the problem of adaptive thermogenesis and muscle loss, despite very low-calorie intakes.

- The long-term success of a diet depends on compliance.

As you can see, the relationship of how many calories you consume per day to the number you expend per day is the single most important factor when it comes to determining whether you lose fat.

Now, whenever someone says this, someone else tries to refute it by bringing up the fact that the quality or composition of the calories you eat matters. They present it as an either/or proposition. But this relationship doesn't discount that some calories are more nutrient dense than others. (After all, we've all heard the term "empty calories.") It simply demonstrates that one can be both well nourished and overfed. Food quality and food quantity are important factors that should be considered together; as important as it is to eat high-quality, nutrient-dense foods for general health, you can still gain fat from eating "healthy" if you eat too many calories relative to what you're expending.

That said, focus on the quality of the foods you eat. Emphasize fruits and vegetables and high-quality meats, eggs, and fish (or protein substitutes, for vegetarians and vegans), while limiting refined foods, simple sugars, hydroge-

A Calorie Isn't a Calorie: The Truth

The people who like to say that "a calorie isn't a calorie" usually do so because (a) some foods are more nutrient dense than others and (b) different nutrient profiles affect the *thermic effect of food*, a term used to describe the energy expended by our bodies in order to consume (bite, chew, and swallow) and process (digest, transport, metabolize, and store) food in different ways. Although both points are true, that explanation still doesn't validate the claim that a calorie isn't a calorie. To understand why it doesn't, we must first establish what a calorie is.

A calorie is a unit of energy equal to the amount of heat needed to raise the temperature of 1 gram of water by 1 degree Celsius. In short, a calorie is a unit of heat. With this definition in mind, for a "calorie isn't a calorie" to be accurate, some type of food would have to provide calories that *aren't* a unit of energy equal to the amount of heat needed to raise the temperature of 1 gram of water by 1 degree Celsius. Name a food that provides calories, whether it be a nutrient-poor or nutrient-dense food, that *aren't* a unit of heat. The fact that you cannot name a food (because there aren't any) proves that a calorie *is* a calorie because *all* calories are units of heat.

This highlights the fundamental problem with saying that a calorie isn't a calorie. It conflates the nutrition of the food with its energy-producing value. This certainly isn't just semantics; it's why we have terms like "nutrient-poor foods" and "nutrient-dense foods" to delineate the nutrition in the food from its energy-producing value. Some foods are more physiologically filling than others, and some deliver more nutrients with those calories.

nated oil, and alcohol. Fruits, veggies, and lean proteins are generally lower in calories than things like fast food and candy. Don't overeat. Stop before you feel bloated and stuffed. You'll likely end up taking in fewer calories without even actually counting them.

You don't just want to be well fed; you want to be well nourished. Emphasizing the quality (i.e., nutrient density) of the foods you eat over the quantity (i.e., number of calories) is an easy approach. Try it and see where that gets you. It spells success for most people.

But it's certainly possible to eat too many calories from nutrient-dense, high-quality foods. Don't think for a second that you can't gain fat from eating "healthy." While you can first emphasize the quality of the foods you eat and see where that strategy gets you, it may only take you so far. You may need another strategy as well. The next step is to focus on the caloric quantity of the food you're eating and put yourself into a caloric deficit. The ways to create a caloric deficit involve eating fewer calories, increasing your activity level to expend more calories, or a combination of both.

What's the Best Type of Diet?

Multiple dietary approaches will result in fat loss if protein intake is sufficient. The most effective strategies state that diets should be individualized and take into account lifestyle habits, medical history (including diabetes, insulin resistance, other diseases, and medical concerns), dietary history, and food preferences. Above all, the most important factor that will help a person lose fat and improve health—no matter what diet plan is followed—is adherence. Choose the diet plan that (a) ensures you get plenty of protein and (b) that you can stick with.

The fact is, when you strip away the big claims and different formulas, the different popular diets get people to eat more lower-calorie, nutrient-dense foods while consuming fewer higher-calorie, nutrient-poor foods (junk foods). The reason you can find people who swear by just about every fad diet *isn't* because of a diet dogma and special eating formula this or that special diet promotes, but because it simply got people to change their lifestyles by eating more nutritious foods more frequently than they were before.

Lifestyle is a factor in diet success. Many people fail when attempting to improve their eating habits, even though they change their lifestyles, because the lifestyle changes they make are unrealistic and misguided. They try to change too many diet behaviors too fast. This is why it's important to (a) choose a healthier eating style that's realistic for you to stick with and (b) gradually implement it by making small changes in your eating behaviors, turning them into positive habits before changing other eating behaviors.

In every fad diet, there's always a specific "enemy." If it's not a type of macronutrient (fat, carbohydrate, etc.), it's a type of food or a list of what's off limits. Interestingly, some of the foods that are on the no-no list of one magic cure-all diet are emphasized as "good" in a different diet. If this isn't enough to highlight why these types of restrictive diets are based mainly on great marketing, keep in mind that—just like workout trends—every few years, there's a new diet claiming to be better than the last. It's no wonder these diets never seem to gain any credibility in the legitimate medical and scientific community.

Additionally, although some supplements have been scientifically validated to aid in health and performance, you don't need to take a specific supplement to improve your general health and physical appearance. There are three things you do need to do:

- Consume a diet that emphasizes whole foods (i.e., fruits, vegetables, and high-quality proteins), while limiting junk food and alcohol.
- Eat plenty of protein.
- Participate regularly in some form of physical activity. Strength training is a great one!

You most likely already knew these things, but the goal of marketing is to make you think you need something more—like a special diet formula or magic supplement. This explains why just about every physique competitor or figure model I've ever trained has told me about the countless times they are asked what they eat or what supplements they take, as if they know secrets about nutrition or looking good that aren't readily available. I've jokingly recommended telling the people who ask them these questions something crazy like, "I eat reticulated python meat for muscle and put powdered bumblebee urine on my thighs and belly before I work out to accelerate fat loss in those areas." Of course, this is nonsense, but it demonstrates how we often think we need to use exotic exercise and nutrition practices and make the process more complicated and unrealistic than it needs to be. Sometimes everyone just needs to be reminded to keep it simple.

It often seems that contradictory scientific conclusions about nutrition appear almost daily. Remain skeptical of "magic" and "miracle" claims and avoid being taken in by marketing hype. You will see that most legitimate studies amount to no more than tinkering with the basic nutritional principles and simple advice provided previously.

Safety and Potential Side Effects of a High-Protein Diet

Spend enough time in the fitness or nutrition field, and you're sure to see someone wave a caution flag, warning you that a high-protein diet is dangerous to your kidneys. However, again, it's not what this or that so-called expert claims; it's what the weight of the scientific evidence dictates.

In a 2000 study, researchers looked at bodybuilders and other well-trained athletes whose protein intake was judged to be either high or medium relative to their body weights. They took blood and urine samples to see if there were signs of kidney problems.

The researchers found that the athletes' nitrogen balance became positive (that is, they had enough protein to build new muscle tissue) when their daily intake exceeded 0.57 grams per pound (1.26 grams per kilogram) of body weight. They saw no link between protein intake and creatinine clearance, albumin excretion rate, or calcium excretion rate, any of which, if elevated, would suggest that a high-protein diet was potentially dangerous. Their conclusion: "Protein intake under 2.8 grams of protein daily per kilogram (2.2 lb) of body weight does not impair renal function in well-trained athletes, as indicated by the measures of renal function used in this study" (2).

In a 2005 study, the researchers suggested that "while protein restriction may be appropriate for treatment of existing kidney disease, we find no significant evidence for a detrimental effect of high protein intakes on kidney function in healthy persons after centuries of a high-protein Western diet" (3).

Another question that arises: Is a high-protein diet harmful to your bones? Not only is that statement based on a myth, it's a completely backward myth. A 2002 study concluded that "excess protein will not harm the skeleton if the calcium intake is adequate" (4). And a review study published in 2003 showed that people with chronically low protein consumption were at higher risk for having a lower bone density and more bone loss (5).

A 1998 study found that protein supplements help elderly folks heal faster from bone-related injuries. They looked specifically at femoral fractures—the large leg bone that connects with the pelvis to create the hip joint—and found that supplementing with 20 grams of protein a day reduced bone loss and allowed seniors to return home sooner from rehabilitation facilities (6).

The takeaway is that, in general, more protein in your diet is better than less, especially when your primary goal is body composition—maximum muscle, minimum fat. A good daily target is 1 gram of protein per pound of body weight. Unless you have kidney disease, there's no reason to think a high-protein diet is dangerous. The real danger to your health comes from a low-protein diet. It's bad for your body composition, bone density, and metabolism.

The Best Exercise Method for Fat Loss: Metabolic Resistance Training

A 2015 systematic review and meta-analysis—one of the most powerful forms of scientific evidence because it's essentially a study of studies—came to two conclusions when it comes to exercise and fat loss:

- Resistance training was *more* effective than aerobic endurance (cardio) training or a combination of resistance and aerobic endurance training, particularly with utilizing whole body and free-weight exercises at around two to three or more sets per exercise performed at an intensity of ≤75 percent 1RM. This equates to using heavy enough loads so you can't do more than about 10 reps per set. It's important to note that using loads that enable you to perform more than 10 reps per set before reaching fatigue are still beneficial for fat loss, but this research highlights the importance of incorporating heavier lifting into your fat loss training efforts.

- When training to maximize fat loss, the focus of the exercise training "should be on producing a large metabolic stress," induced by emphasizing the resistance training parameters or intense levels of cardio training, such as high-intensity intervals (7).

When your main exercise goal is to maximize fat loss, you don't want to focus on using traditional strength training methods. Instead, you want to emphasize metabolic resistance training modalities like *circuits* (a continuous series of exercises using multiple pieces of equipment) and *complexes* (a continuous series of exercises using the same piece of equipment). These metabolic resistance training methods create a higher metabolic demand than traditional resistance training methods do and require more extended, high-intensity, total-body effort than traditional strength training methods (8).

Research looking at the effects of aerobic and strength training on fat mass in overweight or obese adults concluded that "a program of combined aerobic training and strength training did not result in significantly more fat mass reductions over aerobic training alone." Of course, results like these will often make the rounds in the media, along with the claim that "science shows that cardio is better for fat loss than strength training." (9) That the scientific evidence of exercise on fat loss shows that resistance training is *more* effective over the long-term than cardio training or a combination of resistance and aerobic endurance training has been discussed previously.

That said, there's a simple explanation for how cardio can *appear* to be the more effective exercise method for fat loss. It's true that cardio does burn more calories during the workout than resistance training. We've already established that fat loss comes from being in a caloric deficit. Here's the rub: Instead of spending your extra time, which is limited and valuable, doing cardio to expend, let's say, 300 calories, you can simply cut 300 calories out of your diet each day and end up with the same result without having to bother with cardio. In other words, you essentially eliminate the need for doing cardio (from a fat-loss perspective) when you simply eat fewer calories to create a deficit.

Now we must address the other reality. Many people don't just want a "lean" body. They also want a stronger and athletic looking body. To achieve that,

Spot Reduction: The Myth That Won't Die

A zombie idea is something that no matter how many times it's killed, it just keeps rising up again. Spot reduction (i.e., localized fat loss through specific exercise) is a zombie idea.

Some have attempted to use the results of a study that said "an acute bout of exercise can induce spot lipolysis and increased blood flow in adipose tissue adjacent to contracting skeletal muscle" (16), portraying it as scientific evidence showing that targeted fat mobilization is physiologically possible. They then assert that spot reduction is a valid training method.

Here's the problem: Even if targeted fat mobilization is a real physiological phenomenon that can be taken advantage of by contracting the muscles in the fatty area to increase blood flow, if you're following a comprehensive resistance training program, you're already benefiting from the targeted fat mobilization benefits of strength training.

To substantiate claims that a certain training method (e.g., certain exercises with certain set/rep/rest ranges) is more effective than other training methods for spot reduction, a person would have to demonstrate that in a scientifically controlled and comparative environment. The person would also have to refute the studies already done on men and women that show spot reduction does *not* occur because of resistance training (17). For example, one study that investigated spot reduction in the legs found the training program was effective in reducing fat mass, but this reduction was not specifically achieved in the legs (18). Further, two studies that examined the effect of abdominal exercise on abdominal fat found that it did not preferentially reduce adipose (fat) cell size or subcutaneous fat thickness in the abdominal region compared to other adipose sites (19,20).

In short, while you may be able to mobilize the fat nearest to the working muscle, fat is not lost in the *specific* area you're targeting.

---

strength training is necessary. This is why the researchers in the study previously mentioned also stated that a program including strength training is needed for increasing lean muscle (9).

In short, the point of this chapter and the subsequent workout programs in the book is that when fat loss is your main goal, focus on strength training to improve your muscle, which makes up the shape of your body, and watch your diet (instead of doing lots of extra cardio) to reveal your shape.

Don't get it wrong! There's nothing wrong with incorporating cardio into your workouts to reap its aerobic benefits and expend some additional calories in the process. But keep your focus on resistance training over cardio. You don't have to go nuts on the cardio, which can be time consuming and boring, if fat loss if your main exercise goal.

Losing Fat and Gaining Muscle

You won't find a more commonly asked question about exercise than "Can I lose fat and gain muscle at the same time?" The answers often have many different

Muscle Weighs More Than Fat: Clarifying the Confusion

It's obvious that 10 pounds is 10 pounds, regardless of what it is. So, 10 pounds of fat weighs the same as 10 pounds of muscle. However, this doesn't debunk the myth that muscle weighs more than fat, as many people think.

Pound for pound, muscle tissue takes up less space than fat because muscle is denser. This difference in density makes muscle weigh more than fat if you compare same-size portions. Density is the quantity of matter packed into a measured volume. The denser an object is, the more particles compressed together within the same space, and the heavier it is compared to something of equal size but less dense.

The density of an object is often measured in grams per milliliter (g/ml). The density of skeletal muscle is 1.06 grams per milliliter (14), whereas the density of adipose tissue (fat) is about 0.9 grams per milliliter (15). A liter is a metric unit of volume, and 1 liter of muscle weighs 2.3 pounds (1.06 kg), compared to 1 liter of fat, which weighs 1.98 pounds (0.9 kg).

Therefore, the trouble with saying that "muscle weighs more than fat" is that it implies the terms *heavy* and *light*, which, on their own, refer to mass, not density. Density is mass or volume, and weight is mass under the effect of gravity. The density of something stays the same wherever you take it—Earth, Mars, or anywhere in the universe.

The statement "muscle weighs more than fat" needs to be reworded to something like "since muscle is denser than fat, muscle does weigh more than fat if you compare same-size portions." That doesn't sound as sexy, but it's certainly more clear and accurate.

opinions. But it's about what the *scientific evidence* says. To date, there are several studies showing that, yes, you can simultaneously build muscle and lose fat.

Research has demonstrated this in variety of populations:

- Overweight, sedentary adult males (10)
- Older men and women (11)
- Physically active healthy men (12)
- Young women (13)

From a nutritional perspective, although a caloric deficit is needed to lose fat, a caloric surplus isn't necessarily needed to build muscle. This is because stored fat is stored energy. The stored fat calories are available for the body to use as fuel for the muscle-building process.

But hold on. Get this part straight: Your body can't turn fat into muscle or vice versa. Fat is fat, and muscle is muscle. If you're overweight, your body can use your stored energy (fat) to fuel the muscle-building process when the needed calories to build muscle isn't coming from additional food intake.

Science tells us that the more fat and the less muscle you have, the greater your ability to gain muscle and lose fat at the same time. This doesn't mean you should get fat. It just means your biology is working in your favor when you want to pack more muscle on, but have some fat to lose.

It's also important to understand that the leaner you are, the harder it becomes to lose fat while gaining muscle. If you're already lean, a large caloric deficit will make you lose some muscle even with resistance training and adequate protein intake. The goals, especially when you're not overweight but just looking to lose that extra bit of fat, are to make sure your diet delivers enough protein and that you're doing regular resistance training. When you do that, you'll limit any muscle loss to a very small amount.

Although you can't spot reduce with resistance exercise, you sure as heck can spot enhance by building muscle with strength training. The next chapter is all about building muscle. You don't have to be a bodybuilder to want to build your body. You have to know the principles and methods behind building muscle to make the most out of your valuable time and energy. In the next chapter, you'll learn those principles and methods.

4 { Physique

This chapter highlights some of the biggest muscle-building workout mistakes even personal trainers can make.

If you want to get the most out of workouts that focus on building muscle, you need to understand these principles. Use the simple, practical training strategies that this chapter provides. You'll avoid mistakes and get better results.

Building Muscle: The Science of Size and Strength

Making sure you eat proper amounts of protein is important, and to maximize muscle development, you need to create a training stimulus that uses the three mechanisms for increasing muscle hypertrophy (1):

- *Mechanical tension*—This tension is created from movement and external loads on the muscle to produce (concentrically), reduce (eccentrically), or control (isometrically) force.
- *Metabolic stress*—Practically speaking, this is associated with that burning sensation you get in the muscle during fatiguing exercise, and it's otherwise known as achieving the muscle pump.
- *Muscle damage*—This refers to microtears in muscle tissue. They trigger the body to repair the damaged muscle and grow it back bigger and denser. The microtears occur when you're either performing an exercise with heavier weights or doing more reps than you did before. Other causes are performing an unfamiliar exercise variation, stretching your muscles while they're being activated, or accentuating the eccentric (lowering) portion of the exercise. Although this damage often leads to delayed-onset muscle soreness (DOMS) after an intense exercise session, soreness is not needed for muscle development (1).

It's important to note that without mechanical tension, you don't create muscle damage or metabolic stress. Mechanical tension drives muscle growth, and muscle damage or metabolic stress are just the physiological effects of it. This explains why research shows that lifting a lighter load to failure produces gains in muscle size like that produced by lifting a heavy load to failure (2).

From a practical perspective, the scientific evidence on rep ranges tells us that there is no magical rep range for maximizing muscle size; therefore, you can incorporate both heavy-load and low-rep sets (1-5 reps) along with medium-load and high-rep (15-20+ reps) sets if you'd like.

But most people focused on building muscle are usually not interested in using weights so heavy that they can only do five reps or less with it. And that's fine. Performing some sets in the six to eight rep range serves as a nice middle ground between sets with heavy loads and fewer reps (1-5 reps) and sets with medium loads and more reps. This is why the muscle-building workouts in this book don't involve exercises performed for five reps or less.

The heavier the weight, the fewer reps you'll be able to do. The amount of weight you're using also determines the quality of reps you're performing. If the weight load is too heavy, you may not be able to do good, quality reps.

Questions to Ask Yourself Before the Lift

Evaluating your lifting program gives you the chance to see if you could be doing things more effectively. The following details a variety of questions to ask yourself before you lift along with what you need to know in order to avoid the common mistakes and get the most out of your workouts.

Are You Lifting Too Much?

At any given time at any big-box gym, you'll see at least one guy doing biceps curls or shoulder raises, and he has to throw his lower back into it each time he brings the weight up. If you don't see that dude at your gym, it may be because it's you.

It's easy to make this mistake. After all, you're in the gym to lift weights, and the previous section did mention that lifting heavy loads is an effective stimulus for muscle growth, right? Well, sort of. Training to maximize muscle is not about becoming a "weightlifter." It's about using weights as a tool to increase your muscle size. Simply throwing as much weight around as you can move to boost your ego and impress the people around you is the wrong approach.

When you use weights that are too heavy, here's what happens:

- You reduce the time under (mechanical) tension because you're forced to use momentum to cheat.
- You're unable to lower the weight slowly and with control, further reducing your time under (mechanical) tension.
- You utilize more muscles, which reduces the accumulated pump (i.e., metabolic stress) in muscles you intend to target.

Training to maximize muscle isn't just about moving the weight—that's weight-lifting—but about controlling the weight through the entire range of motion involved in the exercise you're doing. The point of emphasis on each repetition is to avoid swinging the weight up or "cheating" by using other areas of your bodyweight to move the load.

Do Cheat Reps Work?

There is research showing that using moderate momentum (cheating) increases the torque of the target muscles even without an increase in the load. That moderate increase in load and using momentum allows the torque to be increased even further. While an excessive use of momentum results in lower demands on the target muscles, an excessive increase of the load reduces the total hypertrophy stimulus by virtue of the decreased number of repetitions that can be performed successfully. The time under tension is shortened dramatically (3).

It can appear as if the results of this study validate cheating by incorporating momentum into the sets, but it doesn't. The results of this study shouldn't surprise you, because mechanical tension on the muscles is still present during cheat reps. However, this *doesn't* mean that cheating with momentum is just as effective as not cheating by avoiding momentum. Cheating is basically only applying mechanical tension in part of the range of motion and using momentum to get through the rest of the range. Although cheating may still have you moving through the full range of motion involved in the exercise, from a mechanical tension perspective, it's essentially a partial rep performed by target muscles. We have good evidence demonstrating that a partial range of motion rep creates less muscle growth than a full range of motion rep (4,5,6).

How Are You Lowering the Lift?

Controlling the weight while minimizing momentum in exercises to maximize muscle gains also applies to the eccentric portion of each rep. People who cheat the weight up (on the concentric portion of the rep) normally also let the weight come crashing back down (on the eccentric portion of the rep) instead of maintaining deliberate control by slowing the weight down when they lower it. Not controlling the weight on the way down could be less effective. We have evidence demonstrating that a slower (4 second) eccentric lowering action during biceps curls produced superior increases in arm growth than did a one-second eccentric action (7). This makes perfect sense. A slower eccentric action causes more time under tension, which creates more mechanical tension on the working muscles than a shorter eccentric portion does.

Additionally, from a training safety perspective, since cheating creates an overload of mechanical tension in a small piece of the range of motion involved in an exercise, it is more likely that you'll use a weight that's too heavy for you, making the muscles deal with forces that exceed the structural integrity of your tendons and ligaments and increasing your risk of injury.

If you want to maximize your gains in muscle size, maximize your time under (mechanical) tension on every rep by using strict form as well as controlled eccentric (lowering) movements of around three to five seconds.

Are You Avoiding Machines?

The whole idea of pitting free weights against machines is like pitting fruits against vegetables. Both training modalities offer a unique benefit the other misses, so it makes sense to do them both to make your muscle-building workouts more comprehensive, just like eating both fruits and vegetables will make your diet more nourishing.

Free weights excel by requiring you to stabilize and control not just the load being moved but also the path of the movement. However, free weights fall short when it comes to keeping consistent mechanical tension on the working muscles throughout the range of motion involved in most exercises. That's where machines excel and therefore offer distinct benefits for building muscle.

All free-weight exercises have one disadvantage that a machine doesn't—gravity! Free weights use a single load vector, gravity, to create resistance. If you use a pulley cable machine, you're also working against a single load vector, which is the line of the cable itself. When you work against a single load vector, you're going to have points within the range of motion involved in the exercise where the lever arm is long, creating high levels of mechanical tension on the involved muscles, and ranges where the lever arm is short, resulting in little to no mechanical tension on those same muscles.

Example: During any style of biceps curl, the point at which your biceps is being maximally loaded (stimulated) is range of motion when your forearm is at a 90-degree angle with the load vector. If you're using free weights, gravity is your load vector. The point of maximal mechanical tension on the biceps would be when your elbow reaches 90 degrees of flexion or when your forearm is parallel to the floor. If you're doing biceps curls using a cable machine, however, the cable itself is the load vector. The point of maximal mechanical tension to your biceps is when your forearm makes a 90-degree angle with the cable.

Here's the kicker: The farther away you move from a 90-degree angle in either direction of the load vector, the shorter the lever arm and the less work your biceps have to do; therefore, your biceps experience less mechanical tension. That's why, in a free-weight biceps curl, the closer you move toward the bottom or top of the range of motion, the less work your biceps do because the lever arm is shortening. People tend to rest between reps at the top and bottom positions when doing barbell or dumbbell curls.

This applies to any free-weight exercise in that they're all being loaded by a single load vector (gravity or a pulley cable). On the other hand, selectorized machines have a cam system, which isn't dependent on a single load vector like free weights or cables. Instead, the cam is set up to offer you a much more consistent resistance throughout a larger portion of the range of motion. This gives you much more time under tension because your working muscles don't get the same chance to rest at the bottom or top position of the range like they do when you are using free weights.

While you can absolutely build plenty of muscle size exclusively using free weights, there's no reason to avoid machines if you have access to them. Both types of exercises have advantages, so don't let popular misconceptions blind you to machines' unique muscle-building benefits. For muscle gains (and strength gains, which are discussed in the Function and Performance chapter), machines can be very beneficial when used with free weights.

Should Men and Women Train Differently?

It's common to see men stampede toward the free weights, while women pack into the Pilates and yoga studios and line up on cardio and weight machines. Should men and women train as differently as they do? There's a lot of confusion, and here's the truth.

I've written workout programs that were featured in major men's exercise magazines, only to see those exact programs later printed in the same publisher's

Might Doesn't Always Make Right:
Who's Your Best Source for Training Advice?

One of the most prolific training myths—another zombie idea that will stay alive, no matter how many times you try to kill it—is that the biggest, strongest, or leanest people in the gym are always the most qualified to give smart, safe, and reliable training advice information. Sometimes they are, but often they're not!

Those people have often achieved their results despite what they (think) they know and what they don't know, not because of it. They're gym rats who focus on organizing their lives around gyms and kitchens. Although they might be a great resource to you on the emotional and psychological aspects of disciplined training and dieting, and can share the experiences they've had in doing so, they're often not so great to rely on for the intellectual aspects of training, such as an understanding of the principles of biomechanics and physiology (along with the current research) that determine how to best individualize a training program based on your goals, abilities, and medical profile.

Never forget that most, if not all, of the training myths that continue to swirl around gyms are perpetuated by the biggest, strongest, and fittest people in them. The fact that these people keep believing this nonsense demonstrates my point. Thinking that those people are the best source of exercise and diet info simply because of how much they lift or how they look keeps the myth alive. However, when you consider that the more time you spend in gyms and kitchens (i.e., on keeping your own gym rat card), the less time you're able to spend on learning the technical and tactical aspects of programming necessary to make you qualified to provide reliable advice and information to other people.

Another way to think about this is to think of astronauts versus astronomers. Astronauts are great to talk with when you want to learn about the mental and emotional aspects of going into and being in space. These experiences are often very individual to them. However, an astronomer is the one to talk to about what you'd have to do to get into space and back to Earth, something that's is based on scientific principles that are universal to everyone.

The world of fitness and conditioning is full of highly trained bodies but poorly trained minds. For example, people often judge the training or nutrition information someone is providing based on how the person providing it looks or how much they can lift. Sure, that seems to make sense on the surface, but here's the problem: What if a person who doesn't possess impressive lifting numbers writes up information on strength training and then gives it to a record-setting powerlifter to read to the rest of us? Is it now better, more reliable strength training information? Or, what if a person who has 20 percent body fat authors a course on fat loss and gives it to a person who has 10 percent body fat to teach? Is it now better, more reliable fat loss information? Of course not, because the information stands or falls on its own merits, which is exactly how it should be judged and discussed.

So, when people with a great physique are making a claim about training or nutrition, they should certainly get your attention based on that, but without good scientific evidence to support what they're telling you, their claims must be taken with a grain of salt. The smartest approach is to think less about what a person looks like and more about the validity and reliability of what they're claiming.

women's exercise magazines. The only thing that changed was the terminology. In the men's version, it said something like, "Use this workout program to build a stronger and more ripped body," whereas in the women's version, it said something like, "Use this workout program to shape the tight and toned body of a goddess."

Despite what it might seem, this common practice is not dishonest or misleading. After all, even the best workout won't do anyone any good if it's not put into practice.

The publishers of these exercise magazines are merely trying to reach their readers using the goals they commonly hear them expressing. Put another way: If exercise is medicine, then we're much more likely to take our daily dose when it tastes good to us. If you do a quick Internet search for body-part specific exercises for the glutes, arms, chest, and shoulders, you'll see many of those terms are commonly followed with "for women" or "for men." This isn't by accident. People are including those words in their Internet searches.

The truth is, there are no exercises for men or exercises for women. There are just exercises. We're different sexes, but our bones, connective tissues, nerves, and muscles fibers are all made of the same raw material and function in the same way. There's nothing inherently male about a barbell exercise or nothing inherently female about machine exercises. They're both effective resistance training methods, and each can be used safely and effectively depending on your ability and goals—not your sex.

Don't be afraid of a machine or resistance exercise. The entire gym is open to you, so learn how to use it to your advantage. This book is designed to help you do that.

This, and the previous three chapters have provided simple and straightforward information that both men and women should keep in mind to get the most out of their exercise time when they're focused on improvements in their fitness, function and performance, fat loss and physique. The next five chapters will detail how to properly and safely perform a wide variety of exercises that are utilized in the workout programs for each goal provided later in the book, beginning with the next chapter on warm-up and mobility exercises.

PART II

Exercises

5 { Warm-Up and Mobility Exercises

This chapter provides five different warm-up sequences you can choose from to begin each workout session. These sequences do far more than just boost your body temperature. They include a variety of mobility exercises to help you develop a more well-rounded body that's not just stronger and better looking but also more mobile. These exercises can help you maintain and increase your overall joint mobility, which can improve joint health. The mobility exercises in the following warm-up sequences complement the workout programs later in this book because they require your joints to move into their end range of motion, whereas the strength training exercises you'll be performing in the workout programs discourage that to maximize safety in handling heavy loads. These mobility exercises also help you perform lifts with more comfort and less restriction.

Each warm-up sequence is designed to be done in place, so they require little space. They have a smooth transition from exercise to exercise, which makes them easy to memorize.

It's important to understand that the warm-up sequences in this chapter are just that: warm-ups. They're not supposed to make you tired. They're intended to complement your workouts by serving as a transition that helps you to feel more prepared to take on the demands of your training session.

The sequences are divided into two major categories: warm-ups that involve holding a small weight plate or medicine ball and bodyweight sequences using no equipment. Each is designed to address the entire body and involve a variety of movement patterns, and which warm-up sequences you do is up to your discretion and equipment availability. Don't always repeat the same one or two sequences. Every one to three workouts, change which sequence you use to make your training more diverse and interesting.

Weight Plate or Medicine Ball Warm-Ups

The following sequences use either a weight plate weighing 5 to 10 pounds (2-4 kg) or a medicine ball weighing about 4.5 to 6.5 pounds (2-3 kg). Select one of the two sequences to begin your workout.

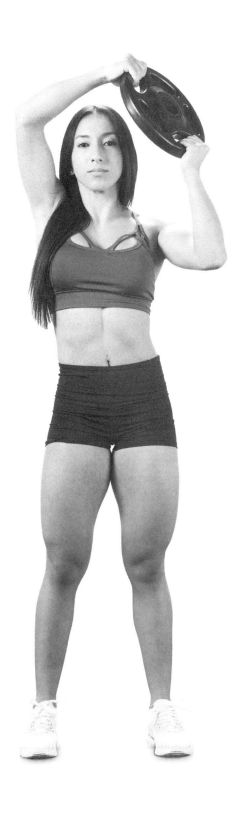

Weight Plate or Medicine Ball Warm-Up 1

This sequence includes the following exercises performed back-to-back for one set each.

 Halo

Setup

Stand with your feet shoulder-width apart and hold the weight plate or medicine ball behind your head.

Action and Coaching Tips

Rotate the weight plate or medicine ball around your head in a horizontal, clockwise pattern (see figures *a* and *b*). Move your arms smoothly, in a coordinated manner, while keeping the center of the medicine ball or weight plate nearly level with your eyes. Perform 8 to 10 reps in one direction, then reverse the motion and perform another 8 to 10 reps.

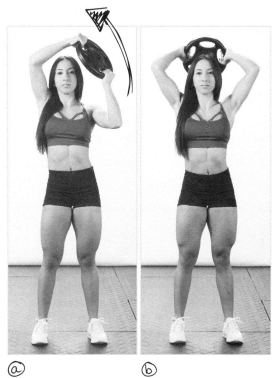

ⓐ ⓑ

 Figure Eight with Hip Rotation

Setup

Stand tall, with your feet slightly wider than shoulder-width apart. Using both hands, hold the weight plate or medicine ball just above your right ear, with your elbows bent a little.

Action and Coaching Tips

Move the weight plate or medicine ball diagonally across your body, toward your left knee, by shifting most of your weight onto your left leg and rotating your torso to the left side while raising your left heel off the ground (see figure *a*). Without stopping the motion, move the plate or ball up to just above your

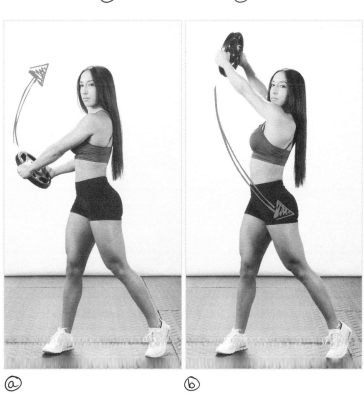

ⓐ ⓑ

right ear (see figure *b*). Repeat on the other side by moving the plate or ball diagonally toward your right knee while shifting most of your weight onto your right leg and rotating your torso to the right side as you raise your left heel off the ground. Again, without stopping motion, move the plate or ball up to just above your right ear. That's one rep! Continue moving dynamically through this action until you've performed 10 to 12 reps of full figure eights.

As the name implies, this exercise involves moving the medicine ball through a figure eight pattern. The cross portion of the figure eight is made in the middle of this exercise, between rotating and shifting your weight from right to left. Do not pause at any time during this exercise; move fast and with control. Move smoothly, with good rhythm and timing in your arm movements and while shifting your weight. Be sure to rotate your hips and shoulders together at the same rate while looking straight ahead.

Reverse Lunge with Twist

Setup

Stand with your feet hip-width apart and hold the weight plate or medicine ball at your chest (see figure *a*).

Action and Coaching Tips

Step backward with your left foot and drop your body so that your knee lightly touches the floor or is right above the floor as you rotate your torso to the right (see figure *b*). Reverse the movement by coming out of the lunge and bringing your left foot forward so that you are back to the starting position, your torso facing forward. Do the same movement with the other leg while turning to the other side. Continue to alternate sides; perform 6 to 8 reps on each side.

Do this exercise smoothly and with a consistent rhythm, coordinating your upper body and lower body in the lifting and lowering phases of each repetition. Keep your head facing forward throughout; in other words, your shoulders rotate, but your head does not. This technique keeps you from getting dizzy and helps maintain range of motion in your neck.

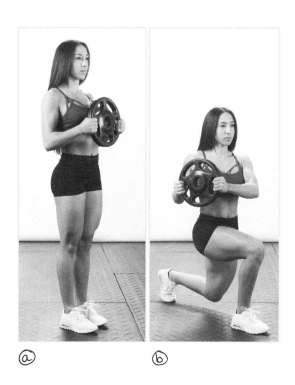

ⓐ   ⓑ

④ Around the World

Setup

Stand in a wide stance, with your feet about 12 inches (about 30 cm) wider than your shoulders. Hold the weight plate or medicine ball directly above your head, with your elbows slightly bent (see figure a).

Action and Coaching Tips

Keeping your elbows bent, use your entire body to make the biggest circles (more like horizontal ovals) that you can make (see figures b and c). Be sure to bend your knees at the bottom aspects of the movement and shift your weight to the same side the ball is on. Also, reach high at the top parts of this exercise. Perform 6 to 8 reps in one direction, then reverse the motion and perform another 6 to 8 reps.

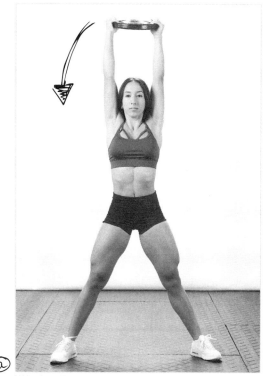

a

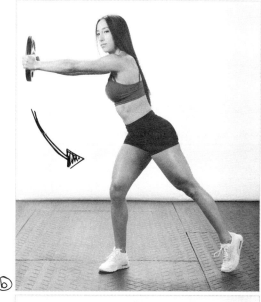

b

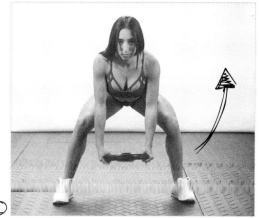

c

Weight Plate or Medicine Ball Warm-Up 2

This sequence includes the following exercises performed back-to-back for one set each.

Rotation

Setup

Stand tall while holding the weight plate or medicine ball at chest height. Your feet should be slightly wider than shoulder-width apart (see figure a).

Action and Coaching Tips

Rotate your torso to the right side while raising your left heel off the ground and rotating on the ball of your foot as you turn (see figure b). Rotate your hips and shoulders together, at the same rate, while looking straight ahead. Quickly reverse the motion and repeat on the other side. Do not pause at any time during this exercise; move fast while using deliberate control. Continue moving dynamically until you've performed 15 to 20 reps on each side. Your nonrotating foot should point nearly straight ahead on each rep.

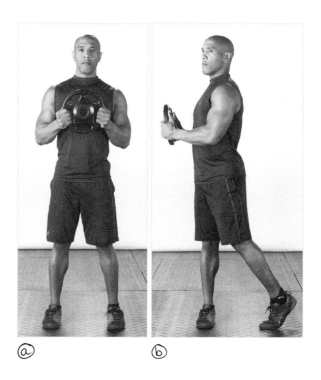

ⓐ　　　　ⓑ

Lateral Ribbon Lunge

Setup

Stand with your feet positioned about 3 feet (about 1 m) apart. Keeping your left leg straight and both feet flat on the floor, shift your weight onto your right leg while slightly bending your right knee and sitting back at your hips (see figure a). Hold the weight plate or medicine ball in front of your right shin.

Action and Coaching Tips

Push your left foot into the ground. Move your right foot toward the midline of your body and place it down so your feet are now hip-width apart. As you step in, simultaneously swing the plate or ball in a circular motion to the left. Continue swinging the plate or ball until it is overhead (see figure b). Repeat by stepping out laterally with your left leg as you swing the plate or ball out to your left shin, then reverse the motion, once again finishing with the plate or ball overhead. Continue to alternate sides; perform 6 to 8 reps on each side.

This exercise gets its name because it involves moving the plate or ball in a ribbon-shaped pattern, with the round portion of the loop occurring as you swing the plate or ball overhead; the X of the ribbon occurs each time you swing the plate or ball across your torso, and each end of the ribbon stops at the bottom of each lunge.

Move smoothly with good rhythm and timing in your arm movement and stepping. Do not allow your back to round out at the bottom of each lunge, and keep your feet flat on the floor throughout.

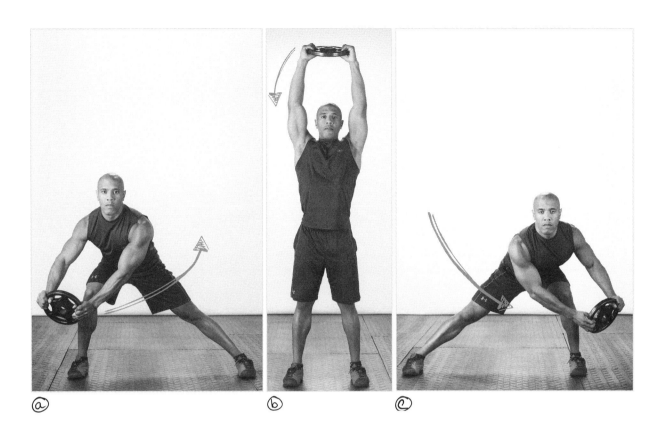

@   ⓑ   ©

③ Overhead Side Lean

Setup

With your feet roughly hip-width apart, hold the weight plate or medicine ball directly above your head, with your elbows slightly bent (see figure a).

Action and Coaching Tips

While keeping the weight plate or medicine ball directly above your head, lean your body laterally to one side and shift your hips to the opposite side until you feel a mild stretch (see figure b). Reverse the motion and repeat, leaning your torso and hips to the opposite direction. Perform 10 to 12 reps per side, alternating sides on each rep.

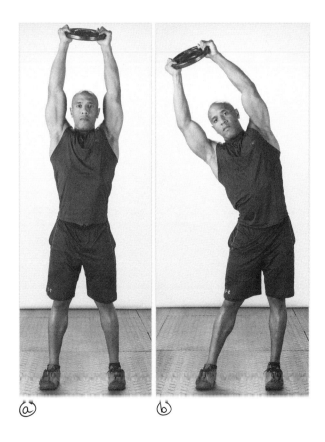

@   ⓑ

Weight Plate or Medicine Ball Warm-Up 2   *>continued*

Swing

Setup

With your feet roughly hip-width apart, hold a weight plate or medicine ball with both hands, your arms straight and in front of your body (see figure *a*).

Action and Coaching Tips

Hinge forward at your hips, keeping your knees bent at roughly a 15- to 20-degree angle. Drive the weight plate or medicine ball between your legs, as if hiking a football (see figure *b*). Once your forearms contact your thighs, quickly reverse the motion

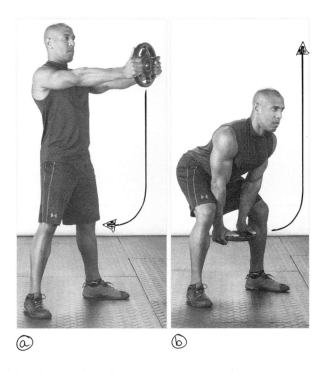

ⓐ   ⓑ

by simultaneously driving your hips forward and swinging the weight plate or medicine ball upward. Finish with the plate or ball at eye level or above your head (if it's not uncomfortable for your shoulders). Reverse the motion to complete one rep. Move dynamically, without pausing at any point. Do 12 to 14 reps.

Do this exercise smoothly and with a consistent rhythm, coordinating your upper body and lower body in the lifting and lowering phases of each repetition. Do not allow your back to round out at the bottom of each rep.

Bodyweight Warm-Ups

As the name implies, these don't involve any additional equipment, except a mat if you want one for the exercises performed on the floor. Select one of the three sequences to begin your workout.

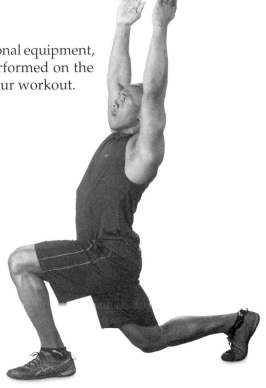

Bodyweight Warm-Up 1

This sequence includes the following exercises performed back-to-back for one set each.

Arm Circles

Setup

Stand tall, with your arms reaching out and your feet hip-width apart (see figure *a*).

Action and Coaching Tips

Keeping your arms straight, swing your arms dynamically toward the back and then up and around to make circles in a smooth and rhythmic action (see figures *a* and *b*). Although your arms are straight, do not lock your elbows. Make the biggest circles you can without any discomfort. Perform 10 to 12 backward rotations and 10 to 12 forward rotations.

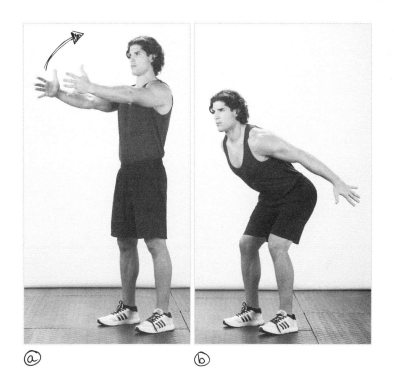

ⓐ　　　　　ⓑ

Hip Circles

Setup

Stand with your feet shoulder-width apart, your feet pointed straight ahead, and your hands on your hips.

Action and Coaching Tips

Keeping your legs straight, rotate your hips, making the biggest horizontal circles you can make without discomfort (see figures *a* and *b*). Perform 6 to 8 reps clockwise and another 6 to 8 reps as you move counterclockwise.

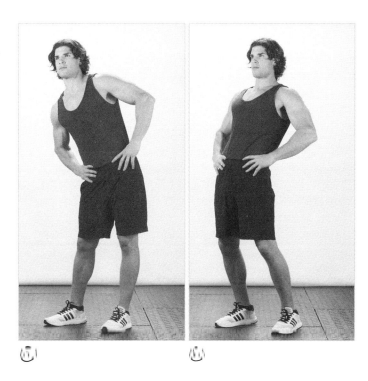

ⓐ　　　　　ⓑ

③ In-Place High Kicks

Setup

Stand tall, with your feet hip-width apart and your arms at your sides (see figure *a*).

Action and Coaching Tips

Kick your right leg up toward the sky, keeping your knee slightly bent (see figure *b*). Simultaneously, reach your left arm out in front of you at shoulder level. Quickly lower your right leg back down to the floor, then kick your left leg up toward the sky, keeping your knee slightly bent. Simultaneously, reach your right arm out in front of you at shoulder level. Then, lower your left leg back down to the floor. Continue alternating legs and using the opposite arm with each kick.

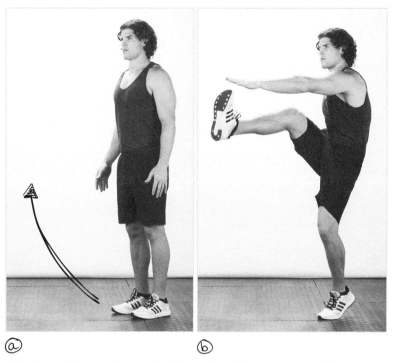

ⓐ   ⓑ

Keep your torso upright and your ankle flexed throughout. Perform 4 to 6 reps on each leg.

④ Zombie Squat with Reach-Through

Setup

Stand with your feet slightly farther than shoulder-width apart and your toes pointed outward. Reach your arms through your legs, keeping your knees slightly bent (see figure *a*).

Action and Coaching Tips

As you bring your torso upright, simultaneously bend your hips and drop them into a squat (see figure *b*). Keep your heels flat on the floor and do not allow your knees to drop toward the midline as you squat. Finish with your arms outstretched in front of you at shoulder level. Reverse to return to the starting position. Perform 6 to 8 reps. Squat as deep as you can on each rep.

For a more advanced variation, perform the exercise in the same manner but place your

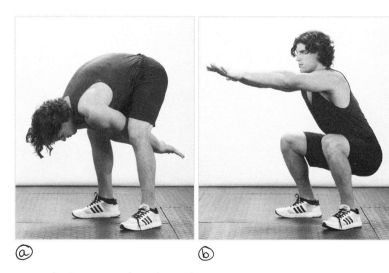

ⓐ   ⓑ

arms overhead, in line with your torso, each time you drop into the squat.

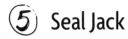 **Seal Jack**

Setup

Stand with your feet together and your arms extended in front of you at shoulder level, your hands together (see figure *a*).

Action and Coaching Tips

As you open your arms horizontally to the side, jump up just enough to spread your feet wide (see figure *b*). Without pausing, quickly reverse the movement. Do the exercise smoothly, opening and closing your legs and arms simultaneously. Be as light on your feet as possible, minimizing the time that your feet are in contact with the ground. Perform 20 to 25 reps.

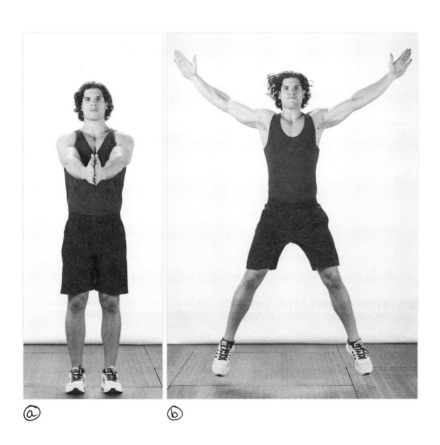

ⓐ   ⓑ

Bodyweight Warm-Up 2

This sequence includes the following exercises performed back-to-back for one set each.

Arm Crossover

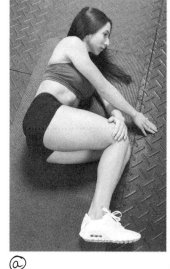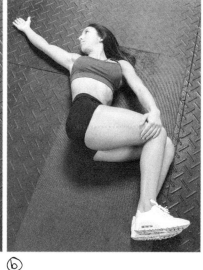

Setup

Lie on your left side, with your knees and hips bent a little more than 90 degrees. Straighten your right arm, palm facing down (see figure *a*).

Action and Coaching Tips

While keeping your bottom arm and both legs in position, rotate your torso to the right as far as you can (without forcing anything) until your right hand and upper back are flat on the floor (see figure *b*). Hold for one or two seconds, then return to the starting position. Perform 6 to 8 reps on each side. Do all reps on one side before switching sides.

If you're unable to get close to touching the other side of the floor when you're rotating, perform this exercise with a small medicine ball or rolled towel between your knees to allow for a greater range of motion.

Yoga Lunge to Same-Side Torso Rotation and Hamstring Stretch Combo

Setup

Begin in a push-up position, with your wrists underneath your shoulders and your feet hip-width apart. Bring your left foot up so that it's flat on the floor just outside of your left hand. Form a nearly straight line with your torso and right leg (see figure *a*).

Action and Coaching Tips

While keeping your torso in a fairly straight line with your back leg, rotate your torso to the left as you reach your left arm toward the ceiling (see figure *b*). Reverse the action and place your left hand back down, but now put it on the floor, just outside of your left foot (see figure *c*). Then, simultaneously shift your weight backward as you try to straighten your left leg while flexing your left ankle toward you (see figure *d*). Reverse the action and place your left hand back down on the floor to the inside of your left foot. Repeat this sequence for 4 to 6 reps on the same side before switching sides by stepping your right foot up so it's just outside of your right hand.

Do not pause for more than a second at any point; maintain a constant flow. If you're unable to place your foot flat next to your hand when you step forward, you can make the exercise easier by elevating your hands on a platform (e.g., an aerobic step).

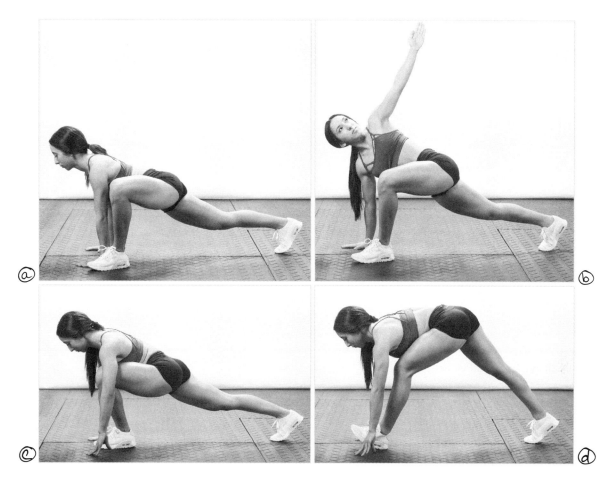

③ Prisoner Squat with Hip Rotation

Setup

Stand tall, with your feet slightly more than shoulder-width apart and your toes turned out about 10 degrees. Interlace your fingers behind your head, with your elbows pointed out to the sides.

Action and Coaching Tips

Squat by bending your knees and sitting back at your hips (see figure a). Go down so that your thighs are almost parallel to the floor. Don't allow your lower back to round out. As you squat down, your knees should track in the same direction as your toes. Do not allow your heels to come off the ground or your knees to come together toward the midline of your body. Reverse the action by extending at your legs and hips, and as you rise, simultaneously rotate your torso to one side while allowing your other foot to rotate freely by elevating your heel and turning on the ball of your foot (see

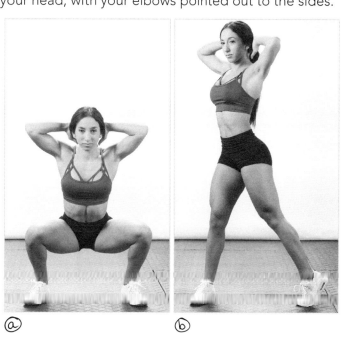

figure *b*). Rotate your hips and shoulder simultaneously, moving them at the same rate. Return to the starting position and repeat the same motion by squatting back down, then rotating to the other side at the top. Perform 5 to 7 reps on each side, which is 10 to 14 total squats.

④ Lateral Lunge with Zombie Arm Reach and Air Row

Setup

Stand with your feet hip-width apart and your arms pulled in to the sides of your body with palms facing toward the front (see figure *a*).

Action and Coaching Tips

Step to one side and lower into a side lunge while keeping your trailing leg straight and both of your feet flat. As you step, stretch your arms to the front at shoulder height (see figure *b*). Reverse the motion by stepping back to the middle as you pull your arms back to your sides. Repeat on the other side. Continue to alternate sides while maintaining good rhythm and timing, both when stepping and when reversing the action; the movement should not look choppy. Perform 4 to 6 reps on each side.

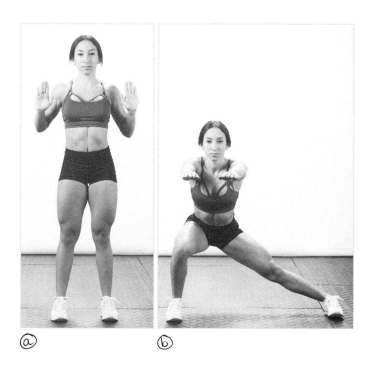

ⓐ   ⓑ

⑤ Jumping Jack

Setup

Stand with your feet hip-width apart and your hands at your sides (see figure *a*).

Action and Coaching Tips

As you raise your arms above your head, jump up just enough to spread your feet wide (see figure *b*). Without pausing, quickly reverse the movement. Do the exercise smoothly, moving your legs and arms simultaneously when opening or closing. Be as light on your feet as possible and minimize the time that your feet are in contact with the ground. Perform 20 to 25 reps.

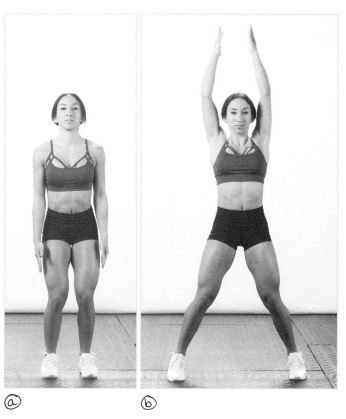

ⓐ   ⓑ

Bodyweight Warm-Up 3

This sequence includes the following exercises performed back-to-back for one set each.

 ## Dynamic Pigeon

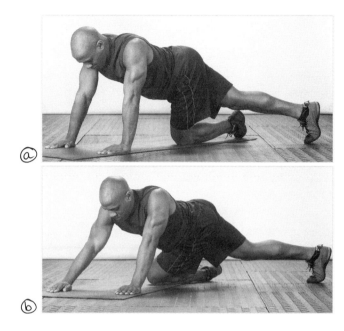

Setup

This is a dynamic (more active) version of a yoga position known as pigeon pose. Get on all fours, with your hands underneath your shoulders and your knees under your hips.

Action and Coaching Tips

Extend your right leg straight at a 45-degree angle across your left leg (see figures a and b). Shift your hips backward as you drive your right leg back at a 45-degree angle as far as you can without lifting your hands off the floor. As you shift your hips backward, allow your arms to extend fully but keep your hands on the floor. Reverse the motion, bringing your right knee back down underneath your right hip. After bringing the right knee back, extend your left leg behind you at a 45-degree angle to perform the same action. Alternate legs while keeping your shoulders parallel to the floor throughout. Do each rep smoothly, with control, without pausing at any time. Perform 6 to 8 reps with each leg.

 ## Downward Dog to Yoga Lunge and Opposite-Side Torso Rotation Combo

Setup

Begin in a push-up position, with your wrists underneath your shoulders and your feet positioned roughly 6 inches (15 cm) farther to each side than shoulder-width apart.

Action and Coaching Tips

Perform the downward dog portion of this drill by shifting your weight backward while raising your hips toward the sky and dropping your heels downward (see figure a). Then, reverse the action while stepping forward on your right foot, keeping it flat on the ground just outside of your right arm so that your torso now forms a straight line with your left leg (see figure b). Rotate your torso to the left as you reach your left arm toward the ceiling (see figure c). Reverse the motion and place your left hand back down on the floor, just underneath your left shoulder. Then, shift your hips backward again into the downward position. As you reverse the motion this time, step forward on your left foot, keeping it flat on the ground just outside your left arm so that your torso now forms a straight line with your left leg. Now, rotate your torso to the right as you reach your right arm toward the ceiling. Reverse the motion and place your right hand back down on the floor, just underneath your right shoulder. That's one rep! Perform 3 to 5 total reps, alternating legs each and each step.

Do not pause for more than a second at any point; maintain a constant flow.

If you're unable to place your foot flat next to your hand when you step forward, you can make the exercise easier by elevating your hands on a platform (e.g., aerobic step).

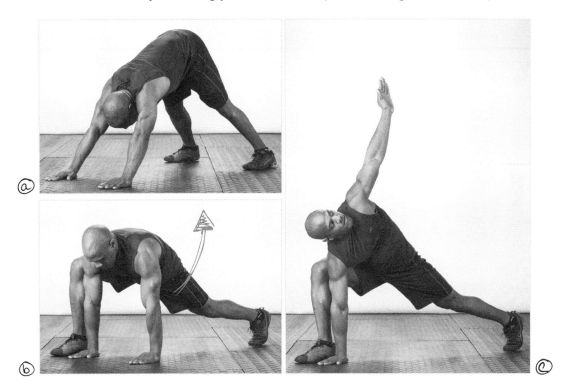

③ Reverse Lunge with Overhead Reach

Setup

Stand tall, with your feet together and arms out to the front with palms down (see figure a).

Action and Coaching Tips

Step backward with one leg, dropping into a lunge position while reaching both arms overhead and leaning backward a little (see figure b). Return to the standing position with your feet together and repeat by stepping back with the other leg. Repeat for 4 to 6 reps per side, alternating legs on each rep.

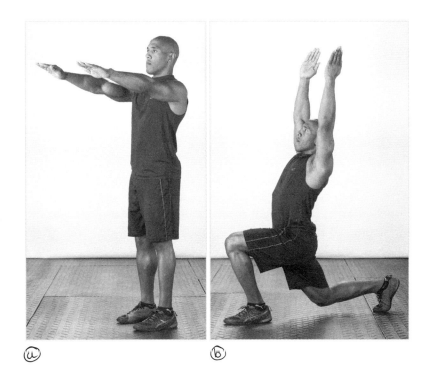

④ Rotational Arm Swing

Setup

Stand tall, with your feet hip-width apart, and reach your arms straight out in front of your shoulders, palms facing in (see figure a).

Action and Coaching Tips

Quickly rotate your torso to the left side, driving both your left hip and your left arm behind you while allowing your right foot to rotate freely by elevating your heel and turning on the ball of your foot. Rotate your hips and shoulder, moving them at the same rate (see figure b). Return to the starting position and repeat the same motion to the other side. Make your motions fast and dynamic. Perform 6 to 8 reps on each side.

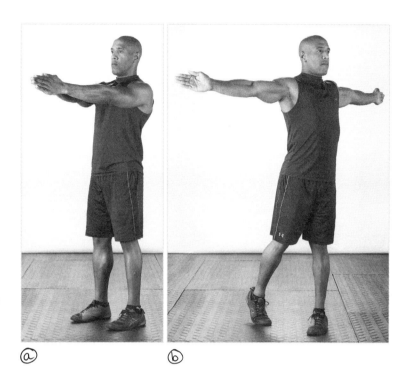

ⓐ　　　ⓑ

⑤ In-Place High-Knee Skip

Setup

Stand tall, with your feet hip width apart and your elbows bent roughly 90 degrees.

Action and Coaching Tips

Lift your left knee to a point just above your hip while also lifting your right arm and moving your left arm back (see figures a and b). Quickly reverse your arm positions as you drive your left leg down to the ground and elevate your right knee. Much like jumping rope, skipping requires a double foot strike pattern, or right-right hops, followed by left-left hops. Unlike running in place, to skip in place, you must coordinate your arm pumping with your double foot strikes. Perform 20 to 25 reps per leg, keeping your torso upright throughout.

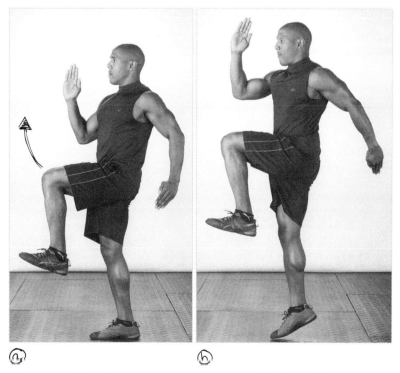

ⓐ　　　ⓑ

Once you've become proficient at using each warm-up sequence in this chapter, you can mix and match the exercises to develop your own personalized warm-ups that best fit you. Just be sure to keep your warm-ups short and not fatiguing, Again, it's supposed to be a warm-up, not a workout.

The following three chapters describe how to perform a variety of exercises utilized in the workout programs later in this book for building muscle, improving function and performance, fat loss, and general fitness and health. No matter which workout program from chapters 10-14 you choose, the warm-ups you've learned in this chapter will help you get ready for action!

6 { Upper-Body Exercises

This chapter covers a variety of exercises designed to strengthen and develop your upper-body musculature. These exercises involve pushing and pulling loads in either a horizontal, diagonal, or vertical plane (direction) from a variety of stances and body positions and using both single-arm (unilateral) and double-arm (bilateral) actions. Although the upper-body pulling motion of moving something—such as an object or opponent—closer to you is the opposite of pushing something away from you, these two movements are often used together, such as in actions like sawing and punching (i.e., a one-two combination in which a left jab is followed immediately by a right cross). Torso muscles maintain your body position and posture while you perform the pushing or pulling action.

Some of the exercises in this chapter distribute the loading challenge through several upper-body muscles. For example, the pushing exercises integrate the chest, shoulder, and triceps muscles. The pulling exercises integrate efforts by the lats, midback, posterior shoulders, and biceps muscles. Other exercises are more targeted and provide a more focused resistance challenge to certain muscle groups in the upper body.

Basic Upper-Body Exercises: PERFECTED

The following section provides basic upper-body exercises and shows you how to do them better than how they are commonly performed. This will help you train smarter, more safely, and efficiently. All it takes is a couple of small tweaks.

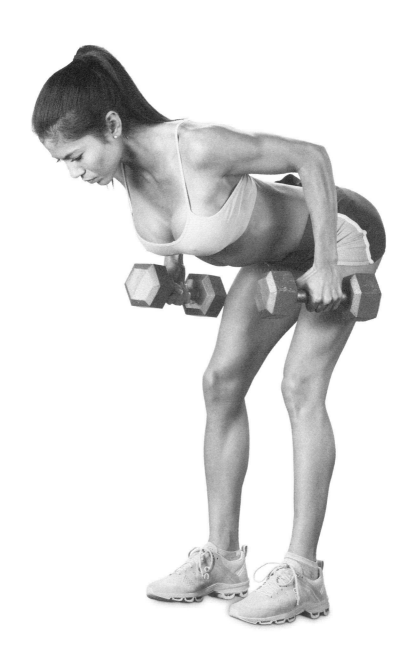

Seated Row

Use a shoulder-width grip on a bar instead of using the narrow V-shaped handle

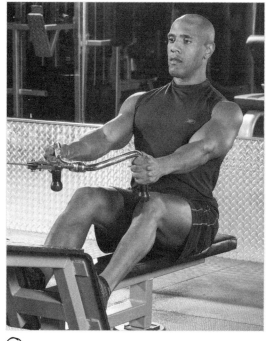

(a)

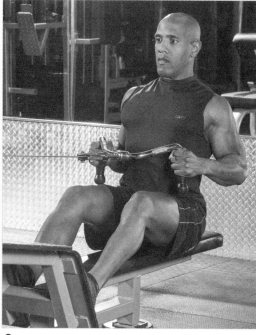

(b)

Setup

Sit on a cable row bench with your feet firmly planted on the foot plate. Grab the neutral-grip handle attached to the cable pulley that places your hands roughly shoulder-width apart (see figure *a*). Keep your knees slightly bent and your back straight. Maintain a slight arch in your lower back and keep your chest out.

Action and Coaching Tips

Pull the handle toward your midsection, focusing on driving your elbows back until the handle touches your lower abdomen (see figure *b*). Do not allow the front of your shoulders to round forward at the end of each repetition. After squeezing your shoulder blades together at the peak of the contraction, slowly return to the starting position.

WHY IT'S BETTER

You use a shoulder-width grip on a bar instead of using the narrow V-shaped handle. This is *not* to say that using the close-grip V-shaped bar is incorrect or somehow inherently dangerous. However, when using a close grip, your hands are stuck in a more narrow position, cutting off the final two to three inches in your range of motion. If you prefer the close-grip method, there is nothing wrong with continuing to use it. With a wider grip, you are allowing your muscles to reach the maximum level of contraction through a greater range of motion that in turn affects muscle recruitment of the midback.

Benefits

- Maximize your range of motion.
- Complete muscle contraction of the midback muscles.

Lat Pull-Down

Setup

Position yourself just behind a traditional lat pull-down bar and hold it with an overhand grip over your head (see figure *a*).

Action and Coaching Tips

Pull the bar down to the top of your chest while keeping your back straight and your elbows following a straight line (see figure *b*). Slowly reverse the motion, keeping control. You can also add variety to this exercise by performing it using an underhand grip, with your palms facing you at roughly shoulder-width apart.

WHY IT'S BETTER

You place hands in an overhand grip a few inches outside shoulder-width, instead of very wide on the bar. The belief that a wider grip on the pull-down bar activates the lats more than a narrow one does originates in bodybuilding dogma, but it also appears to be based in science. One study found that the wide-grip pull-down produced greater muscle activity than pull-downs using a closer, underhand grip. The problem is that this study didn't compare different overhand grip widths (1).

Luckily, another study compared a 6-rep max (6RM) load and muscle activity using three different overhand (i.e., pronated) grip widths. Lifters performed 6RM in the lat pull-down with narrow, medium, and wide grips—1, 1.5, and 2 times the biacromial distance, a measure of shoulder width. This study found that, aside from a bit more biceps involvement in the medium-grip width, all three grips produced similar lat activation (2).

You can mix up grip widths to add subtle variety to your lat pull-downs without feeling as if you're missing out on the "special" lat building benefit of using a wide grip. That said, if your objective is to add in some extra biceps work while also doing lat pull-downs, a medium-width grip is just what the muscle doctor ordered.

Benefits

- Less awkward grip
- Same lat muscle recruitment with more biceps recruitment

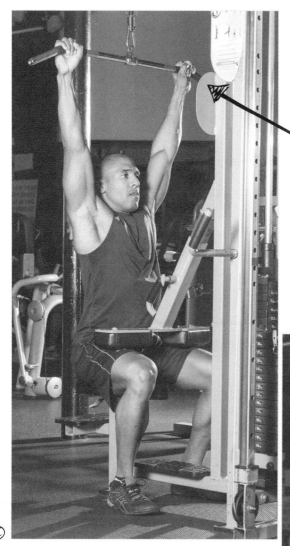

Place hands in an overhand grip a few inches outside shoulder-width, instead of very wide on the bar

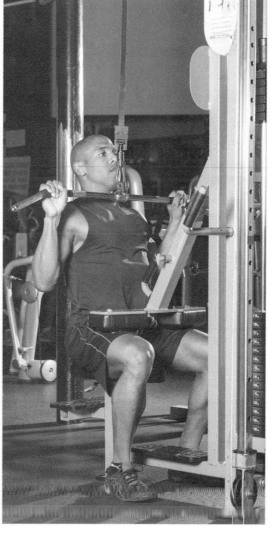

Leaning Lat Pull-Down

Setup

This exercise is performed in the same manner as the lat pull-down, except you lean backward slightly instead of remaining upright. Position yourself just behind a traditional lat pull-down bar and hold it with an overhand grip over your head, then lean back at roughly 25 degrees from upright (see figure a). Find a grip width somewhere outside of shoulder width that feels most comfortable to you.

Action and Coaching Tips

While leaning your torso backward, pull the bar down to the top of your chest while keeping your elbows pointed in the same direction as your line of pull (see figure b). Slowly reverse the motion, keeping control.

For variety, you can use an underhand grip with your palms facing you. Or, you can use a neutral grip by exchanging the straight bar for a handle that allows your palms to face one another, spaced roughly shoulder-width apart.

WHY IT'S BETTER

You lean backward at roughly 25 degrees from upright. Most personal trainers, strength coaches, and exercise enthusiasts think that upper-body pushing must involve some type of flat pressing movement, some type of incline pressing movement, and some type of overhead pressing movement. They're on the right track because pressing in each direction creates a slightly different loading stimulus.

There's no reason this shouldn't also apply to pulling movements, just like how horizontal pushing movements (i.e., bench press, push-ups, etc.) are complemented by horizontal pulling movements (i.e., adding row variations). And, just like how vertical pushing movements (i.e., shoulder presses) are complemented by vertical pulling movements (i.e., pull-ups and pull-downs), diagonal pushing movements (i.e., incline presses, angled barbell presses) are complemented by exercises like the leaning lat pull-down or the one-arm half-kneeling angled cable row, both of which are featured later in this chapter.

Benefits

- Provides a different loading stimulus than with an upright torso
- Adds training variety

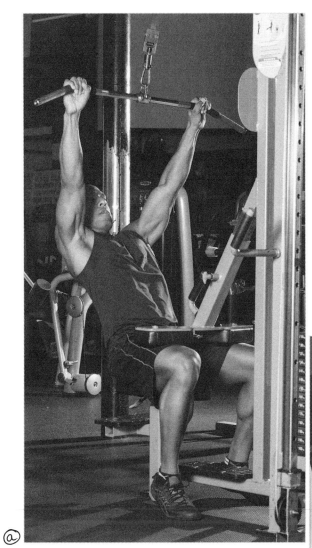

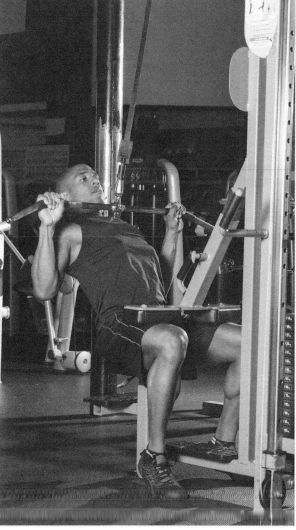

Lean backward at roughly 25 degrees from upright

Push-Up

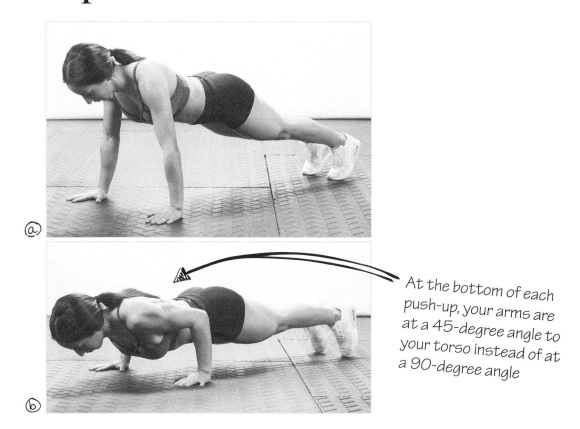

At the bottom of each push-up, your arms are at a 45-degree angle to your torso instead of at a 90-degree angle

Setup
Place your hands on the floor just farther than shoulder-width apart, with your elbows straight. Turn your hands outward so that your fingers point at roughly 45 degrees (see figure a).

Action and Coaching Tips
Lower your body to the floor while keeping your elbows directly above your wrists (see figure b). Once your elbows are almost at a 90-degree angle, reverse the motion by pushing your body up so that your elbows are straight again. At the top of each push-up, do not finish with your shoulder blades pinched together; instead, protract (push apart) your shoulder blades while keeping your body in a straight line.

WHY IT'S BETTER
At the bottom of each push-up, position your arms at a 45-degree angle to your torso instead of at a 90-degree angle. From an overhead view, your arms will form the shape of an arrow instead of a T with your torso. The T position makes the exercise easier and therefore creates a lesser effective training stimulus because it requires less muscle activation (as measured by EMG) in the pecs and the triceps. Plus, in the T position, shoulder horizontal abduction flexibility is limited, so you're not making the most of the range of motion you can train through (3).

Benefits
- Maximize your range of motion
- Better involvement of the chest and triceps muscles

Barbell Bent-Over Row

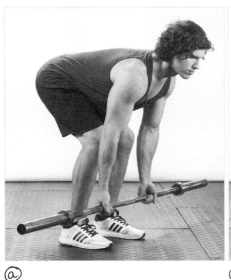 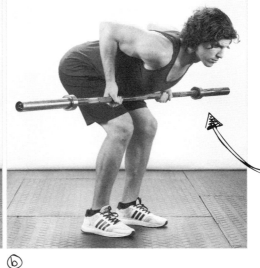

Select a weight you can hold for a few seconds at the top of the range of motion

ⓐ ⓑ

Setup

Stand with your feet roughly hip-width apart. Hold a barbell with an underhand grip and keep your hands just outside shoulder-width apart. You can also perform bent-over rows with an overhand grip, which many people find to be a weaker gripping option. Bend over at your hips, keeping your back straight so that your torso is roughly parallel to the floor (see figure a). Keep your knees bent 15 to 20 degrees.

Action and Coaching Tips

Row the bar into your body, just above your belly button (see figure b). Pause for one second and pinch your shoulder blades together at the top. Do not allow the fronts of your shoulders to round forward at the top of each repetition. Slowly lower the bar to complete the rep. Do not allow your back to round out at any time.

WHY IT'S BETTER

To ensure you can control the weight throughout the entire range of motion, select a weight you can hold for a few seconds at top of the concentric portion of the range of motion (i.e., with the barbell pulled into your body) while maintaining good technique. If you can't hold it for a few seconds, then the weight is too heavy to perform a full set while maintaining control on each rep. This is an important deviation from the way most people choose the weight for this exercise, which is usually based on how heavy it feels at the beginning (i.e., bottom portion) of the row instead of at top portion.

When performing the barbell bent-over row, the lever arm is at its longest—you have the least mechanical advantage—when your humerus (your "biceps bone") is parallel with the floor (in line with your torso). This is at or very close to the end of concentric portion of the range of motion. This is why you often see lifters pull the weight halfway with good form, then jolt it the rest of the way when performing exercises like barbell bent-over rows and one-arm dumbbell rows. Using a weight based on what you can move during the most difficult part of the range of motion, instead of at the easier portion of the ranges, like most people commonly do, ensures that you're not just moving the weight, but controlling the weight through the entire range of motion involved in the exercise.

Benefits

- Maximize your range of motion
- Complete muscle contraction of the midback muscles

63

One-Arm Dumbbell Row

Setup

Stand parallel to a traditional weight bench with your left hand and left knee on top of the bench and a dumbbell in your right hand. Your right foot is on the floor, and the right knee is slightly bent. Keep a straight back that is roughly parallel to the floor. Rotate your torso slightly to the right so that your right shoulder—the same side you're holding the dumbbell on—is slightly below the level of your left shoulder (see figure *a*).

Action and Coaching Tips

While keeping your right shoulder slightly below the level of your left shoulder, perform the row by pulling the dumbbell toward your body so that your right elbow ends up at roughly a 90-degree angle while you drive your left shoulder blade toward your spine (see figure *b*). Do not allow your rowing-side shoulder to move forward at the top of each rep. Slowly lower the dumbbell toward the floor until your arm straightens, without allowing the dumbbell to touch the floor.

WHY IT'S BETTER

You rotate the shoulder toward the side you're holding the dumbbell. Instead of keeping your shoulders parallel to the ground, rotate it slightly toward the same side you're holding the dumbbell on.

When performing one-arm dumbbell rows, people usually pull the weight halfway with good form and then pull it the rest of the way up by turning the torso toward the rowing arm. As discussed previously, as you get closer to the concentric end of the range of motion in rowing exercises, you're getting weaker as the weight is getting heavier (because the lever arm is getting longer). Turning your torso upward on the side you're rowing with is a "cheat" that may be good for the ego, but it reduces the involvement of your midback muscles. Keeping your torso rotated slightly toward the same side you're holding the dumbbell on prevents this cheat and ensures better use of your midback muscles through the full range of motion involved in the exercise.

Benefits

- Avoid cheating through the top portion of the range of motion
- Improved muscle contraction of the midback muscles

Rotate your shoulder toward the side you're holding the dumbbell

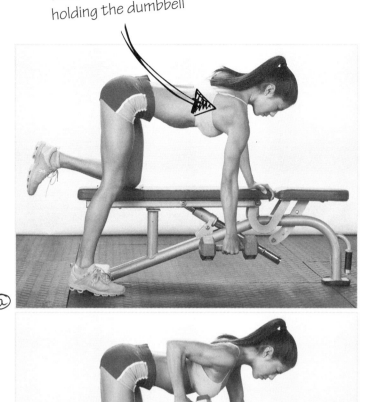

(a)

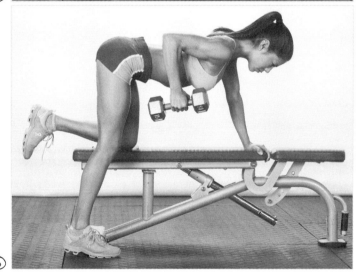

(b)

Two-Arm Dumbbell Bent-Over Row

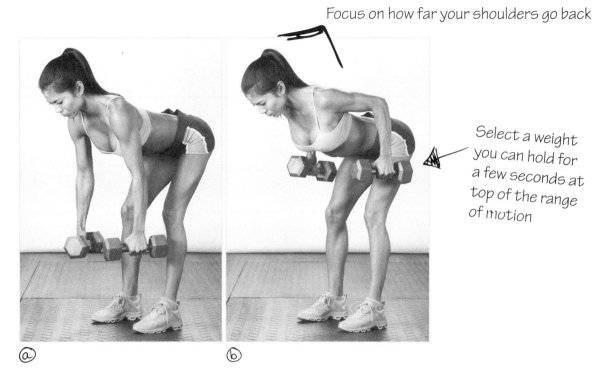

Focus on how far your shoulders go back

Select a weight you can hold for a few seconds at top of the range of motion

(a)   (b)

Setup

Stand with your feet hip-width apart and hold a dumbbell in each hand. Bend over at your hips, keeping your back straight so that your torso is roughly parallel to the floor (see figure a). Keep your knees bent 15 to 20 degrees.

Action and Coaching Tips

Row the dumbbells toward you while keeping your arms at a 45-degree angle to your torso; at the top, pinch your shoulder blades together (see figure b). Pause for one second at the top of each repetition. Slowly lower the dumbbells without allowing them to contact the floor until the set is completed. Do not allow your back to round out at any time. At the top of each repetition, do not allow your wrists to bend or the fronts of your shoulders to round forward.

WHY IT'S BETTER

To ensure you can control the weight throughout the entire range of motion, select a weight you can hold for a few seconds at top of the concentric portion of the range of motion (i.e., with the dumbbells pulled into your body) while maintaining good technique. If you can't hold it for a few seconds, then the weight is too heavy to perform a full set while maintaining control on each rep. This is an important difference from the way most people choose the weight for this exercise, which is usually based on how heavy it feels at the beginning (i.e., bottom portion) of the row instead of at top portion.

Also, when performing the row, focus on how far your shoulders go back. A good row isn't about how far your elbows go back. It's about how far your shoulders go back since the target back muscles control your shoulder. At the end of the concentric portion of each rep, your elbow should be bent at roughly a 90-degree angle. Bending it more makes the row more biceps-dominant, which takes work away from your back musculature.

Benefits

- Increased activation of your back musculature
- Reduces cheating

Dumbbell Rear Delt Fly

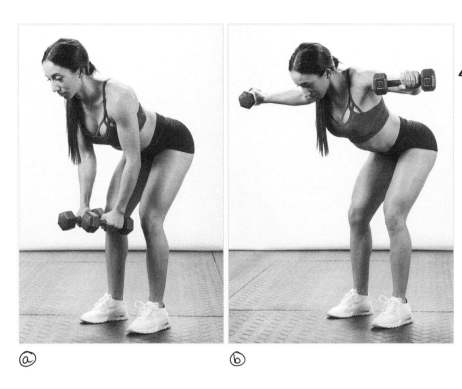

Use a neutral grip with your palms facing each other

(a)   (b)

Setup
Stand with your feet hip-width apart and hold a dumbbell in each hand. Bend over at your hips, keeping your back straight so that your torso is roughly parallel to the floor and your knees are bent 15 to 20 degrees (see figure *a*).

Action and Coaching Tips
Keeping a small bend in your elbows, raise your arms out to your sides (see figure *b*). Your arms should be at a 90-degree angle relative to your torso at the top of each repetition, thus forming a *T* shape with your torso at the top of each rep. Do not swing the dumbbells up. Pause for one second at the top of each repetition and pinch your shoulder blades together, then slowly lower the dumbbells in front of your torso. Do not allow your back to round out at any time.

WHY IT'S BETTER
You use a neutral grip, with your palms facing each other, instead of a thumbs-down grip or an offset grip where you hold the dumbbells all the way to the pinky side. Research has shown that using a neutral grip when doing a rear delt fly increased the activity of the posterior delts compared to using a thumbs-down grip (4). This also makes sense from an anatomy perspective because the neutral hand position is more externally rotated than the pronated position, as both the posterior deltoid and infraspinatus muscles are also external rotators of the shoulder (5). Gripping the dumbbell all the way to the pinky finger side forces you to resist shoulder internal rotation (by using more of your posterior delts as external rotators).

Benefits
- Better targeting and recruitment of the rear deltoids
- More efficient

Dumbbell Biceps Curl

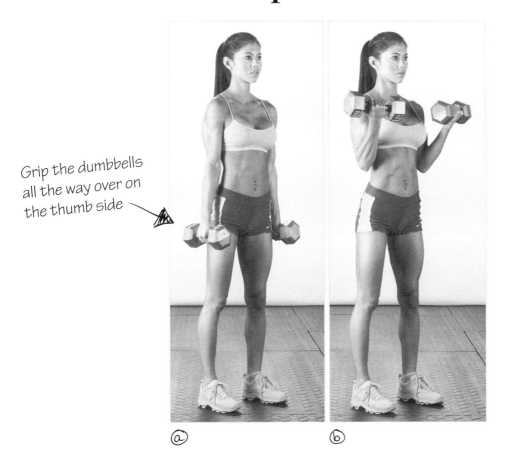

Grip the dumbbells all the way over on the thumb side

(a)   (b)

Setup

Stand tall, with your feet hip-width apart. Hold a dumbbell in each hand next to your hips (see figure a).

Action and Coaching Tips

Curl the dumbbells up toward your shoulders by bending at your elbow without allowing your elbow to move forward or backward (see figure b). Do not swing the weight up by overextending at your lower back. Once your hands are up in front of your shoulders, reverse the motion by slowly lowering the dumbbells back to your side.

WHY IT'S BETTER

Instead of gripping the dumbbell from the middle in the traditional manner, grip it all the way over on the thumb side. The biceps are not only elbow flexors but also wrist and forearm supinators. If we want to achieve maximal biceps recruitment when doing dumbbell curls, we must involve both elbow flexion and forearm supination. You can do this by holding the handle all the way over on the thumb side. This small change makes a huge difference because this grip forces you to resist forearm pronation. The biceps are forced to act as supinators while also serving as elbow flexors.

Benefits

- Better targeting and recruitment of the biceps
- More efficient

Dumbbell Upright Row

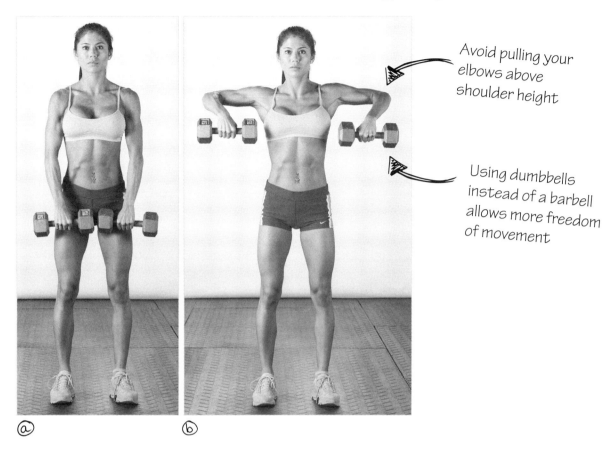

Avoid pulling your elbows above shoulder height

Using dumbbells instead of a barbell allows more freedom of movement

(a)　(b)

Setup
Stand tall, with your feet hip-width apart. Hold a pair of dumbbells, resting them on your thighs (see figure a).

Action and Coaching Tips
Pull the dumbbells toward the sky, outside of your torso, until your elbows reach shoulder height (see figure b). Then lower the dumbbells back to your thighs in a controlled fashion to reset and begin your next repetition.

WHY IT'S BETTER
You use a wider grip, with dumbbells instead of a barbell, and avoid pulling your elbows above shoulder height. Using dumbbells instead of a barbell allows more freedom of movement. Your arms can move apart as your lift the weight. A wider grip has been shown in studies to increase deltoid and trapezius activity and reduce biceps brachii activity (6). In addition to maximizing recruitment of the muscle we're trying to develop, we need to also consider exercise safety. Avoid pulling the elbows above shoulder height.

Research indicates that impingement typically peaks between 70 and 120 degrees of glenohumeral elevation. Research has recommended that asymptomatic individuals elevate their arms during the upright row to just under 90 degrees (shoulder height) (7). Other authors have made similar recommendations, so at least in this case, don't listen to the full range of motion gods.

Benefits
- Increased shoulder muscle recruitment
- Potentially safer on the shoulder joints

69

Dumbbell Front Shoulder Raise

Setup

Stand tall, with your feet hip-width apart. Hold a pair of dumbbells at your sides (see figure a).

Action and Coaching Tips

With your elbows slightly bent, raise your arms out in front of your body until your elbows go just above your forehead (see figure b). Do not swing the weight up. Slowly lower the dumbbells back to your sides. Use deliberate control on the lifting and lowering portion of each rep.

WHY IT'S BETTER

You increase range of motion when lifting your arms up during this exercise. Stopping when your arms are parallel to the floor is like stopping a biceps curl when your forearm is parallel to the floor.

Many lifters say they don't lift their arms above shoulder level—even keeping them slightly below shoulder level—when doing shoulders raises to minimize the involvement of the upper traps. Interestingly, many of these same people do shrugs, upright rows, and other trap-oriented exercises.

Now, if for some reason you're avoiding upper trap exercises and do not want activity in your upper traps, just know that research has found that, out of 16 commonly used shoulder training and rehabilitation exercises—such as seated row, knee push-up plus, or biceps curl—all but one exercise showed moderate to low activity in the upper traps (8). And none of the 16 exercises investigated in this study were a shoulder shrug or upright row. The one exercise mentioned here is commonly known as the full can, which is where you're standing with your arm at your side in external rotation. Then you lift your arm in the scapular plane (at a 30-degree angle to your torso) until your arm is 90 degrees to the floor. In short, it's very much like a side shoulder raise.

The point is, don't have the delusion that your upper traps aren't being activated in upper-body exercises that you didn't think involved that muscle group.

Benefits

- Greater range of motion
- More comprehensive shoulder training

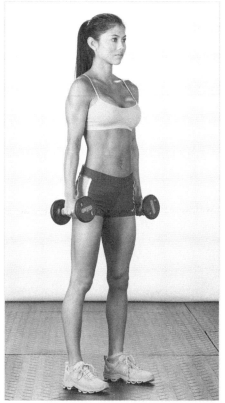

@

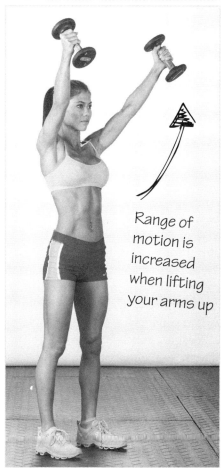

Range of motion is increased when lifting your arms up

ⓑ

Dumbbell Side Shoulder Raise

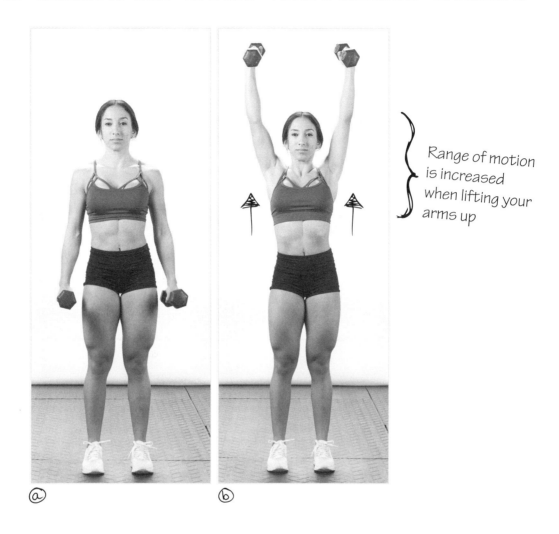

Range of motion is increased when lifting your arms up

Setup
Stand tall, with your feet hip-width apart. Hold a pair of dumbbells at your sides (see figure a).

Action and Coaching Tips
With your elbows slightly bent, raise your arms out to the sides at roughly a 30-degree angle in front of your torso until your elbows go just above your forehead (see figure b). Do not swing the weight up. Slowly lower the dumbbells back to your sides. Use deliberate control on the lifting and lowering portion of each rep.

WHY IT'S BETTER
You increase range of motion versus what is conventionally done. You lift your arms in the scapular plane, at roughly a 30-degree angle to the torso, instead out to the sides. Research shows that doing shoulder exercises in the plane of the scapula creates the same demands on the shoulder musculature, but reduces the unwanted stress on the rotator cuff tendon (9,10).

Benefits
- Potentially safer on the shoulder joints
- More natural path of movement

Dumbbell Overhead Press

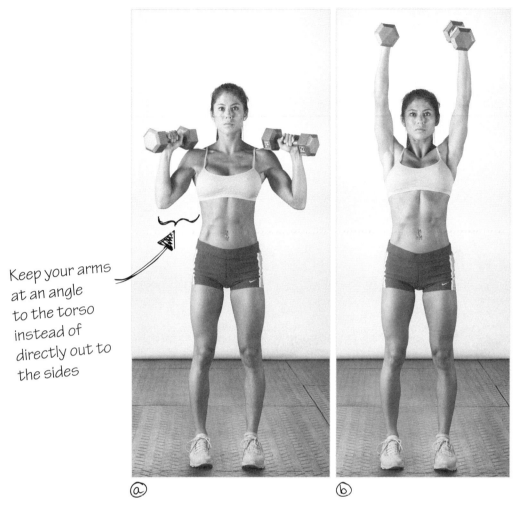

Keep your arms at an angle to the torso instead of directly out to the sides

(a)　(b)

Setup

Stand tall with your feet hip-width apart. Hold a dumbbell in each hand just above your shoulder, with your elbows at roughly a 30- to 45-degree angle to your torso (see figure a).

Action and Coaching Tips

Press the dumbbells directly overhead until your arms are almost straight (see figure b). Slowly reverse the motion, bringing the dumbbells back down to the starting position, outside your shoulders. At the bottom of each repetition, your elbows should be directly underneath the dumbbells; your forearms should remain perpendicular to the floor. Do not allow your wrists to bend backward at any time.

WHY IT'S BETTER

You keep your arms at an angle to the torso, in the scapular plane, instead of directly out to the sides. Just like with the lateral raises, doing this exercise in the plane of the scapula will create tension in the delts but decrease joint stress.

Every time you raise your arm overhead, there's some level of contact of the rotator cuff on the acromion, so there's always some level of impingement with arm elevation (11). But you don't want excessive contact that causes irritation and inflammation, because that can lead to shoulder impingement syndrome. Doing the dumbbell overhead press in the plane of the scapula is one strategy to minimize joint stress.

Benefits

- Potentially safer on the shoulder joints
- More natural path of movement

Dumbbell Triceps Skull Crusher

Hold two dumbbells parallel to one another instead of using both hands to hold one dumbbell

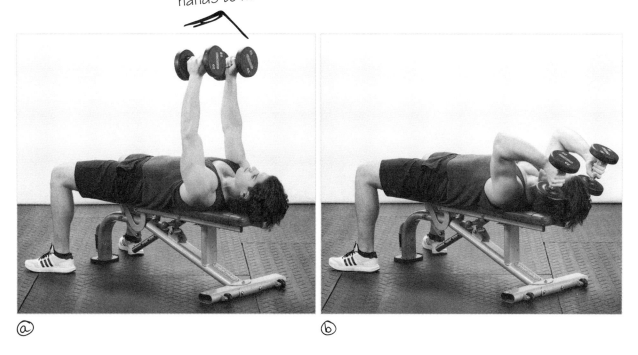

ⓐ   ⓑ

Setup

Lie supine on a weight bench while holding a dumbbell in each hand, with your arms outstretched above your shoulders, toward the sky (see figure a).

Action and Coaching Tips

Bend your elbows, lowering the dumbbells toward your forehead while keeping your palms facing one another (see figure b). Once your elbows almost reach a 90-degree angle, reverse the motion and extend your elbows until they're almost straight again to complete the rep. To avoid getting hit in the head by the dumbbells, lower them slowly with deliberate control.

WHY IT'S BETTER

You hold two dumbbells parallel to one another instead of using both hands to hold one dumbbell. Holding two dumbbells is universally more comfortable and less awkward on the shoulders while also making it easier to avoid flaring your elbows out to the sides.

Benefits

- Less awkward
- More natural to maintain arm position

Cable Rope Face Pull

Grab rope handles from the outside instead of from the inside

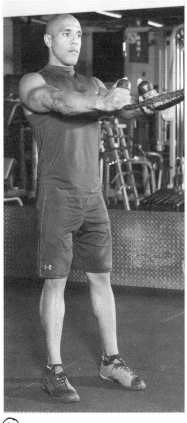

(a)

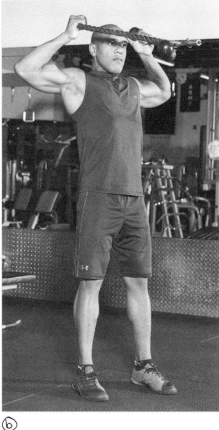

(b)

Setup

Stand in front of an adjustable cable column with a rope attached at or above your eye level. Hold one end of the rope in each hand, your palms facing one another and your elbows pointed out to the sides (see figure a).

Action and Coaching Tips

Pull the rope toward your face, without overarching your lower back, as you drive your arms apart so that your hands end up just outside your ears (see figure b). At the end of each repetition, your elbows should be slightly higher than your shoulders, and the middle of the rope should end up just in front of your forehead. Slowly reverse the movement back to the starting position.

WHY IT'S BETTER

Here, you grab rope handles from the outside instead of from the inside, as is commonly done. Grabbing the rope handles from the outside not only is less awkward on your wrists but also allows you to move through a greater range of motion when performing this exercise.

Benefits

- Increased range of motion
- Less awkward on the wrists

Additional Upper-Body Exercises

The exercises in this section also focus on helping you maximize the strength and development of your upper-body musculature. There aren't unique adjustments for doing them, so they don't warrant the same level of description as the exercises in the previous section. You also may find some not-so-common upper-body exercises here to help you incorporate some variety into your workouts.

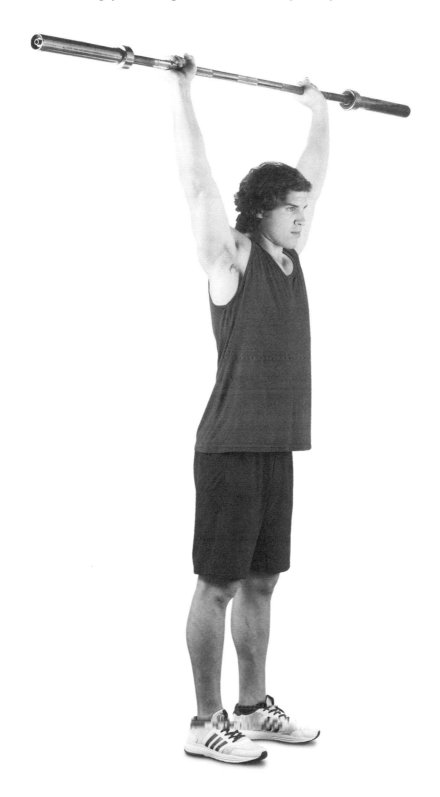

Barbell High Pull

Setup

Stand with your feet shoulder-width apart. Pick up a barbell, your hands a few inches outside shoulder-width apart. Slightly bend your knees and hinge forward at your hips, with the barbell resting just above your knees (see figure a).

Action and Coaching Tips

Explode your body upward, using your arms and legs to pull the bar toward the sky until your elbows reach shoulder height (see figure b). To initiate the movement, use your lower body, not your arms. When you lift the bar, do not allow your lower back to overextend. Then lower the bar back to your thighs with control to reset and begin your next repetition.

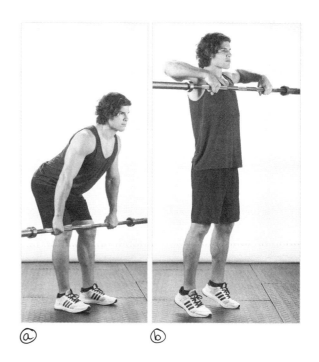

ⓐ　　　ⓑ

Angled Barbell Press and Catch

Setup

Stand with your feet shoulder-width apart. Place one end of a barbell in a corner or inside a landmine device and hold on to the other end (see figure a).

Action and Coaching Tips

Explosively press the barbell up and away from you, allowing it to leave your hand by a few inches (see figure b). Then catch it with your other hand (see figure c) and control

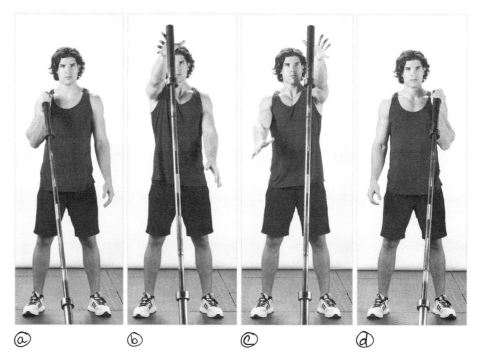

ⓐ　　　ⓑ　　　ⓒ　　　ⓓ

it on the way down to your shoulder (see figure d). Explode the barbell up again, throwing it a few inches in front of your hand. Then catch it with your other hand and lower it with a controlled motion back to the original side to complete a full repetition. It's okay to allow your torso to rotate a bit each time you catch and throw the barbell.

Each time you catch the barbell, do so as if catching an egg. Use your entire body, simultaneously bending your knees (slightly) and arms to absorb the fall and keep the egg from breaking.

Angled Barbell Shoulder to Shoulder Press

Setup

Stand tall, with your feet parallel to one another and a little wider than shoulder-width apart. Hold on to the end of the barbell with both hands stacked one over the other and with the end of the barbell in front of your right shoulder (see figure a).

Action and Coaching Tips

Press the barbell out and away from you so that when your arms reach full extension, the barbell is directly in line with the center of your body (see figure b). Slowly reverse the motion and lower the barbell to your left shoulder. Press it out and away again so that it ends up in the middle of your body. Make sure you do not allow your shoulders or hips to rotate throughout this exercise.

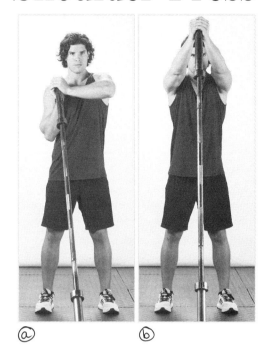

ⓐ ⓑ

One-Arm Angled Barbell Press

Setup

Stand with one leg in front of the other, splitting your stance. Place one end of a barbell in a corner or inside a landmine device and hold on to the other end of the barbell (see figure a). If the barbell is in your right hand, your right leg is your back leg.

Action and Coaching Tips

Press the barbell up and away from you while keeping your torso upright and stable (see figure b). Do not press the barbell toward the midline of your body; keep it in line with your same-side shoulder as you press it up and out. Slowly reverse the motion and lower the barbell back in front of your shoulder. At the bottom

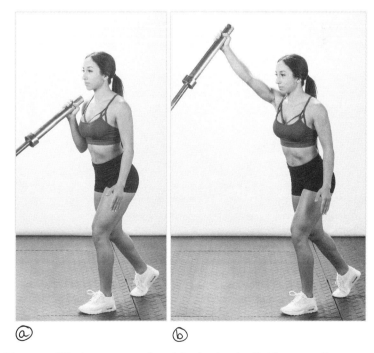

ⓐ ⓑ

of each repetition, your forearm should form a 90-degree angle with the barbell. Do not allow your wrists to bend backward at any time; keep your wrist straights throughout this exercise.

Barbell Overhead Push Press

Setup

Stand with your feet shoulder-width apart. Hold the barbell at the top of your chest, with your hands just outside shoulder-width apart.

Action and Coaching Tips

Holding the barbell at your chest, slightly bend your knees (see figure a), then quickly reverse the motion, exploding into the bar and driving it overhead with your arms and legs in a coordinated fashion (see figure b). Do not allow your lower back to overextend as you press the barbell overhead. Once the bar is completely overhead, slowly reverse your motions to complete a full repetition. Keep your wrists straight; do not allow them to bend backward at any time.

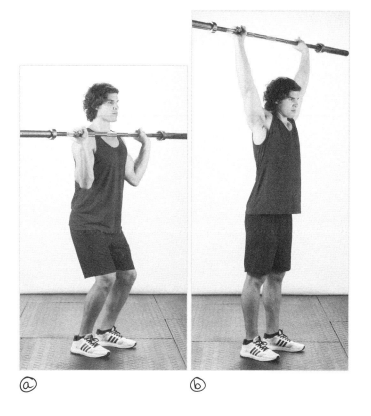

ⓐ　　　　　ⓑ

Barbell Overhead Press

Setup

Stand with your feet shoulder-width apart. Hold the barbell at the top of your chest, with your hands just outside shoulder-width apart (see figure a).

Action and Coaching Tips

Press the barbell overhead until your elbows are almost fully straight (see figure b). Do not allow your lower back to overextend as you press the barbell overhead. Once the bar is completely overhead, slowly reverse your motions to complete a full repetition. Keep your wrists straight; do not allow them to bend backward at any time.

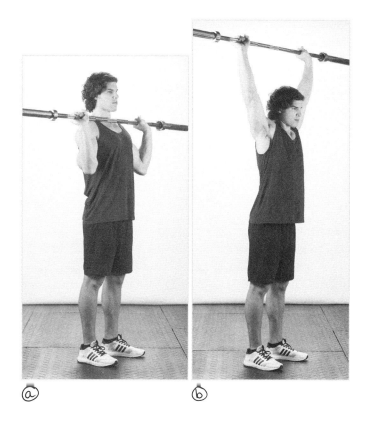

ⓐ　　　　　ⓑ

Barbell Bench Press

Setup

Lie on a weight bench with your feet flat on the floor, pressing them firmly into the ground to keep you stable. Hold an Olympic barbell above your head using a grip that places your hands outside your shoulders (see figure a).

Action and Coaching Tips

Slowly lower the bar toward your chest until your elbows reach just below your torso (see figure b). Keep your elbows at roughly a 45-degree angle relative to your torso. Press the bar up to the sky above your chest. Keep your elbows directly under your wrists throughout, and do not allow your wrists to bend backward at any time.

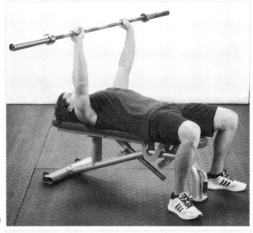

(a)

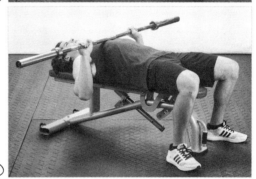

(b)

Barbell Incline Bench Press

Setup

Lie on a weight bench angled at about 45 degrees, with your feet flat on the floor, pressing them firmly into the ground to keep you stable. Hold an Olympic barbell overhead using a grip that places your hands outside your shoulders (see figure a).

Action and Coaching Tips

Slowly lower the bar toward your chest until your elbows reach just below your torso (see figure b); keep your elbows at roughly a 45-degree angle relative to your torso. Press the bar up to the sky above your chest. Keep your elbows directly under your wrists throughout, and do not allow your wrists to bend backward at any time.

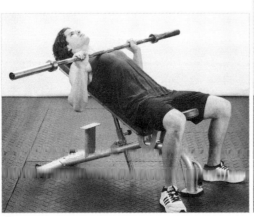

(a)

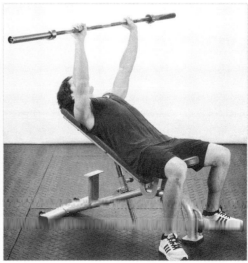

(b)

Wide-Grip Barbell Bent-Over Row

Setup

Stand with your feet shoulder-width apart. Hold a barbell with your hands roughly 1 foot (0.3 m) outside your hips. Bend over at your hips, keeping your back straight so that your torso is roughly parallel to the floor (see figure a). Keep your knees bent 15 to 20 degrees.

Action and Coaching Tips

Row the bar into the middle of your torso just below your chest, pinching your shoulder blades together at the top (see figure b). As you pull the bar, keep your elbows directly above your hands, and do not allow your wrists to bend. At the top of each repetition, pause for a second, keeping the barbell as close to the lower part of your chest as possible without allowing the fronts of your shoulders to round forward. Slowly lower the bar without allowing it to contact the floor until the set is completed. Do not allow your back to round out at any time.

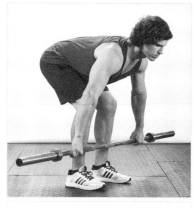

ⓐ

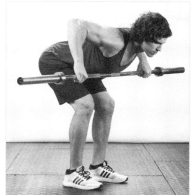

ⓑ

Dumbbell High Pull

Setup

This exercise is performed in the same way as the barbell high pull except that the dumbbells allow your arms to begin closer and then move apart at the top of each rep. Stand with your feet shoulder-width apart. Hold a dumbbell in each hand, just in front of your thighs. Slightly bend your knees and hinge forward at your hips with the dumbbell handles resting just above your knees (see figure a).

Action and Coaching Tips

Explode your body upward, using your arms and legs to pull the dumbbells slightly outward and toward the sky until your elbows reach shoulder height (see figure b). To initiate the movement, use your lower body, not your arms. When you lift the dumbbells, do not allow your lower back to overextend. Then lower the dumbbells back to your thighs in a controlled fashion to reset and begin your next repetition.

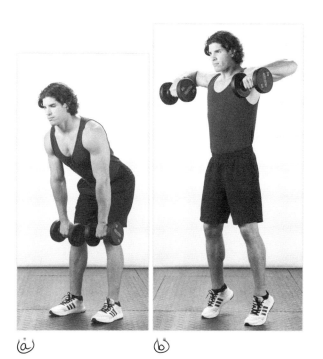

ⓐ   ⓑ

Dumbbell Bench Press

Setup

Lie on a weight bench with your feet flat on the floor, pressing them firmly into the ground to keep you stable. Hold a dumbbell in each hand above your shoulders, with your arms straight (see figure *a*).

Action and Coaching Tips

Slowly lower the dumbbells outside your body at a 45-degree angle to your torso, stopping when your elbows go just below your torso level (see figure *b*). Press the dumbbells back up toward the sky, above your shoulders.

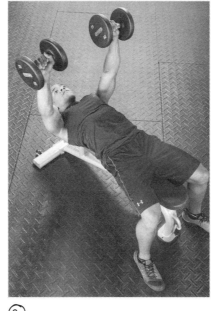

ⓐ

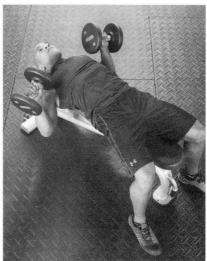

ⓑ

One-Arm Dumbbell Overhead Push Press

Setup

Stand tall, with your feet roughly shoulder-width apart. Hold a dumbbell in front of one shoulder.

Action and Coaching Tips

Slightly bend your knees (see figure *a*), then quickly reverse the motion, exploding into the dumbbell and driving it overhead with your arm and legs in a coordinated fashion (see figure *b*). Do not allow your lower back to overextend as you press the dumbbell overhead. Once the dumbbell is completely overhead, slowly reverse your motions to complete a full repetition. Keep your wrists straight; do not allow them to bend backward at any time.

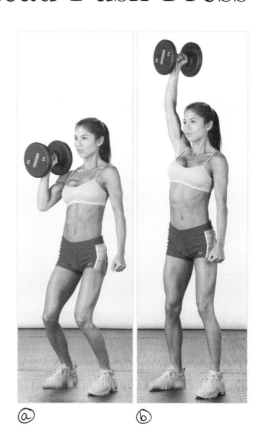

ⓐ   ⓑ

Dumbbell Incline Bench Press

Setup

Lie on a weight bench angled at about 45 degrees with your feet flat on the floor, pressing them firmly into the ground to keep you stable. Hold a pair of dumbbells above your head, outside your shoulders (see figure a).

Action and Coaching Tips

Slowly lower the dumbbells outside your body at a 45-degree angle to your torso, stopping when until your elbows go just below your torso level (see figure b). Press the dumbbells back up toward the sky, above your shoulders.

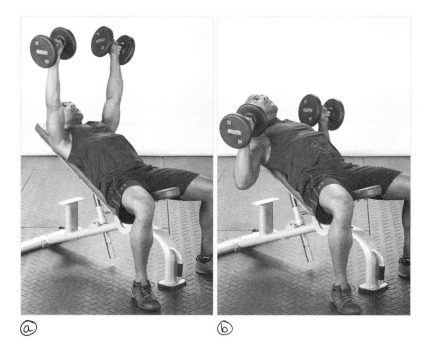

ⓐ ⓑ

One-Arm Dumbbell Overhead Press

Setup

Stand tall with your feet roughly shoulder-width apart while holding a dumbbell in front of one shoulder (see figure a).

Action and Coaching Tips

Press the dumbbell overhead without allowing your lower back to overextend (see figure b). Once the dumbbell is completely overhead, slowly reverse your motions to complete a full repetition. Keep your wrist straight; do not allow it to bend backward at any time.

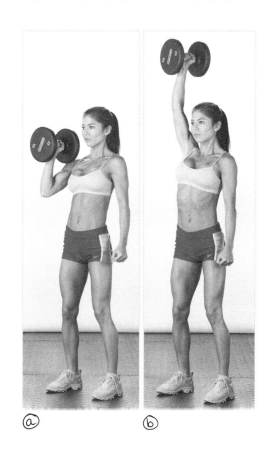

ⓐ ⓑ

Dumbbell Rotational Shoulder Press

Setup

Stand tall, with your feet roughly shoulder-width apart. Hold a dumbbell in front of each shoulder (see figure *a*).

Action and Coaching Tips

Press one dumbbell into the air directly over your same-side shoulder as you rotate to the opposite side (see figure *b*). To better allow your hips to rotate, raise your heel off the ground as you turn. Lower the dumbbell in a smooth, controlled manner as you bring your torso back to facing straight ahead. Then turn to the opposite side to perform the rep with the other arm.

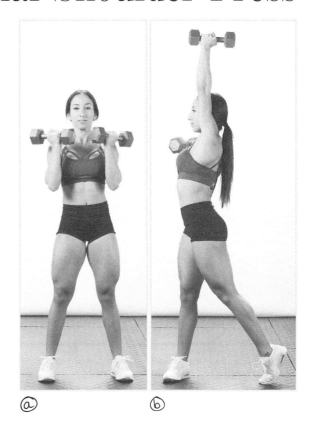

ⓐ   ⓑ

One-Arm Dumbbell Off-Bench Row

Setup

Stand facing a traditional weight bench, with your left hand on top of the bench and a dumbbell in your right hand. Keep a straight back that is roughly parallel to the floor. Stand in a slightly staggered stance, with your right leg behind your left leg (see figure *a*). You can also stand in a parallel stance with your feet hip-width apart and your knees slightly bent.

Action and Coaching Tips

Perform the row by pulling the dumbbell toward your body so that your right elbow ends up at roughly a 90-degree angle while you drive your right shoulder blade toward your spine (see figure *b*). Do not allow your rowing-side shoulder to move forward at the end of each rep. Slowly lower the dumbbell toward the floor until your arm straightens, but don't allow the dumbbell to touch the floor. Repeat all reps on the same side before switching sides.

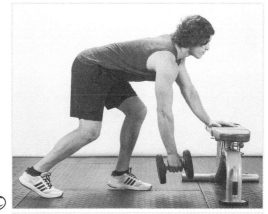

ⓐ

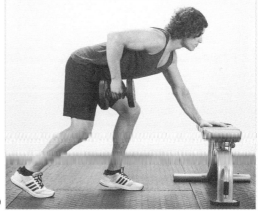

ⓑ

One-Arm Freestanding Dumbbell Row

Setup

Assume a split stance, with your left leg in front of your right leg and both knees slightly bent. With your right hand, hold the dumbbell in a neutral position so that your palm faces the opposite side of your body; your left hand hangs near the front knee. Hinge at your hips, keeping your back straight so that your torso becomes roughly parallel with the floor (see figure a). Keep your back heel raised off the ground to ensure that most of your weight is on your front leg.

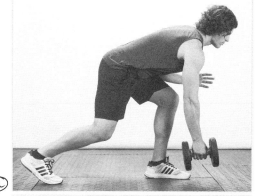

Action and Coaching Tips

Perform a row by pulling the dumbbell toward your body, without rotating your shoulders or hips more than a few degrees, while pulling your scapula toward your spine in a controlled manner as your arm moves (see figure b). Do not allow your rowing-side shoulder to move forward at the end of each rep. Slowly lower the dumbbell without letting it touch the floor. Maintain a stable spinal position, keeping your back straight throughout the exercise. Complete all reps on one side before switching sides.

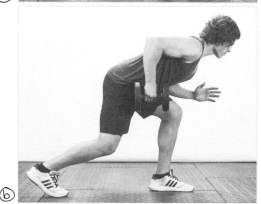

Dumbbell Pec Fly

Setup

Lie on a weight bench with your feet flat on the floor, pressing them firmly into the ground to keep you stable. Hold a dumbbell in each hand above your shoulders, with your arms straight and your palms facing each other (see figure a).

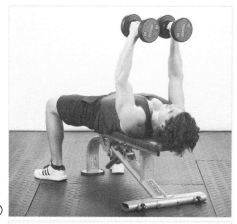

Action and Coaching Tips

Keeping your elbows slightly bent, slowly open your arms out to your sides until your elbows go just below your torso and you feel a stretch in your chest (see figure b). Reverse the motion by driving the dumbbells back up in a motion similar to that of hugging a tree. For additional isometric work, you can squeeze the dumbbells together for one or two seconds at the top of each rep.

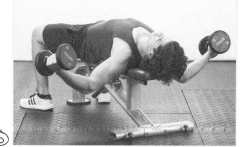

Dumbbell Chest Squeeze Press

Setup

Lie on a weight bench with your feet flat on the floor, pressing them firmly into the ground to keep you stable. While holding a dumbbell in each hand above your shoulders with your arms straight and your palms facing each other, squeeze the dumbbells together (see figure a).

Action and Coaching Tips

While continuing to squeeze the dumbbells together as hard as you can, bend at your elbows and lower the dumbbells down to your chest as your elbows go out to the sides (see figure b). Reverse the motion by pressing the dumbbells back up while squeezing them together.

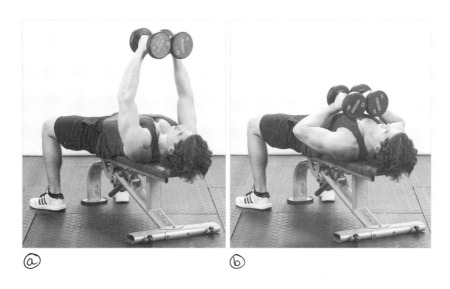

(a)　　　　(b)

Dumbbell Bent-Over Back Shrug

Setup

Stand with your feet hip-width apart. Hold a dumbbell in each hand. Bend over at your hips, keeping your back straight, so that your torso is parallel to the floor (see figure a). Keep your knees bent 15 to 20 degrees.

Action and Coaching Tips

Pinch your shoulders blades together while allowing your elbows to bend slightly (see figure b). Pause for two to three seconds before slowly reversing the motion by protracting your shoulder blades at the bottom of each rep. Do not allow your back to round out at any time.

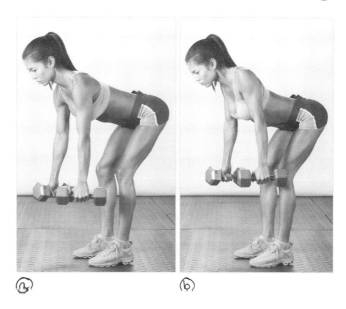

(a)　　　　(b)

One-Arm Dumbbell Overhead Triceps Extension

Setup

Stand with your feet hip-width apart. Hold a dumbbell with one arm extended above your head and your elbow directly above your shoulder (see figure a).

Action and Coaching Tips

While keeping your elbow above your shoulder, bend your elbow and slowly lower the dumbbell behind your head until your elbow is fully bent (see figure b). Reverse the motion by extending at your elbow to press the dumbbell back up and complete the rep.

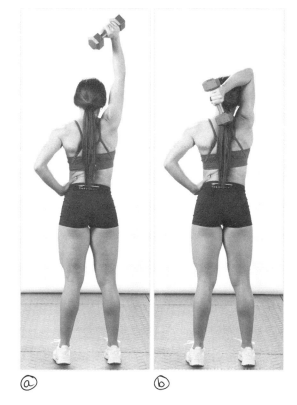

ⓐ　　　　ⓑ

Dumbbell Triceps Kickback

Setup

Stand with your feet hip-width apart. Hold a dumbbell in each hand. Bend at your hips, keeping your back straight so that your torso is parallel to the floor. Keep your knees bent 15 to 20 degrees. Pull the dumbbells up into your torso as if performing a row, keeping your elbows bent to a 90-degree angle (see figure a).

Action and Coaching Tips

Keeping your torso and biceps bone parallel with the ground, extend your elbows until they're straight (see figure b). Pause for one or two seconds. Slowly reverse the motion by allowing your elbows to bend back to a 90-degree angle to complete one rep.

ⓐ　　　　ⓑ

E-Z Bar Biceps Curl

Setup

Stand tall with your feet hip-width apart, holding an E-Z bar with both hands, using an underhand grip, next to your hips (see figure a).

Action and Coaching Tips

Curl the bar up toward your shoulders by bending at your elbows without allowing your elbows to move forward (see figure b). Do not swing the weight up by overextending at your lower back. Once your hands are up in front of your shoulders, reverse the motion by slowly lowering the bar back down.

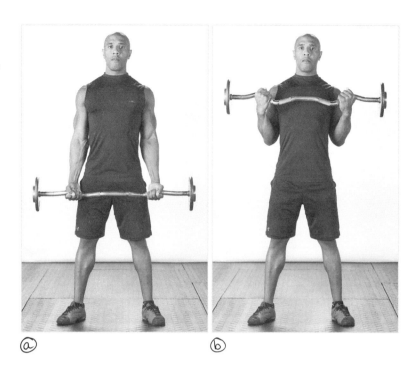

ⓐ ⓑ

E-Z Bar Preacher Biceps Curl

Setup

To perform this exercise, you'll need to use the apparatus that's commonly known as the preacher curl. Sit on the seat of the preacher curl with your spine upright and your feet hip-width apart. Place your chest and arms against the pad while holding an E-Z bar with both hands roughly shoulder-width apart with an underhand grip (see figure a).

Action and Coaching Tips

Without allowing your shoulders to round forward, curl the bar up toward your shoulders by bending at your elbows (see figure b).

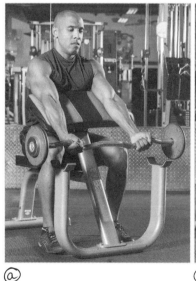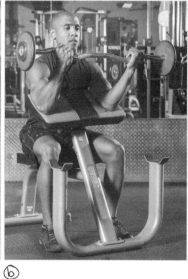

ⓐ ⓑ

Once your hands are above your elbows, reverse the motion by slowly lowering the bar back down. You can also perform this exercise with an overhand grip.

Dumbbell Incline Bench Biceps Curl

Setup

Lie on a weight bench angled at about 45 degrees, with your feet flat on the floor, pressing them firmly into the ground to keep you stable. Hold a pair of dumbbells below your shoulders and keep your arms straight (see figure a).

Action and Coaching Tips

Curl the dumbbells up toward your shoulders by bending at your elbows without allowing your elbows to move forward (see figure b). Once your hands are up in front of your shoulders, reverse the motion by slowly lowering the dumbbells back down. You can also perform this exercise with a neutral grip.

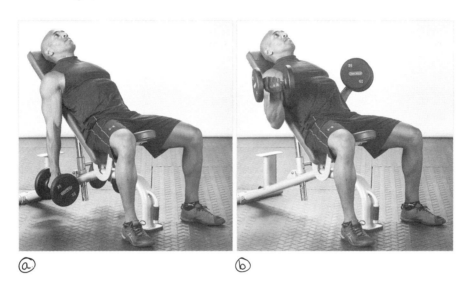

ⓐ　　　　　　ⓑ

Dumbbell Shoulder A

Setup

Stand with your feet hip-width apart and hold a dumbbell in each hand. Bend over at your hips, keeping your back straight so that your torso is parallel to the floor. The arms hang down below the shoulders (see figure a). Keep your knees bent 15 to 20 degrees.

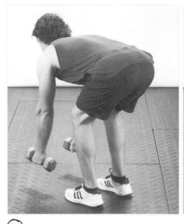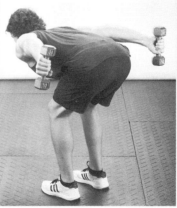

ⓐ　　　　　　ⓑ

Action and Coaching Tips

Keeping a small bend in your elbows, raise your arms backward, just outside your hips, pointing your thumbs toward the floor (see figure b). Do not swing the dumbbells up. Your arms should be at a 15-degree angle relative to your torso at the top of each repetition, thus forming an A shape with your torso. Pinch your shoulder blades together and pause for one second at the top of each repetition, then slowly lower the dumbbells in front of your torso. Do not allow your back to round out at any time. Pinch your shoulder blades together at the top of each rep.

Dumbbell Shoulder W

Setup

Stand with your feet hip-width apart. Bend over at your hips, keeping your back straight so that your torso is parallel to the floor and your knees are bent 90 degrees. Holding a dumbbell in each hand, bend your arms against your torso, with palms facing up (see figure a).

Action and Coaching Tips

Raise your arms out to your sides just outside your torso, keeping your thumbs pointed toward the sky (see figure b). At the top of each repetition, your arms should form a W shape. Pause for one second at the top of each repetition and then slowly lower your arms back down in front of your torso.

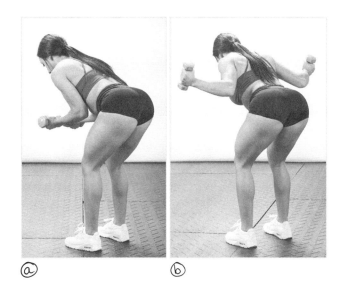

ⓐ　　　　　ⓑ

Dumbbell Shoulder Y

Setup

Stand with your feet hip-width apart. Bend over at your hips, keeping your back straight so that your torso is parallel to the floor and your knees are bent 15 to 20 degrees. Holding a dumbbell in each hand, your arms hang down toward the floor with palms facing in (see figure a).

Action and Coaching Tips

Keeping a small bend in your elbows, raise your arms out to shoulder height, pointing your thumbs toward the sky (see figure b). Do not swing your arms up. Your arms should be at a

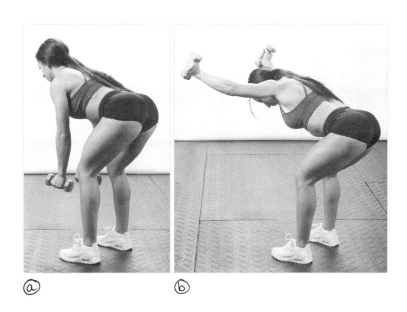

ⓐ　　　　　ⓑ

45-degree angle relative to your torso at the top of each repetition, thus forming a Y shape with your torso. Pause for one second at the top of each repetition, then slowly lower your arms in front of your torso. Do not allow your back to round out at any time.

Dumbbell Shoulder T

Setup

Stand with your feet hip-width apart. Bend over at your hips, keeping your back straight so that your torso is parallel to the floor and your knees are bent 15 to 20 degrees. Holding a dumbbell in each hand, your arms hang down toward the floor with palms facing up (see figure a).

Action and Coaching Tips

Keeping a small bend in your elbows, raise your arms out to your sides, pointing your thumbs toward the sky (see figure b). Do not swing your arms up. Your arms should be at a 90-degree angle relative to your torso at the top of each repetition,

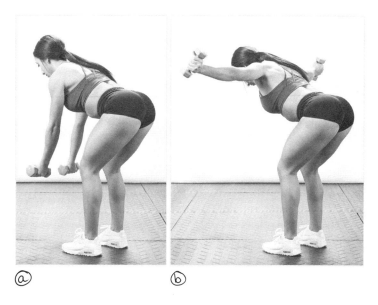

thus forming a *T* shape with your torso. Pinch your shoulder blades together and pause for one second at the top of each repetition, then slowly lower your arms down in front of your torso. Do not allow your back to round out at any time.

Dumbbell Shoulder L

Setup

Lie prone on a weight-bench with your head above the top of the bench and feet placed on each side with your knees bent and legs relaxed. Holding a dumbbell in each hand, raise your arms out to the sides to shoulder height, bending your elbows 90 degrees so that your hands point down toward the ground (see figure a). This exercise can also be performed from a standing, bent-over position with your torso parallel to the floor.

Action and Coaching Tips

Without moving your elbows, rotate your arms up as far as you can to bring your hands toward the ceiling (see figure b). Pause for a second or two at the top of each rep. Slowly reverse the motion to return to the starting position.

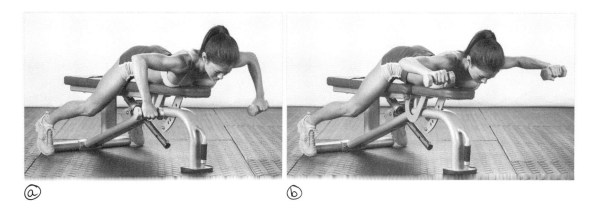

Dumbbell Pullover

Setup

Lie supine on a weight bench while holding a dumbbell in each hand with your arms outstretched above your shoulders toward the sky with your palms facing each other (see figure a).

Action and Coaching Tips

Keeping your elbows slightly bent, reach your arms overhead lowering the dumbbells toward the floor while keeping your palms facing one another (see figure b). Once your arms are roughly parallel to the ground, reverse the motion and raise the dumbbells back up until they're almost straight again to complete the rep.

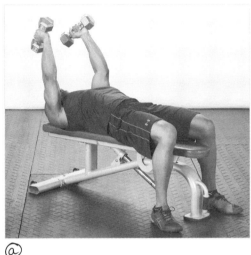
@

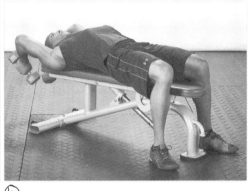
ⓑ

Lat Pull-Down with Neutral Grip

Setup

Position yourself just behind neutral grip handles that are attached to the lat pull-down machine. Hold the handles so your arms are roughly shoulder-width apart over your head (see figure a).

Action and Coaching Tips

Pull the handles down to the top of your chest while keeping your back straight and your elbows following a straight line (see figure b). Slowly reverse the motion, controlling the movement.

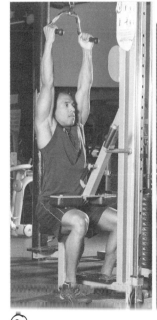
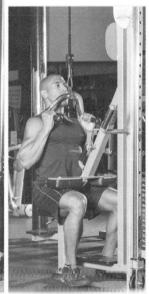

@   ⓑ

Leaning Lat Pull-Down with Neutral Grip

Setup

This exercise is performed in the same manner as the lat pull-down with a neutral grip except that you lean backward slightly instead of remaining upright. Position yourself just behind the neutral grip handles that are attached to lat pull-down machine and lean backward at roughly 25 degrees from upright (see figure a). Your arms should be roughly shoulder-width apart over your head.

Action and Coaching Tips

Pull the bar down to the top of your chest (see figure b). Keep your elbows pointed in the same direction as your line of pull. Slowly reverse the motion, controlling the movement.

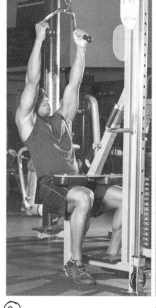 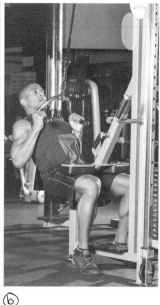

ⓐ　　　　ⓑ

One-Arm Cable Press

Setup

Stand facing away from an adjustable cable column while holding a handle at roughly shoulder height. With the cable handle in your left hand and your elbow at roughly a 45-degree angle from your body, split your stance by putting your left leg behind your right leg (see figure a). Keep your rear foot straight and your back heel off the ground.

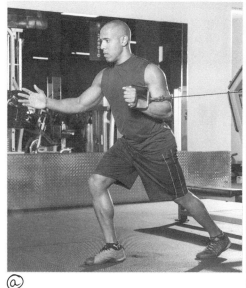 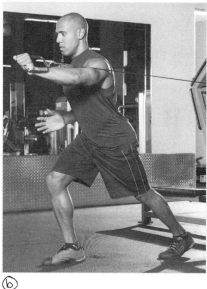

ⓐ　　　　ⓑ

Action and Coaching Tips

Press the cable straight out in front of you (see figure b). Slowly reverse the motion and bring the handle back in to your body as you bring your left arm back toward you in a row-like motion while extending the opposite arm. Don't allow your shoulders or hips to rotate more than a few degrees. Lean slightly forward to allow you to move heavier loads.

To prevent the cable attachment from digging into your arm, you can use an extender strap (which can be purchased at a store that sells rock-climbing gear) between the handle and the cable attachment.

Standing Cable Chest Press

Setup

Stand tall in a split stance with your rear heel elevated off the floor, just in front of the middle of a cable crossover machine. The wider the cables are apart, the farther in front of the apparatus you'll need to stand to properly perform this exercise. Hold the handles in each hand at your shoulder level, with arms out to your sides and your elbows bent 90 degrees (see figure a).

Action and Coaching Tips

Press into the handles by extending your arms and bringing them together toward the midline of your body (see figure b). Slowly reverse the motion until your arms are back out to your sides and your elbows are bent. A slight forward torso lean is okay to use if needed to perform this exercise, especially when using heavier loads relative to your strength level.

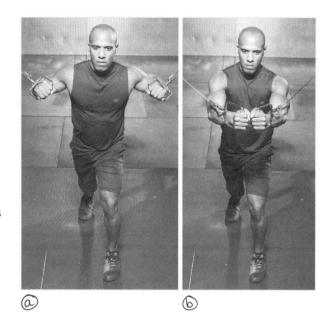

ⓐ　　　　ⓑ

One-Arm Cable Row

Setup

Stand tall, with your spine straight and your knees slightly bent while facing an adjustable cable column adjusted to roughly shoulder height. With your right hand, grab the handle in a neutral grip (i.e., with your palm facing the opposite side of your body) and split your stance so that your right leg is behind your left leg (see figure a). Keep your back heel raised off the ground to ensure that most of your weight is on your front leg.

Action and Coaching Tips

Perform a row by pulling the cable toward your body, driving your shoulder blade back so that it's retracted at the end of the row (see figure b). Do not allow your rowing-side shoulder to move forward at the end of each rep. Maintain a stable spine, without allowing your shoulders and hips to rotate more than a few degrees. Slowly reverse the motion by allowing your scapula to protract while your arm straightens. Perform all reps on one side before doing the other side.

ⓐ　　　　ⓑ

One-Arm Motorcycle Cable Row

Setup

Stand tall, facing a cable machine or a resistance band that's attached at roughly midtorso height to a stable structure or inside a doorjamb (many resistance bands come with an attachment for this). Hold the cable handle or both resistance band handles in your right hand. Stand

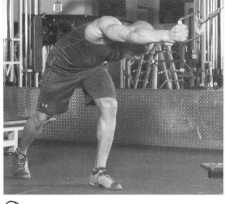 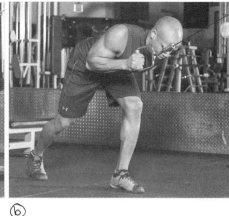

with your feet in a split stance, your right leg behind and your feet roughly shoulder-width apart. Hinge at your hips and lean forward, keeping your knees bent 15 to 20 degrees until your torso becomes parallel with the floor (see figure a).

Action and Coaching Tips

Pull your right arm into your side without allowing your torso to move or your shoulder to round forward (see figure b). Slowly reverse the motion by allowing your arm to straighten to complete one rep. Perform all reps on the same side before switching sides and reversing your stance.

One-Arm Compound Cable Row

Setup

Stand facing an adjustable cable column that's set at your midtorso level. Keep your feet roughly shoulder-width apart in a split stance, with your left leg in front and your knees slightly bent (see figure a). Hold the handle in your right hand using a neutral grip (i.e., with your palm facing the opposite side of your body). Keep your back heel raised off the ground to ensure that most of your weight is on your front leg.

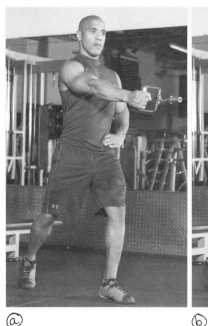 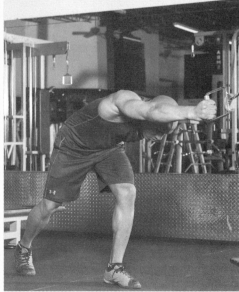

Action and Coaching Tips

Hinge at your hips, reaching your right arm in front of you toward the origin of the cable (see figure b). Do not allow your rowing-side shoulder to move forward at the end of each rep. Reverse this motion while performing a row. Finish the row as you return to the upright standing position. Slowly reverse the motion, hinging at your hips and reaching out; use good rhythm and timing. Perform all reps on one side before switching to the other side.

One-Arm Half-Kneeling Angled Cable Row

Setup

Using a mat or rolled towel for comfort, assume a half-kneeling position with your right knee on the floor in front of a cable column that's set at above the height of your head if you were standing (see figure a). Keep your torso straight and both knees bent at 90 degrees. With your right hand, grab the handle in a neutral grip (your palm facing the opposite side of your body) so your arm and cable are at a 45-degree angle to your body.

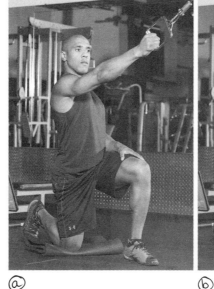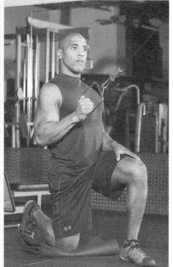

@ ⓑ

Action and Coaching Tips

Perform a row by pulling the cable toward your body, driving your elbow down and into your body as far as you can while keeping your forearm at a 45-degree angle (see figure b). Keep your spine upright and do not allow your rowing-side shoulder to move forward at the end of each rep. Slowly reverse the motion by allowing your arm to extend and your same side shoulder to rotate slightly toward the cable. Perform all reps on one side before doing the other side.

Seated Row Shrug

Setup

This exercise usually requires a specially designed seated-row apparatus that is available in most gyms. Sit with your feet hip-width apart on the platform with your knees slightly bent and your back straight (see figure a). Hold a lat bar in an overhand grip, with your hands roughly 10 inches (25 cm) outside your chest.

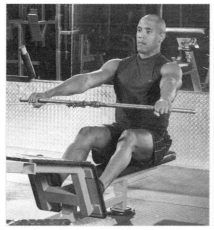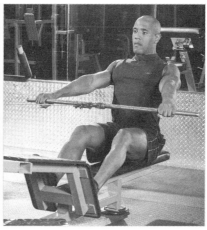

@ ⓑ

Action and Coaching Tips

Keeping your arms almost straight, pinch (retract) your shoulder blades together and pause for a second or two (see figure b). Slowly reverse the movement by allowing your shoulder blades to separate (protract) as far as possible without allowing your spine to round.

Wide-Grip Seated Row

Setup

This exercise usually requires a specially designed seated-row apparatus that is available in most gyms. It can also be done by sitting on the floor in front of a low cable with your feet braced against two dumbbells. Sit with your feet hip-width apart against the platform or dumbbells, your knees slightly bent, and your back straight (see figure a).

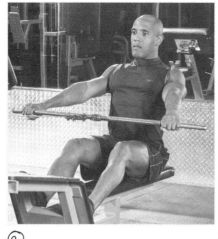

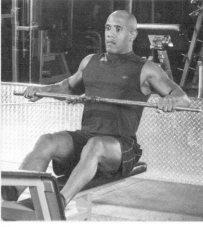

Hold a lat bar in an overhand grip, with your hands roughly 10 inches (25 cm) outside your chest.

Action and Coaching Tips

Pull the bar into your body at chest level, pinching your shoulder blades together at the end (see figure b). Do not allow your wrists to bend as you pull the bar; keep your elbows directly behind your hands throughout. At the top of each repetition, pause for one second, keeping the bar as close to your chest as possible without allowing the fronts of your shoulders to round forward. Slowly reverse the movement.

Fighter's Cable Lat Pull-Down

Setup

You'll need a dual adjustable cable machine for this exercise. Sit between a set of cables above you. Hold a handle in each hand with your arms straight at roughly a 45-degree angle to your torso (see figure a).

Action and Coaching Tips

Pull one arm toward your body, bringing your elbow all the way down to your hip bone. Combine the pull-down motion with a small side crunch in a motion, similar to that of a fighter blocking a body strike (see figure b). Reverse the motion in a controlled fashion. Once your arm becomes straight, repeat the action with the other arm. Do not allow your torso to

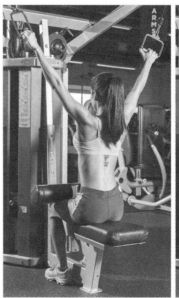

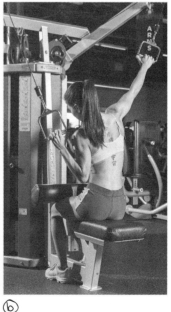

twist, and keep your forearms perpendicular to the floor throughout.

Cable Pec Fly

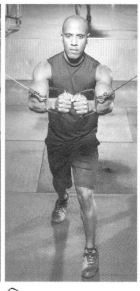

Setup

Stand tall, in either a split stance or a parallel stance, just in front of the middle of a cable crossover machine. In each hand, hold handles attached at shoulder level. Your arms extend out to your sides, with a slight bend in the elbows (see figure a).

Action and Coaching Tips

Bring your arms together in front of you while keeping a soft bend in your elbows, as if you were hugging a tree, until your hands touch in the center (see figure b). Slowly reverse the motion until your arms are back out to your sides and your elbows are just behind your shoulders.

Overhead Cable Triceps Rope Extension

Setup

You'll need an adjustable cable column to perform this exercise. The rope should be attached above your mid-torso level. Stand in front of the column, but face away from where the rope is attached. Stand in a split stance, leaning your torso slightly forward and your rear heel off the ground. Hold each side of the rope in each hand with your arms by your ears and your elbows bent beyond 90 degrees (see figure a).

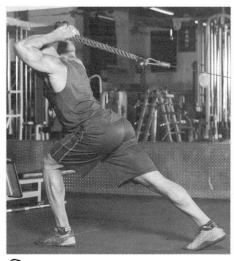

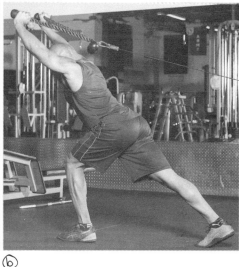

Action and Coaching Tips

Keeping your body in the starting position, extend your elbows until your arms are straight (see figure b). Do not drive your shoulders downward as you extend your arms on each rep. Slowly reverse the motion and repeat.

Cable Triceps Rope Extension

Setup

Stand in front of an adjustable cable column with a rope attached above your eye level. Hold one side of the rope in each hand, with your elbows bent above 90 degrees and your palms facing each other (see figure a).

Action and Coaching Tips

With your knees slightly bent, straighten your elbows until your arms are straight (see figure b). Do not allow your shoulders to round forward as you press the rope downward on each repetition. Slowly reverse the motion to complete the rep. Keep your elbows by your sides throughout.

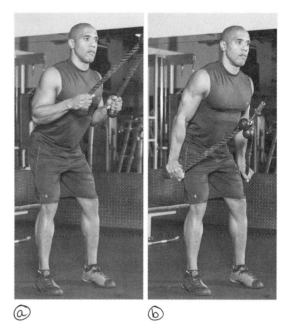

a   b

Low-Cable One-Arm Rear Delt Fly

Setup

Stand with your feet roughly hip-width apart next to a cable column with a handle that's attached at your ankle level. Grab the handle with your opposite side hand and move a few feet away from the cable. Bend over at your hips, keeping your back straight so that your torso is roughly parallel to the floor. Allow the arm that's holding the handle to reach across your body toward the cable's origin, keeping your elbow slightly bent (see figure a).

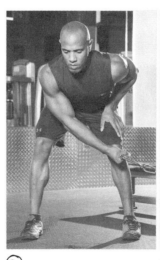
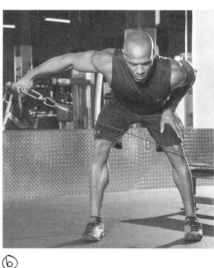

a   b

Action and Coaching Tips

With a slight bend in your elbow and your hand positioned in a neutral grip, lift your arm out to the side until it's roughly parallel to the floor so that it forms a 90-degree angle with your torso (see figure b). Slowly reverse the motion, allowing your arm to reach across your body at the end of each rep. Complete all reps on the same side before switching sides. Do not allow your torso to rotate at any point; keep your shoulders fairly level with the ground throughout.

Cable Compound Straight-Arm Pull-down

Setup

Stand facing an adjustable cable column, with your feet roughly hip-width apart and a rope attached to the column above your eye level. Hold one end of the rope in each hand, your palms facing one another. Hinge at your hips with a slight bend at your knees and extend your arms above your head (see figure a).

Action and Coaching Tips

As you raise your torso to an upright position, pull the rope down, keeping a small bend in your elbows, until the handles touch just outside of your hips (see figure b). Do not round your shoulders forward at the top of

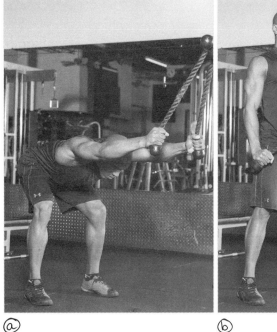
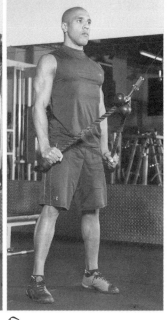

ⓐ   ⓑ

each repetition. Slowly reverse the motion, hinging at your hips and reaching your arms back above your head; use good rhythm and timing. Perform the exercise smoothly, with your arms going down as your torso goes up and vice versa.

Low-Cable Angled Upright Row

Setup

Stand tall, about two feet in front of an adjustable cable column with a lat pull-down bar attached to a cable column below your knees. With your arms straight and at a small angle away from your body, hold each side of the bar a few inches out-side of shoulder width, your palms facing down (see figure a).

Action and Coaching Tips

Pull the bar toward you at a 45-degree angle until your elbows reach just above shoulder height, and don't overarch at your lower-back (see figure b). Pause at the top for one or two seconds before slowly reversing the motion. Do not allow your wrists to bend and keep your elbows and forearms in line with the cable throughout.

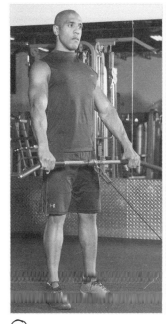
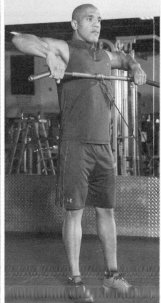

ⓐ   ⓑ

Low-Cable One-Arm Side Shoulder Raise

Setup

Stand tall, with your feet roughly hip-width apart next to a cable column with a handle that's attached at your ankle level. Grab the handle with your opposite side hand and move a few feet away from the cable to allow the arm that's holding the handle to reach across your body toward the cable's origin (see figure a). Your elbow should be slightly bent.

Action and Coaching Tips

Keeping your elbow slightly bent, raise your arm out to the side at roughly a 30-degree angle in front of your torso until your elbow goes just above your forehead (see figure b). Do not overextend at your lower back or side bend at your torso to raise the weight. Slowly lower the handle back down and across your body to complete the rep. Perform all reps on the same side before switching sides.

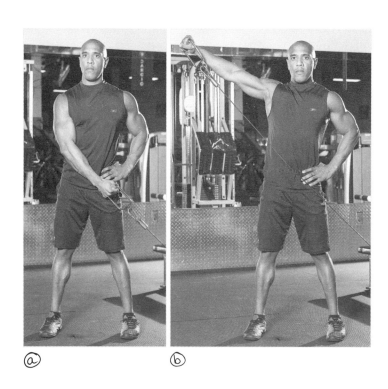

a   b

Cable Biceps Curl

Setup

Stand tall in front of an adjustable cable column with an E-Z Bar handle attached to the column below your knees. Hold each side of the handle, using a neutral grip, your palms facing each other. Keep your arms by your sides and your elbows slightly bent (see figure a).

Action and Coaching Tips

Curl the E-Z Bar up toward your shoulders by bending at your elbows without allowing them to move forward (see figure b). Once your hands are up in front of your shoulders, reverse the motion by slowly lowering the rope until your arms are almost straight.

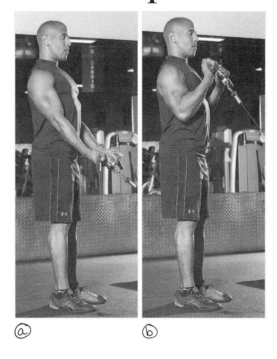

ⓐ ⓑ

Low-Cable One-Arm Face-Away Biceps Curl

Setup

Stand facing away from a cable column, with your feet roughly hip-width apart and the handle attached at your ankle level. Hold the handle in one hand, your arm straight and in line with your torso (see figure a).

Action and Coaching Tips

Curl the handle up toward your shoulder by bending at your elbow without allowing your elbow to move forward (see figure b). Do not cheat the weight up by overextending at your lower back. Once the cable lightly touches your forearm, reverse the motion by slowly lowering the handle back down until your elbow is straight. Perform all reps on the same side before switching sides. Do not allow your elbow to drift in front of or behind your torso throughout.

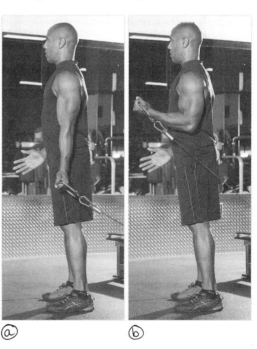

ⓐ ⓑ

Machine Chest Press

Setup

This exercise requires a specially designed machine that is available in most gyms. The machine allows you to push its handles horizontally away your body. Sit tall, with your back in front of the pad. Hold the handles at mid-chest level, with your elbows directly behind the handles with your arms bent (see figure a). Find a comfortable foot placement that best allows you to perform the exercise with proper technique.

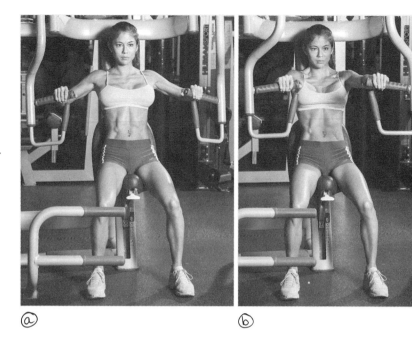

Action and Coaching Tips

Without fully locking out your elbows, press the handles so your arms are straight in front of your shoulders (see figure b). Slowly reverse the motion, bringing the handles back to the starting position.

Machine Back Row

Setup

This exercise requires a specially designed machine that is available in most gyms. It allows you to pull its handles horizontally into your body. Sit tall, with your chest in front of the pad. Hold the handles at around shoulder height with a neutral, overhand, or underhand grip, depending on the gripping options the machine allows (see figure a for an example using the neutral grip). Find a comfortable foot placement that best allows you to perform the exercise with proper technique.

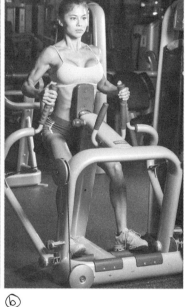

Action and Coaching Tips

Row the handles into your body, pinching your shoulder blades together at the top without allowing the fronts of your shoulders to round forward (see figure b). Slowly reverse the motion until your elbows are straight to complete the rep.

Machine Shoulder Press

Setup

This exercise requires a specially designed machine that is available in most gyms. It allows you to push its handles vertically above your body. Sit tall with your back against pad. Hold the handles at roughly shoulder level, with your elbows directly underneath the handles and your elbows bent (see figure a). Find a comfortable foot placement that best allows you to perform the exercise with proper technique.

Action and Coaching Tips

Press the handles directly overhead until your arms are almost straight (see figure b). Slowly reverse the motion, bringing the handles back down to the starting position outside your shoulders. At the bottom of each repetition, your forearms should remain perpendicular to the floor. Do not allow your wrists to bend backward at any time.

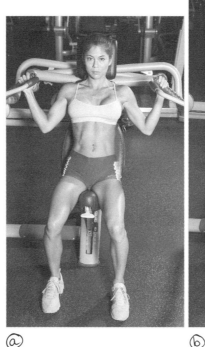
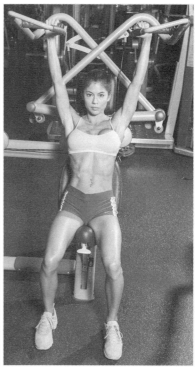

ⓐ   ⓑ

Machine Rear Delt Fly

Setup

This exercise requires a specially designed machine that is available in most gyms. It allows you to pull its handles horizontally to the outside of your body. Sit tall, with your chest in front of the pad. Hold the handles at shoulder height with a neutral, overhand, or underhand grip, depending on the gripping options the machine allows (see figure a for an example using the neutral grip). Find a comfortable foot placement that best allows you to perform the exercise with proper technique.

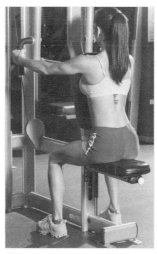
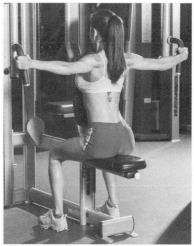

ⓐ   ⓑ

Action and Coaching Tips

Keeping your elbows slightly bent, open your arms out to the sides of your body (see figure b). Slowly reverse the movement. Be sure to keep a stable spine and minimize any overarching in your lower back when performing this exercise.

Machine Chest Fly

Setup

This exercise requires a specially designed machine that is available in most gyms. It allows you to push its handles horizontally to the inside of your body. Sit tall, with your back in front of the pad. Hold the handles at shoulder height with a neutral grip, your palms facing forward (see figure a). Find a comfortable foot placement that best allows you to perform the exercise with proper technique.

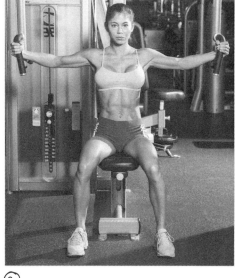
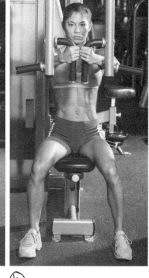

@   ⓑ

Action and Coaching Tips

Keeping your elbows slightly bent, close your arms in front of your body until the handles touch. Slowly reverse the movement, allowing your hands to go out to the sides of your body (see figure b). Be sure to keep a stable spine and minimize any overarching in your lower back when performing this exercise.

Resistance Band Step and Chest Press

Setup

Face away from a heavy-duty resistance band attached at roughly shoulder height to a stable structure or inside a doorjamb (many resistance bands come with a doorjamb attachment). With your knees slightly bent and your feet roughly hip-width apart, hold a handle in each hand, your arms at a 45-degree angle to your sides and your forearms parallel to the floor (see figure a). The band should create enough tension that it forces you to lean slightly forward.

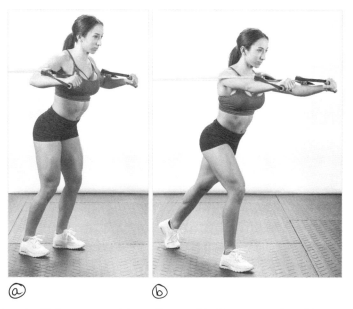

@   ⓑ

Action and Coaching Tips

Step forward with one leg while performing a chest press with both arms; maintain your slight forward torso lean with your rear heel off the ground (see figure b). Step your lead leg back to the starting position while allowing your arms to come back as well. Alternate legs on each repetition. Explode into each repetition, as if you were shoving someone. Be sure to use a resistance band that creates enough tension to make you work to hold your position from the start of each repetition—not just at the end, when your arms are extended.

Resistance Band Loop Push-Up

Setup

Place a Superband around your upper back and place your fingers (but not your thumbs) inside the bands from the bottom up (see figure a). Position your hands on the floor shoulder-width apart, with your elbows straight (see figure b). Turn your hands outward so that your fingers point at roughly 45 degrees.

Action and Coaching Tips

Perform a push-up by lowering your body to the floor while keeping your elbows directly above your wrists (see figure c). At the bottom of each push-up, position your arms at a 45-degree angle so your torso forms the shape of an arrow. Once your elbows are almost at a 90-degree angle, reverse the motion by pushing your body up so that your elbows are straight again. At the top of each push-up, do not finish with your shoulder blades pinched together; instead, protract (push apart) your shoulder blades while keeping your body in a straight line. Keep your body in a straight line from your head to your hips to your ankles; do not allow your head or hips to sag toward the floor at any point.

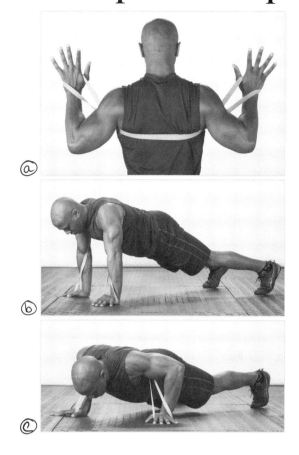

Resistance Band Triceps Extension

Setup

Stand in front of a resistance band attached at above your eye level to a stable structure or inside a doorjamb (many resistance bands come with a doorjamb attachment). Hold one handle in each hand, with your elbows bent above 90 degrees. With your knees slightly bent, hinge forward at your hips to position your torso at roughly a 45-dgree angle while keeping your back straight (see figure a).

Action and Coaching Tips

Straighten your elbows toward the sides of your body until your arms are straight (see figure b). Do not allow your shoulders to round forward as you press the handles downward on each repetition. Slowly reverse the motion to complete the rep. Keep your elbows by your sides throughout.

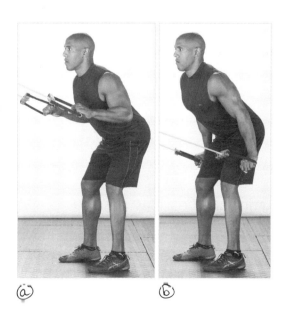

Resistance Band Overhead Triceps Extension

Setup

Stand in a staggered stance facing away from a resistance band attached at below your torso level to a stable structure or inside a doorjamb (many resistance bands come with a doorjamb attachment). Hold one handle in each hand and lean your weight forward with your arms extended at roughly a 45-degree angle above your head, with your elbows bent above 90 degrees (see figure a).

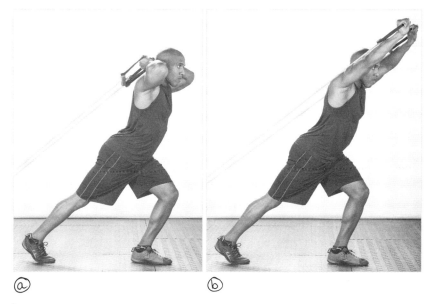

ⓐ　　　ⓑ

Action and Coaching Tips

Without allowing your elbows to flare out to the sides, extend your elbows toward the front of your body until your arms are straight (see figure b). Slowly reverse the action to complete the rep.

Resistance Band One-Arm Incline Press

Setup

Face away from a resistance band that's attached at a low position (below knee level) to a stable structure or inside a doorjamb (many resistance bands come with an attachment for this). Lean slightly forward and stand in a split stance, with your left leg in front. Hold both handles of the band in your right hand (see figure a).

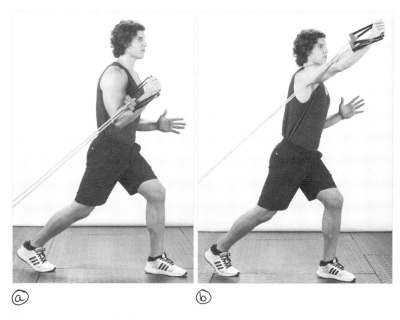

ⓐ　　　ⓑ

Action and Coaching Tips

Without allowing your torso to rotate or overextending at your low back, drive your arm straight out at a 45-degree angle (see figure b). Be sure to keep your arm at the same angle as the band. Slowly bring your arm back to complete one rep. Perform all reps on one side before switching arms and reversing your stance.

Resistance Band Side Shoulder Raise

Setup

Stand tall with your feet hip-width apart with the middle of a resistance band underneath the middle of your feet. Cross the resistance band in front of you by grabbing the handle that's on your right side with your left hand, and grab the handle that's on your left side with your right hand. Hold the handles by your sides with your elbows slightly bent (see figure a).

Action and Coaching Tips

With your elbows slightly bent, raise your arms out to the sides at roughly a 30-degree angle in front of your torso until your elbows go just above your forehead (see figure b). Do not overextend at your lower back to raise the weight up. Slowly lower the handles back to your sides.

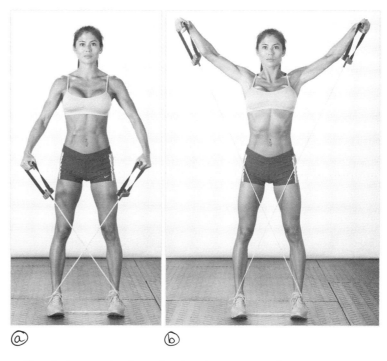

a   b

Resistance Band Bent-Over Row

Setup

Stand tall, facing a resistance band that's attached at a low position (just above the ground) to a stable structure or inside a doorjamb (many resistance bands come with an attachment for this). Holding one handle in each hand, lean at a 45-degree angle, keeping your knees soft and your back straight (see figure a).

Action and Coaching Tips

Pull the band toward your body so that your wrists come by your ribs, ensuring that you squeeze your shoulder blades together every time you pull your arms in without allowing the fronts of your shoulders to round forward (see figure b). Reverse the motion by extending your arms back out, without allowing your lower back to round out or losing your torso.

a   b

Resistance Band One-Arm Bent-Over Row

Setup

Stand in a split stance, with your right leg in front while facing a resistance band that's attached at a low position (just above the ground) to a stable structure or inside a doorjamb (many resistance bands come with an attachment for this). Holding both handles of the band in your left hand, lean forward at a 45-degree angle, keeping your knees soft and your back straight (see figure a).

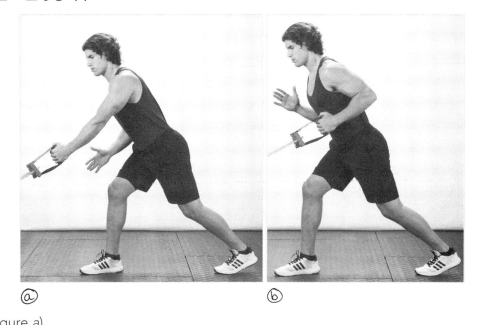

Action and Coaching Tips

Pull the band toward your body so that your wrists come by your ribs, ensuring that you squeeze your shoulder blades together every time you pull your arm in without allowing the front of your shoulder to round forward (see figure b). Reverse the motion by extending your arms back out, without allowing your lower back to round out or losing your stance. Perform all reps on one side before switching arms and reversing your stance.

Resistance Band Chest Fly

Setup

Face away from a band that's attached at roughly shoulder height to a stable structure or inside a doorjamb (many resistance bands come with an attachment for this). With your feet hip-width apart and in a parallel stance, hold a handle in each hand, keeping your elbows out to your sides and your forearms parallel to the floor (see figure a).

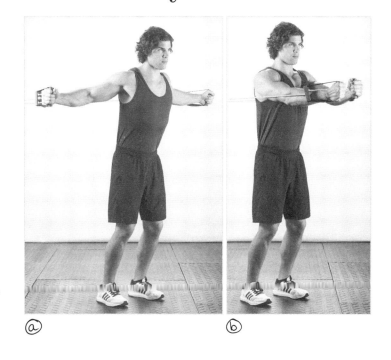

Action and Coaching Tips

Bring your arms together in front of you while keeping a soft bend in your elbows, as if you were hugging a tree, until the bands lightly touch the outsides of your arms (see figure b). Slowly reverse the motion until your arms are back out to your sides and your elbows are just behind your shoulders.

Resistance Band Biceps Curl

Setup

Stand tall, facing a resistance band that's attached at a low position (just above the ground) to a stable structure or inside a door-jamb (many resistance bands come with an attachment for this). Hold one handle in each hand with your arms in line with the band at a roughly 45-degree angle to the floor, elbows straight and palms facing the upward (see figure a).

Action and Coaching Tips

Curl the handles up toward your shoulders by bending at your elbows without allowing your elbows to move upward (see figure b). Do not allow your lower back to overextend as you curl the band into you. Once you cannot bend your elbows any further, reverse the motion slowly until your elbows are straight again.

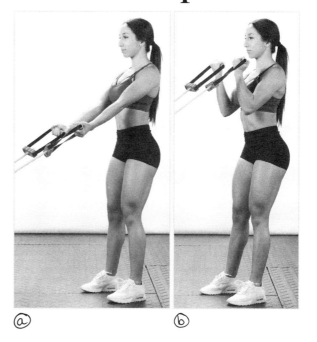

ⓐ   ⓑ

Resistance Band Loop Pull-Apart

Setup

Stand tall while holding a resistance band loop with both hands just outside shoulder-width, keeping your arms extended out in front of you at shoulder height (see figure a). There should be some tension in the band to start each rep.

Action and Coaching Tips

With your elbows slightly bent, pull the band apart until it lightly touches the top of your chest (see figure b). As you pull the band apart, do not extend at your lower back or allow your shoulders to round forward. Slowly reverse the motion, until your arms come back to the width they started at. Keep tension in the band throughout.

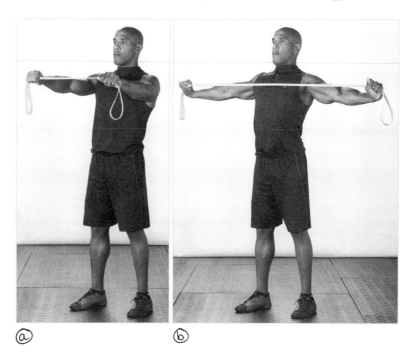

ⓐ   ⓑ

To reduce the resistance, you can either begin with your hands positioned wider or hold one layer of the band instead of both layers as shown.

Supine Resistance Band Shoulder L

Setup

Lie supine on the floor, with your knees slightly bent and your legs raised above you. Wrap the center of a resistance band behind your feet. Holding one handle of the resistance band in each hand, place your arms out to the sides at shoulder height, bending your elbows 90 degrees and

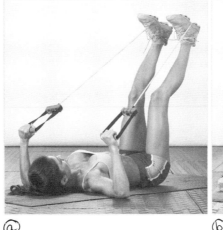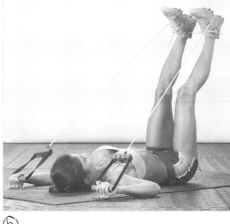

keeping your elbows and the backs of your arms in contact with the ground (see figure a).

Action and Coaching Tips

Without moving your elbows or allowing your arms to lift off the ground, rotate your arms down. Bring your hands toward the floor as far as you can (see figure b). Pause for a second or two at the bottom of each rep. Slowly reverse the motion to return to the starting position.

Resistance Band Pull-Up

Setup

Hang from a pull-up bar using an overhand grip and place one foot inside a resistance band loop that's anchored on the bar you're pulling yourself up to (see figure a).

Action and Coaching Tips

Bring yourself up so that your chin goes above the bar (see figure b). Don't swing your body. Slowly lower yourself with control.

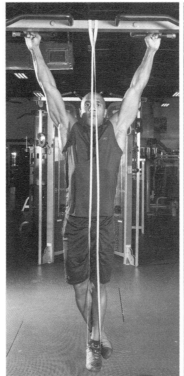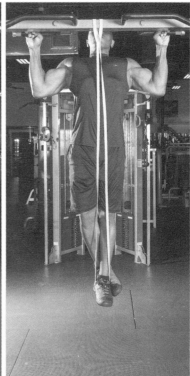

One-Arm Push-Up

Setup

Assume a one-arm plank position, with your feet spread several inches wider than your shoulders (see figure a). Your weight-bearing arm should be positioned so that your wrist is directly under the same-side shoulder. Turn your weight-bearing hand out slightly so that your fingers point at roughly a 45-degree angle away from your body. Your non-weight-bearing arm should be on the opposite hip or behind your back.

Action and Coaching Tips

Drop into a one-arm push-up, allowing your torso to rotate a few degrees away from your weight-bearing arm while keeping your elbow on the working side tight to your body (see figure b). Drive into the floor and push your body back to the top of the push-up to complete a full rep. Perform all repetitions on one side before switching to the other arm. Do not allow your lower back to sag toward the floor at any time.

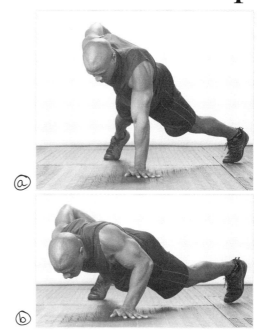

Lockoff Push-Up

Setup

Begin in a low push-up position, with your feet shoulder-width apart, one hand on top of a medicine ball or platform, and your other hand on the floor (see figure a).

Action and Coaching Tips

Press up with one hand on top of the platform or medicine ball. At the top of the push-up, lock off by fully straightening the elbow of the arm resting on the platform or ball (see figure b). Place the other arm at your chest and pause for one or two seconds at the top of each repetition, then slowly lower yourself. Perform half of the repetitions with your right arm elevated and the other half with your left arm elevated. Do not allow your shoulders or hips to rotate at any time; keep your torso parallel to the ground throughout.

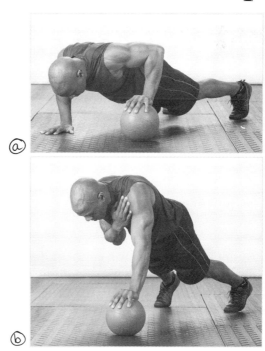

Explosive Push-Up

Setup

Place your hands shoulder-width apart on the floor with your elbows straight (see figure *a*). Turn your hands outward so that your fingers point at roughly 45 degrees.

Action and Coaching Tips

Lower yourself to the floor while keeping your elbows directly above your wrists and at a 45-degree angle to your torso (see figure *b*). Once your elbows are angled at almost 90 degrees, quickly reverse the motion by explosively pushing your body up so that your hands leave the floor (see figure *c*). Land lightly on the floor as you simultaneously lower yourself down to begin the next repetition. Do not allow your hips to elevate before the rest of your body; keep your body in a straight line throughout.

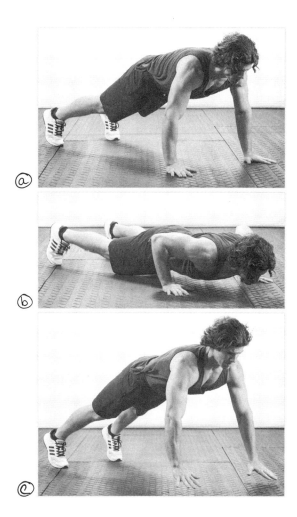

Box Crossover Push-Up

Setup

Begin in a push-up position, with both hands on top of a platform and your feet just outside shoulder-width apart (see figure *a*).

Action and Coaching Tips

Without moving your feet, step one hand off the box or ball to the floor while performing a push-up (see figure *b*). As you come out of the push-up, bring your hand back to the platform or ball. Repeat the same action on the other side. Do not allow your head or hips to sag toward the floor at any point.

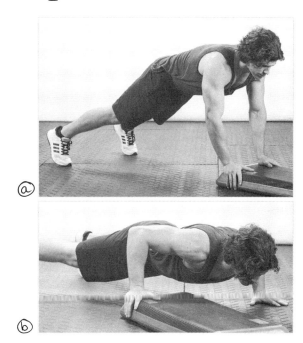

Explosive Box Crossover Push-Up

Setup

Begin in a push-up position with both hands on top of a platform and your feet just outside shoulder-width apart (see figure a).

Action and Coaching Tips

Without moving your feet, step one hand off the box or ball to the floor and lower into a push-up position (see figure b) while raising into an explosive push-up by driving your body up and across the platform as fast as you can (see figure c). Catch some airtime. As you come out of the push-up, bring your opposite hand back to the platform. Repeat the same action to the other side. Do not allow your head or hips to sag toward the floor at any point.

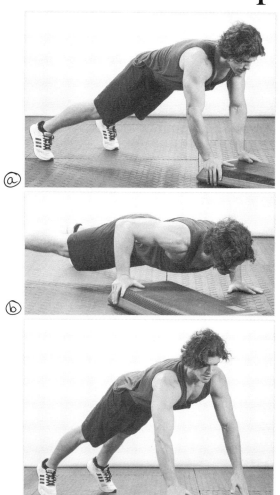

Close-Grip Push-Up

Setup

Begin in a push-up position, with both hands on top of a platform and your feet shoulder-width apart (see figure a). Turn your hands outward so that your fingers point down toward the floor.

Action and Coaching Tips

Perform a push-up by lowering your chest toward the platform until your elbows are angled at almost 90 degrees (see figure b). At the bottom of each push-up, your elbows should be against your sides. Then, reverse the motion by pressing yourself away from the floor until your elbows are straight.

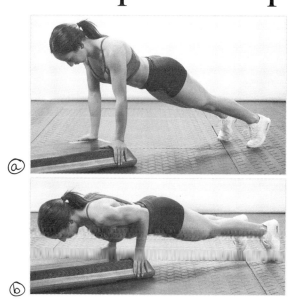

113

Stability-Ball Push-Up

Setup

Assume a plank position with your hands on a (55 to 65 cm size) stability ball and your fingers pointing down toward the floor (see figure a).

Action and Coaching Tips

Perform a push-up by lowering your body to the ball while keeping your elbows directly above your wrist (see figure b). Once your elbows reach an angle just below 90 degrees, reverse the motion by pushing your body up so that your elbows are straight again. At the top of each push-up, do not finish with your shoulder blades pinched together; instead, protract (push apart) your shoulder blades while keeping your body in a straight line. Do not allow your head or hips to sag at any point.

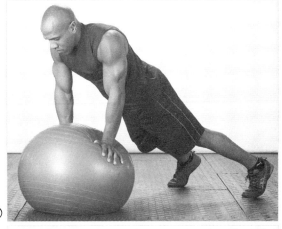

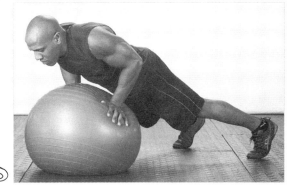

Feet-Elevated Push-Up

Setup

Begin in a push-up position, with your hands shoulder-width apart on the floor and your feet elevated on top of a weight bench or chair (see figure a).

Action and Coaching Tips

Perform a push-up by lowering your body to the floor while keeping your elbows directly above your wrists (see figure b). At the bottom of each push-up, position your arms at a 45-degree angle to form the shape of an arrow with your torso. Once your elbows are almost at a 90-degree angle, reverse the motion by pushing your body up so that your elbows are straight again. At the top of each push-up, do not finish with your shoulder blades pinched together; instead, protract (push apart) your shoulder blades while keeping your body in a straight line.

Keep your body in a straight line, from your head to your hips to your ankles; do not allow your head or hips to sag toward the floor at any point.

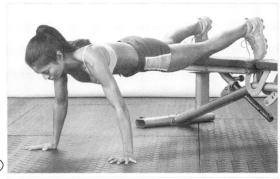

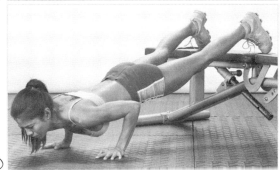

Smith Bar Triceps Skull Crusher

Setup

Using a Smith machine, face a barbell positioned at belly-button height and hold on to the bar with your hands roughly shoulder-width apart. Lean forward with your arms extended (see figure *a*).

Action and Coaching Tips

Bend at your elbows and lower your forehead to your wrists (see figure *b*). Reverse direction and extend your elbows, as in a triceps extension, to complete the rep. Keep your entire body straight throughout the action.

To increase the difficulty, lower your body closer to the floor by lowering the bar; the closer your torso comes to being parallel with the floor, the tougher the exercise is. To decrease the difficulty, use a higher bar placement.

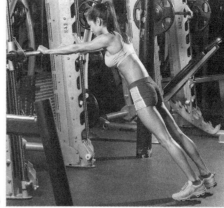

@

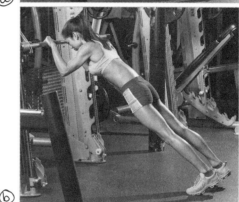

b

Underhand Grip Smith Bar Row

Setup

This exercise is an alternate version of the suspension row. Using a Smith machine, face a barbell positioned at belly-button height. Hold on to the bar using an underhand grip, your arms extended straight in front of your shoulders. Lean back, keeping your body in a straight line from head to toe (see figure *a*).

Action and Coaching Tips

Pull yourself up toward the bar by bending at your elbows, keeping your elbows tight to your sides (see figure *b*). Perform a rowing motion until your midtorso contacts the bar. When pulling yourself up, keep your body in a straight line; do not lead with your hips. At the top of each repetition, pause at the top for a second and do not allow the fronts of your shoulders to round forward. Slowly lower yourself until your elbows are straight.

To increase the difficulty, start the exercise from a more severe backward lean by lowering the bar, thus bringing your body closer to the floor.

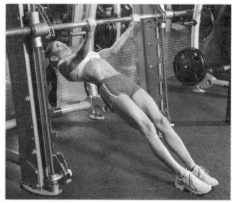

@

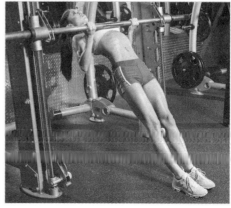

b

Wide-Elbow Smith Bar Row

Setup

This exercise is an alternate version of the wide-elbow suspension row. Using a Smith machine, face a barbell positioned at belly-button height and hold on to the bar using an overhand grip, your hands placed about 5 inches (13 cm) outside of your shoulders. Keeping your arms straight and extended in front of your shoulders, lean back with your body in a straight line from head to toe (see figure a).

Action and Coaching Tips

Pull yourself up toward the bar by bending at your elbows and performing a rowing motion while flaring out your elbows (see figure b). Do not allow your wrists to bend as you pull yourself up; keep your elbows directly behind your hands throughout. Your elbows should be at a 90-degree angle to your torso at the top of each repetition. Pause at the top for a second, then slowly lower yourself until your elbows are straight. Keep your body in a straight line; do not lead with your hips when pulling yourself up.

To increase the difficulty, start the exercise from a more severe backward lean by lowering the bar, thus bringing your body closer to the floor.

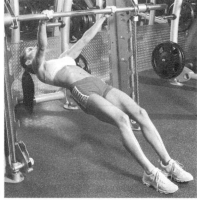

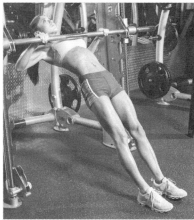

Wide-Elbow Smith Bar Shrug

Setup

Using a Smith machine, face a barbell positioned at belly-button height and hold on to the bar using an overhand grip, your hands placed about 5 inches (13 cm) outside of your shoulders. Keeping your arms straight and extended in front of your shoulders, lean back with your body in a straight line from head to toe.

Action and Coaching Tips

Keeping your arms nearly straight, pinch (retract) your shoulder blades together and pause for one or two seconds (see figure). Slowly reverse the movement by allowing your shoulder blades to separate (protract) as far as possible without allowing your spine to round out.

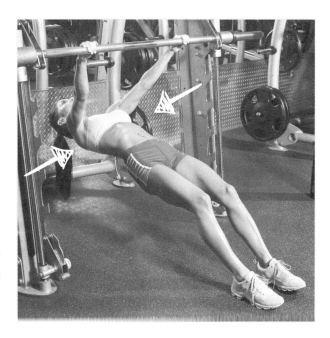

Chin-Up

Setup

Hang from a pull-up bar using an under-hand grip (see figure a). Grip the bar at a width that feels comfortable for you. You can use assistance to perform the movement with less than your bodyweight by either placing your feet on the platform or by placing one foot inside a resistance band loop that's anchored on the bar you're pulling yourself up to.

Action and Coaching Tips

Bring yourself up so that your chin goes above the bar without swinging your body (see figure b). Pause for one second at the top of each rep before lowering yourself. Slowly lower yourself with control.

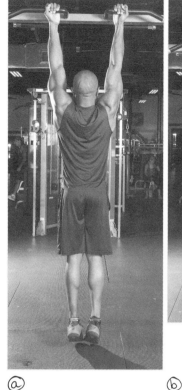
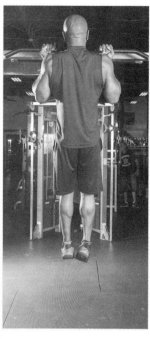

ⓐ   ⓑ

Neutral Grip Pull-Up

Setup

Hang from a pull-up bar using a neutral grip that place your hands around shoul-der-width apart (see figure a). You can use assistance to perform the movement with less than your bodyweight by either placing your feet on the platform or by placing one foot inside a resistance band loop that's anchored on the bar you're pulling yourself up to.

Action and Coaching Tips

Bring yourself up so that your chin goes above the handles without swinging your body (see figure b). Pause for one second at the top of each rep before lowering your-self. Slowly lower yourself with control.

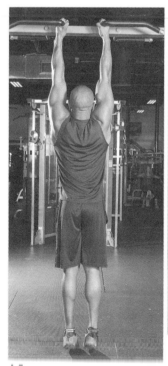
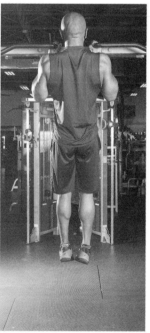

ⓐ   ⓑ

Pull-Up

Setup

Hang from a pull-up bar using an overhand grip. You can use assistance to perform the movement with less than your bodyweight by either placing your feet on the platform or by placing one foot inside a resistance band loop that's anchored on the bar you're pulling yourself up to (see figure a for an example using a resistance band loop).

Action and Coaching Tips

Bring yourself up so that your chin goes above the bar (see figure b). Don't swing your body. Slowly lower yourself with control.

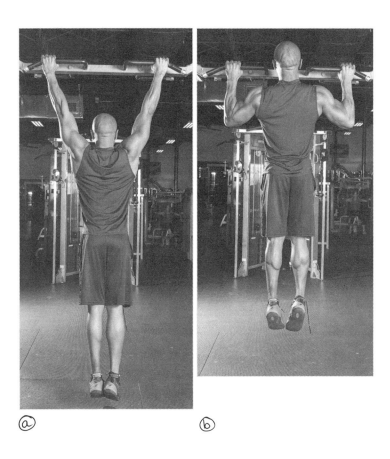

@   ⓑ

7 { Lower-Body Exercises

The exercises presented in this chapter challenge your lower-body musculature—which consists primarily of the glutes, hamstrings, quadriceps, and calves—from a parallel stance, split stance, or single-leg stance.

Some of these exercises distribute the loading challenge through several muscles in the lower body and lower back as the movement is performed, while other exercises provide more focused resistance only to certain muscle groups in the lower body.

Finding Exercises That Are Perfect for You!

The exercises in this chapter, as well as those in the upper-body and core exercise chapters, can be for any goal. The goal dictates how they're structured and utilized within a given program.

An individualized program isn't just about what exercises you do; it's also about what exercises you don't do based on your ability and injury profile. Find exercises that fit you instead of trying to fit yourself to exercises. As mentioned previously (in chapter 2), most people don't have to do a specific exercise to improve. There are only training principles that must be adhered to, and there are many exercise applications and variations that allow people to adhere to the principles and achieve their goals.

Trying to fit the individual to the exercise instead of fitting the exercise to the individual is one of the biggest training mistakes. For example, many personal trainers and strength coaches attempt to fit everyone into the mold of performing deadlifts or squats in the conventional style by using a barbell. Though well intentioned, this approach is misguided.

Bodies vary, and people should not do the same exercises in the same manner. Taking a one-size-fits-all approach to deadlifting, or any other exercise, not only ignores the obvious physiological differences between humans but also can be dangerous. Sure, we're all part of the human species, just like all makes and models of cars are part of the category that we refer to as vehicles. But, as with vehicles, humans come in all shapes and sizes. Your size and shape are determined by your structure, which in turn determines function. A Mini Cooper and

(continued)

> *continued*

a minivan are made up of the same basic parts and can perform the same basic driving functions. But you'd never expect a Mini Cooper to drive and handle in the same way as a minivan because of the different ways in which their (same) basic parts are put together.

This is why it's unrealistic to expect a guy who's built like a football running back to move the same way as a guy built like a lineman. Granted, both can change levels, run, push, pull, twist, and so on; however, they perform the movements in different ways based on their differing structures. Because of these individual variations in the ways that humans move, no given exercise can exactly match everyone's movements.

As I said in chapter 2, resistance exercises are just ways to put force across joints. That's it! When you understand this, you quickly see that no exercise has magical powers; barbells, dumbbells, cables, machines, and bands are all just different tools that allow us to apply force across joints. Choose the exercise variations that best fit how you move.

Basic Lower-Body Exercises: PERFECTED

The following section provides basic lower-body exercises and shows you how to do them better than the way they are commonly performed. This will help you train smarter, more safely, and efficiently. All it takes is a couple of small tweaks.

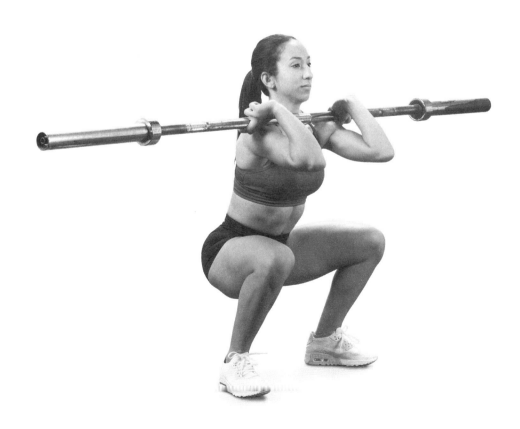

Barbell Squat

Setup

Place a barbell across your shoulders (not on your neck) and stand with your feet just farther than shoulder-width apart and your toes turned out 10 to 15 degrees (see figure a).

Action and Coaching Tips

Bend at your knees and hips and lower your body toward the floor; go as low as you can without losing the arch in your lower back (see figure b). Your heels should not lift off the ground, and avoid allowing your knees to drop in toward the midline of your body; keep your knees tracking in the same direction as your toes. Once you've gone as deep as you can, reverse the motion and stand up.

WHY IT'S BETTER

You adjust your stance (width and foot position) to best fit your body and the way you move. Experiment with wider stances than parallel and with turning your toes out slightly to find the stance that allows you to go down the deepest in the squat while maintaining an arch in your lower back.

Many lifters think a proper squat is a shoulder-width stance with your feet pointed straight forward. The new angle here is to not take such a one-size-fits-all approach to squatting. Research in both Eastern and Western populations has not only found normal variations in femoral neck angles but also asymmetrical differences between the left and rights sides of individuals (1,2). This is in addition to normal anatomical variations in the structure of the hip acetabulum, which can influence how someone is able to perform the squat movement (3,4).

The normal anatomical variations of the hip joint structure and the length of one's torso, femur, and tibia—structure determines function—indicate that an optimal squat is very individual and therefore uses a variety of foot positions, stance widths, depths, and torso angles.

Benefits
- Better range of motion
- Safer, more natural path of movement for your body

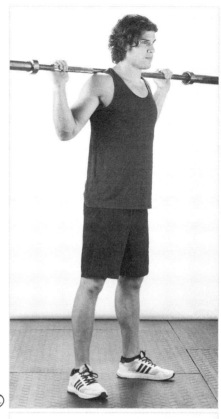

(a)

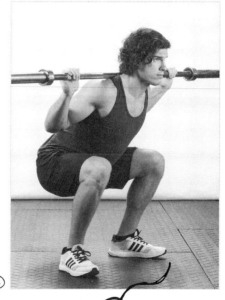

(b)

Adjust your stance to best fit your body

Barbell Front Squat

Setup

The front squat uses the same mechanics as the back squat; the only difference involves the bar placement. Rest an Olympic barbell on the top of your chest, keeping only your thumb, index finger, and middle finger underneath the bar (see figure *a*). Stand with your feet just farther than shoulder-width apart and your toes turned out 10 to 15 degrees. Stay tall and lift your chest to create a rack for the bar instead of trying to hold it up with only your arms. If you feel like front squats bother your wrists or are simply unable to get your wrists into the proper position, loop wrist straps around the bar and hold on tight, keeping upward tension on the straps by pulling them vertically as you perform the front squat.

Action and Coaching Tips

Bend at your knees and hips and lower your body toward the floor as far as you can without losing the arch in your lower back (see figure *b*). As you drop into the squat, keep your elbows lifted high toward the sky. Once you've gone as deep as you can control—without allowing your heels to lift off the ground or your lower back to lose its arch—reverse the motion by extending your legs and returning to the standing position to complete the rep. Be sure to keep your knees wide and tracking in the same direction as your toes throughout; do not allow your knees to drop in toward the midline of your body.

WHY IT'S BETTER

In addition to taking a more individualized approach to finding your optimal squat stance, which was discussed in the section on barbell squats, you're doing three things differently here from the way people often try to perform barbell front squats. The first is using your chest to create a rack for the bar to rest on instead of trying to hold it up with only your arms. The second is allowing your pinky and ring fingers to stay above the bar, which makes it much less awkward on your wrists and hands to hold the bar in place than when trying to keep all your fingers underneath the bar. Third, if the previous two tweaks bother your wrists, or you are simply unable to get your wrists into the position described, you can use wrist wraps.

Benefits
- Easier on your wrists
- Less awkward to hold the barbell in place

Use your chest to create a rack for the bar to rest on

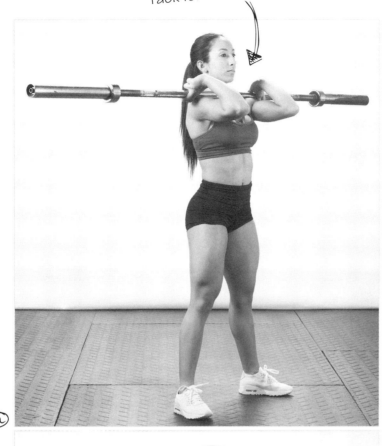

(a)

Allow your pinky and ring fingers to stay above the bar

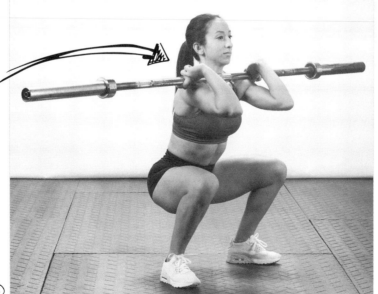

(b)

Barbell Hybrid Deadlift

Setup

Stand in front of a barbell with your feet slightly farther than shoulder-width apart and turned out 15 degrees. Keeping your back straight and maintaining an arch in your lower back, hinge at your hips and bend your knees. Lower your torso to about a 45-degree angle and grab the bar, your hands shoulder-width apart.

Action and Coaching Tips

Keeping your back straight, drive your hips forward toward the barbell and lift it off the ground while straightening your legs (see figures a and b). Reverse the motion and slowly lower the barbell back to the floor to complete the rep. As you hinge forward, drive your hips backward and do not allow your back to round. Lift the bar by extending your hips, not by overextending your lower back. Keep the barbell close to you throughout; it should touch your shins and track against the fronts of your legs as you perform each repetition. Your arms should be close to touching the insides of your legs at the bottom of each lift.

WHY IT'S BETTER

This lift combines the Romanian and sumo deadlifts, which you'd do with a wider stance and a more upright torso. For many, the hybrid deadlift is a smart substitute for traditional deadlifts for two reasons. First, the wider stance is easier and more natural for most lifters to do while maintaining the alignment cues. Second, this starting position keeps the barbell closer to the hip joints than the conventional style, which provides a shorter lever arm. This gives you a greater mechanical advantage while placing less overall stress on the lower back. One study did a biomechanical analysis of straight bar and trap (hex) bar deadlifts and found that the trap bar deadlifts placed less overall load on the lumbar spine because it also involves a shorter lever arm. However, not everyone has access to a trap bar (5).

Benefits

- More universally comfortable and natural
- Less stress on the lower back

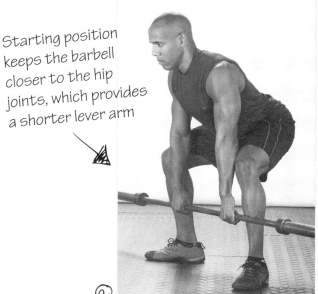

Starting position keeps the barbell closer to the hip joints, which provides a shorter lever arm

ⓐ

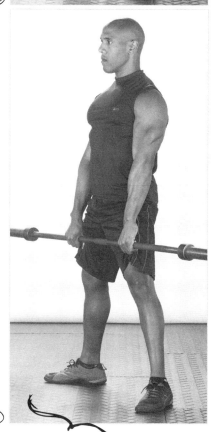

ⓑ

Wider stance is easier and more natural

Elevated Dumbbell Leaning Reverse Lunge

Setup

Stand on the flat side of an Olympic weight plate or on an aerobic step platform, your feet hip-width apart (see figure a). Hold a dumbbell in each hand at your sides. You can also do this exercise using only body weight by allowing your hands to hang down at your sides or by interlacing your fingers behind your head.

Action and Coaching Tips

Step backward on your left leg, placing the ball of your foot on the floor while bending both knees and lowering your body into a lunge. As your knees bend, hinge at your hips and lean forward at roughly a 45-degree angle while keeping your back straight (see figure b). Once your back knee lightly touches the floor, reverse the motion by stepping back up to the platform. Do the same with the other leg.

Use a platform low enough to allow you to touch your back knee to the floor on each repetition. If a reduction in range is needed, you can perform this exercise without standing on a platform.

WHY IT'S BETTER

You lean forward at roughly a 45-degree angle as you perform each lunge off a weight plate or platform. Lunging off the platform increases the range of motion you're able to train through during this exercise. Also, leaning your torso forward increases the recruitment of the glutes and hamstrings. This places less force on your knee joint and therefore demands less activation of the quadriceps. Doing lunges with a forward torso lean can be especially helpful to females since women are more quadriceps-dominant than men are (6), tend to have weaker hamstrings (7,8), and therefore can be more prone to knee injury (9).

Benefits

- Increases the range of motion you're training through
- Increases recruitment of the glute and hamstrings

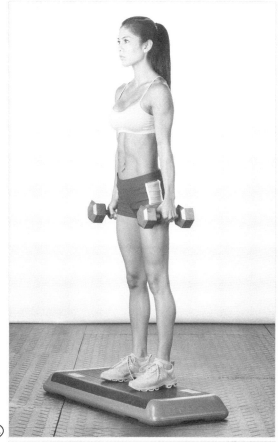

@

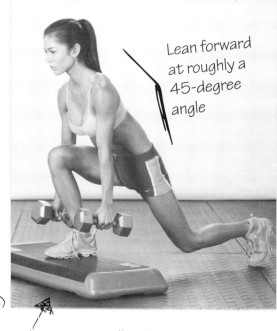

Lean forward at roughly a 45-degree angle

b

Elevated platform allows you to increase the range of motion

125

Elevated Dumbbell Reverse Lunge

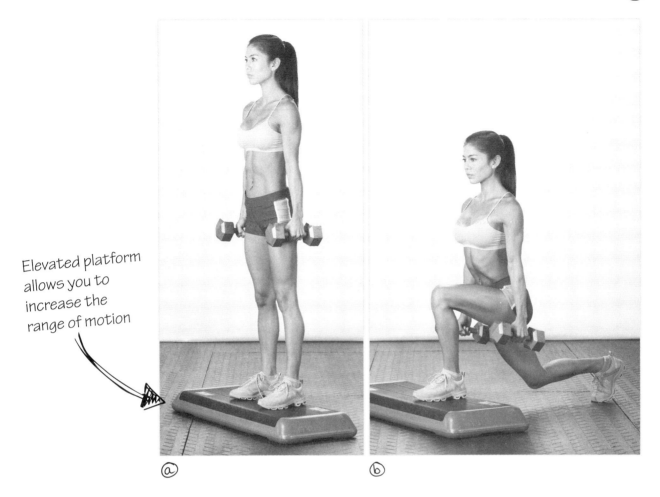

Elevated platform allows you to increase the range of motion

(a)　(b)

Setup

Stand on the flat side of an Olympic weight plate or on a workout step, with your feet hip-width apart (see figure a). Hold a dumbbell in each hand at your sides. You can also do this exercise using only body weight by allowing your hands to hang down at your sides or by interlacing your fingers behind your head.

Action and Coaching Tips

Keeping your torso upright, step backward on your right leg, placing the ball of your foot on the floor while bending both your knees and lowering your body into a lunge (see figure b). Once your back knee lowers toward the floor, reverse the motion by stepping back up to the platform. Do the same with your other leg.

WHY IT'S BETTER

Performing reverse lunges from an elevated platform allows you to increase the range of motion. The platform should be low enough to allow you to touch your back knee to the floor on each repetition.

Benefits

- Increased recruitment of the quadriceps from the leaning version
- Increases the range of motion you're training through

Traveling Dumbbell Leaning Lunge

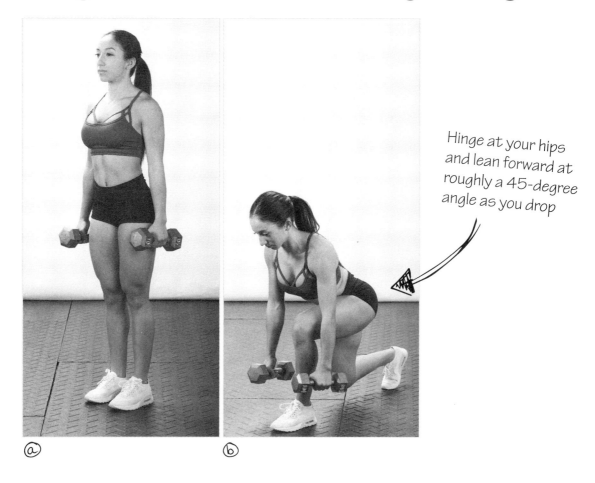

Hinge at your hips and lean forward at roughly a 45-degree angle as you drop

Setup

Stand tall, with your feet hip-width apart (see figure a). Hold a dumbbell in each hand at your sides. You can also do this exercise using only body weight by allowing your hands to hang down at your sides or by interlacing your fingers behind your head.

Action and Coaching Tips

Take a large step forward and drop your body so that your back knee lightly touches the floor. As your knees bend, hinge at your hips and lean forward at roughly a 45-degree angle while keeping your back straight (see figure b). Stand back up tall while bringing your rear leg forward to meet your front leg and step forward with the opposite leg—the one that was behind you on the last rep. Do not step so far out on each lunge that you're unable to do this exercise smoothly and with control. Repeat as you walk down the room.

WHY IT'S BETTER

You hinge at your hips and lean forward at roughly a 45-degree angle as you drop into each lunge. At the bottom of each lunge, the dumbbells end up at each side of your front foot instead of by your hips due to the forward torso lean.

This version of the walking lunge still incorporates the quadriceps, but it reduces the forces placed on the knee joint and transfers more force into the glutes and hamstrings.

Benefits

- Reduced forces on the knee joint
- Increase recruitment of the glute and hamstrings

Dumbbell Leaning Bulgarian Split Squat

Setup

Stand tall while holding a dumbbell in each hand at your sides. Place your left foot on top of a bench or chair behind you (see figure a). Your front leg should be far enough in front of the bench that your shin can stay nearly vertical as you drop into each rep. You can also do this exercise using only body weight by allowing your hands to hang down at your sides or by interlacing your fingers behind your head.

Action and Coaching Tips

Lower your body toward the floor without allowing your back knee to rest on the floor. As you lower your body, keep your back straight and lean forward at about a 45-degree angle (see figure b). Drive your heel into the ground to raise your body to the starting position, thus completing the rep. Perform all reps on one side before switching to the other leg. Keep your weight on your front foot throughout the exercise.

WHY IT'S BETTER

As your knees bend, you hinge at your hips and lean forward at roughly a 45-degree angle while keeping your back straight. At the bottom, the dumbbells are on each side of your front foot instead of by your hips. In addition to targeting your glutes and hamstrings, leaning your torso forward while your rear leg is elevated on something (like a weight bench) at or above your knee height prevents you from overextending your lower back. You won't place unwanted stress on that area to maintain a fully upright torso with this exercise.

Benefits

- Less awkward and more natural to maintain the torso position
- Increase recruitment of the glute and hamstrings

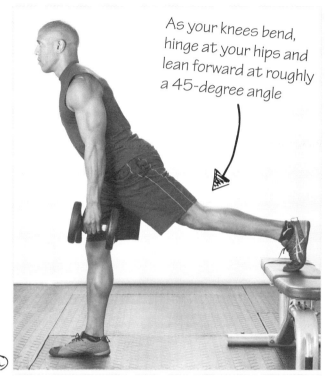

As your knees bend, hinge at your hips and lean forward at roughly a 45-degree angle

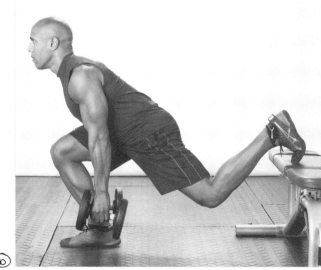

At the bottom, the dumbbells are on each side of your front foot instead of by your hips

Low Foot Bulgarian Split Squat

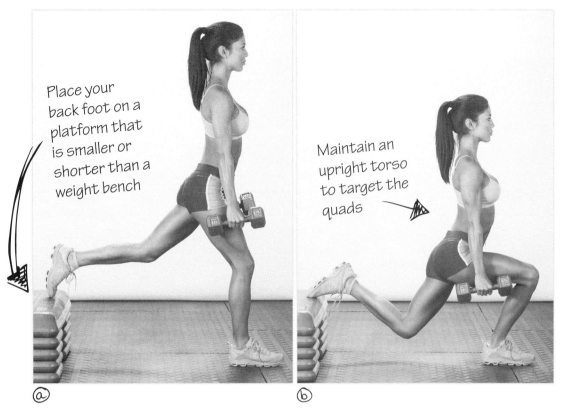

Place your back foot on a platform that is smaller or shorter than a weight bench

Maintain an upright torso to target the quads

(a)   (b)

Setup

Stand tall while holding a dumbbell in each hand at your sides. Place your left foot on a small box or aerobic platform that's behind you and as high as the middle of your shin (see figure a). Your right leg should be far enough in front of the box that your shin can stay close to vertical as you drop into each rep. You can also do this exercise using only body weight by allowing your hands to hang down at your sides or by interlacing your fingers behind your head.

Action and Coaching Tips

Keeping your torso upright, lower your body toward the floor without allowing your back knee to rest on the floor (see figure b). As you lower your body, keep your back straight. Drive your heel into the ground to raise your body to the starting position, thus completing the rep. Perform all reps on one side before switching to the other leg. Keep your weight on your front foot throughout the exercise.

WHY IT'S BETTER

You place your back foot on a platform that's smaller or shorter than a weight bench and is around the height of the middle of your shin. Performing Bulgarian split squats with an upright torso is an effective way to target the quadriceps during this exercise, just like performing lunges with an upright torso also targets these muscles. Placing your back foot on a platform that is smaller or shorter than a weight bench prevents you from overextending your lower back. You won't place unwanted stress in that area to maintain a fully upright torso as you perform this exercise.

Benefits

- Less awkward and more natural to maintain the torso position
- Increased recruitment of the quadriceps from the leaning version

One-Leg Squat

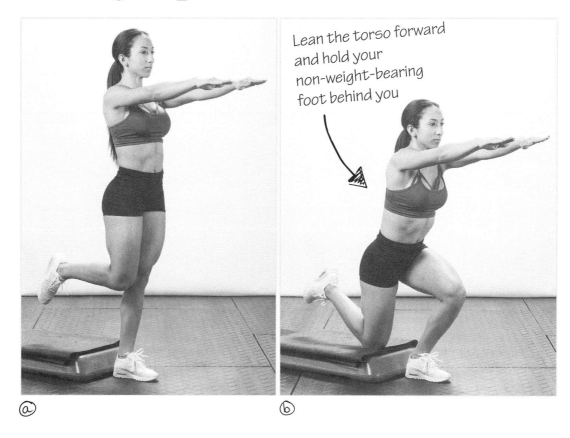

Lean the torso forward and hold your non-weight-bearing foot behind you

ⓐ   ⓑ

Setup

Stand in front of a pad that is two to three inches (about 8-13 cm) thick, a small stack of weight plates with a mat on top, or a workout step. Shift your weight to your left leg and lift the right foot off the floor, with the knee bent and slightly behind your left leg (see figure a). Your hands are outstretched in front of you to serve as a counterbalance. You can also perform the exercise while holding a dumbbell at each shoulder.

Action and Coaching Tips

Slowly lower yourself toward the floor by bending your weight-bearing knee and sitting back at your hips until you lightly tap your back knee on the object (see figure b). Do not allow your back (non-weight-bearing) foot to touch the floor. Reverse the motion and stand up again. Perform all reps on the same side before switching sides.

WHY IT'S BETTER

You lean the torso forward and hold your non-weight-bearing foot behind you instead of in front of you. This position is commonly called a pistol squat, but note that this isn't to say the pistol squat exercise is somehow a bad or dangerous exercise. However, this version of the single-leg squat, called a knee-tap squat, puts you in position that's more common to how we move in life and sport, which is why it feels more natural and less awkward to perform. Plus, leaning the torso forward increases the glute and hamstring muscle involvement, which also makes it easier on the knee joint.

Benefits
- Less awkward
- More universally comfortable and natural

45-Degree Hip Extension

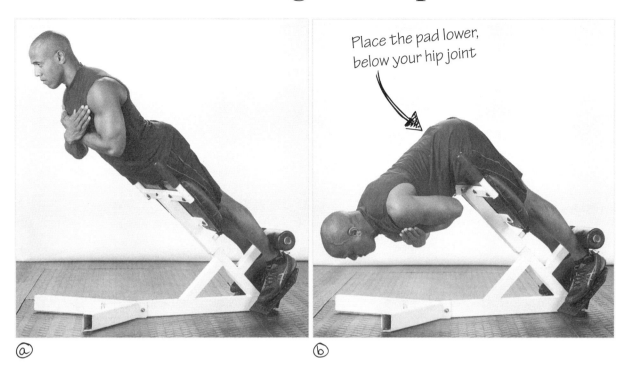

Place the pad lower, below your hip joint

(a)   (b)

Setup
For this exercise, you will need a specially designed apparatus known as a 45-degree back extension. With your feet hip-width apart, rest your thighs against the pad, which is positioned below your hip bones, and keep your back straight (see figure *a*). Cross your arms in front of your chest.

Action and Coaching Tips
Hinge at your hips, keeping your back straight, and lower down (see figure *b*). Reverse the motion by extending at your hips, without arching your lower back too much. Pull yourself up so that your body forms a straight line from shoulders to hips to ankles. To make the exercise more difficult, hold a weight plate at your belly or chest.

WHY IT'S BETTER
You place the pad lower, below your hip joint, so you're able to hinge at your hips without rounding out at your lower back. Although this exercise is commonly referred to as a 45-degree back extension, the focus of this version is to create the extension motion via *hip* extension— hence the name used here. Keeping your spine straight while you perform the motion at your hip joints ensures the maximal involvement from your glute and hamstring muscles instead of your lower back muscles.

Benefits
- Less stress on the lower back
- Increased involvement of the glute and hamstring musculature

Dumbbell Step-Up

Setup

Stand facing a weight bench with your left foot on the bench (see figure a). Hold a dumbbell in each hand by your hips. You can also do this exercise using only body weight by allowing your hands to hang down at your sides or by interlacing your fingers behind your head.

Action and Coaching Tips

Step up by straightening your left knee (see figure b). Once you're on top of the bench, allow your right foot to gently touch the bench to help maintain your balance, then reverse the motion by stepping down with your right foot first. Bring your left foot down to the floor. Place your right foot on top of the bench and repeat the exercise. Switch the working leg (i.e., the stepping leg) on the ground, not when you're on top of the bench.

Move smoothly and with control; avoid jerking your torso forward to initiate each rep. Lean slightly forward while keeping most of your weight on the front leg throughout.

WHY IT'S BETTER

You switch legs on the ground, not on top of the bench, and lean slightly forward as you perform the step-up. As you lean forward, you also raise your back heel off the ground and shift your hips forward so your shoulders, hips, and down leg form a straight line that's at roughly a 45-degree angle to the floor. When most people do step-ups, they switch legs on top of the bench. This is problematic. It can cause you to step up and down using the same leg, and that can be confusing to keep track of, thus causing your workout to be uneven. Changing legs on the floor is easier to count and track.

This exercise is normally performed without this adjustment in body position, so it's very easy to cheat (even while trying not to) by using your back leg to do much of the work and using momentum to propel yourself up. The body positioning involved in performing this version of the step-up forces you to move smoothly and with control so you don't jerk your torso forward to complete each rep.

Benefits

- Better recruitment of the leg and glute musculature
- Prevents cheating

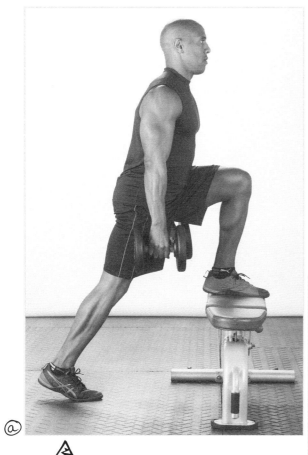

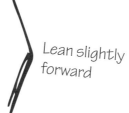

Lean slightly forward

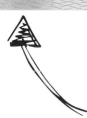

Switch legs on the ground, not on top of the bench

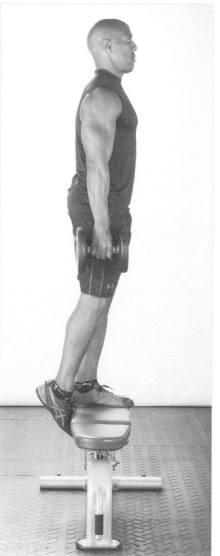

Copenhagen Hip Adduction

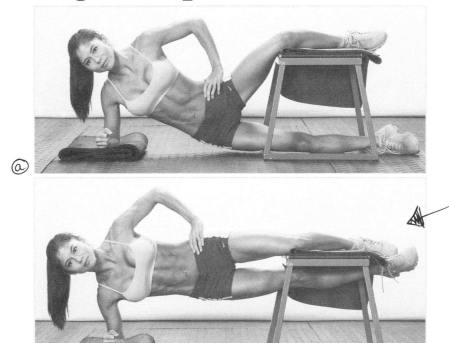

Place the knee on top of a platform

Setup

Lie on the floor on your right side with your elbow directly underneath your right shoulder, your right leg straight, and your left leg bent 90 degrees. Rest your left knee and calf on top of a bench or plyo box that's roughly 17 to 20 inches high (43-50 cm) while your right leg is underneath the box platform (see figure a). You'll want to place a rolled-up towel or mat underneath your left leg and right elbow for comfort.

Action and Coaching Tips

Keeping your right leg straight and your body in a straight line from your left knee to your hips to your shoulders, press your left leg into the top of the platform as you elevate your right hip off the ground and simultaneously lift your right leg up to squeeze the inside of your right thigh against the inside of your left thigh (see figure b). Pause for one or two seconds at the top before reversing the action and lowering your right leg and hip back down to the floor to complete one rep. Do all reps on the same side before switching sides and performing this exercise with your right leg on top of the platform.

WHY IT'S BETTER

The importance of strengthening the adductors with exercises like this is discussed in chapter 2, Function and Performance. This exercise is often shown being done with a training partner holding your top leg underneath your top knee and foot. Without a partner, keeping your top leg straight and placing your top foot on the end of a platform or plyo box exposes you to additional lateral forces through your knee joint that are greatly reduced when the partner is also holding your knee. Here, you don't need a partner, because placing the knee on top of the platform allows you to reap the same benefits while providing more support at your knee joint.

Benefits

- Less unwanted stress on the knee joint
- No need for a training partner to perform

Additional Lower-Body Exercises

The exercises in this section also focus on helping you maximize the strength and development of your lower-body musculature. There aren't unique adjustments for doing them, so they don't warrant the same level of description as the exercises in the previous section. You also may find some not-so-common lower-body exercises here to help you incorporate some variety into your workouts.

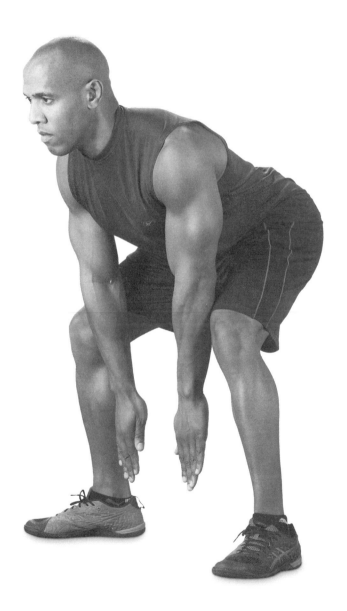

Squat Jump with Arm Drive

Setup

Stand with your feet roughly shoulder-width apart.

Action and Coaching Tips

Squat by bending at your knees and hips so that your thighs are just above/parallel to the ground (see figure a). Reach your arms just behind your hips, keeping your elbows slightly bent. Jump straight up by simultaneously extending your legs and swinging your arms above you (see figure b). Land as lightly and quietly as possible, thus returning to the starting position.

Each time you squat, keep your knees in the same line as your toes; your knees should not come toward one another at any time. Do not allow your back to round out at the bottom position before you jump, and jump as high as you can on each repetition.

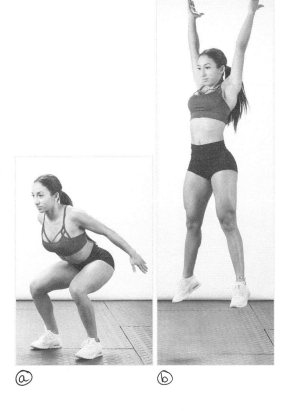

ⓐ ⓑ

Deadlift Jump

Setup

Stand with your feet roughly shoulder-width apart and hands on the front of the legs.

Action and Coaching Tips

Hinge at your hips and bend forward toward the floor (see figure a). Keep your back straight and your knees bent at a 15- to 20-degree angle. Let your arms hang in front of your body by your knees and keep your elbows slightly bent.

Jump straight up by simultaneously extending your hips and knees (see figure b). Land as lightly and quietly as possible, thus returning to the starting position. Do not allow your back to round out at the bottom of each repetition.

Each time you set up for the next jump, keep your knees in the same line as your toes; your knees should not come toward one another at any time. Jump as high as you can on each repetition.

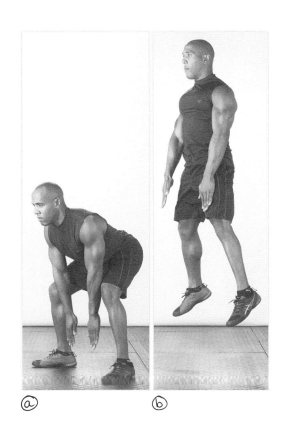

ⓐ ⓑ

Broad Jump

Setup

With your feet roughly shoulder-width apart, hinge at your hips and bend forward toward the floor (see figure a). Keep your back straight and your knees bent at a 15- to 20-degree angle. Reach your arms just behind your hips, keeping your elbows slightly bent.

Action and Coaching Tips

Allow your weight to shift forward. Just before you feel as though you're going to fall, jump forward as far as possible by simultaneously extending your hips and knees and swinging your arms above you (see figure b). Land as lightly as possible. Reset your position to perform the next repetition. If you're working in a small space, turn around after each repetition and jump back to where you were instead of continuing to jump in the same direction.

Each time you drop down to perform the next jump, do not allow your back to round out and keep your knees in the same line as your toes; your knees should not come toward one another at any time.

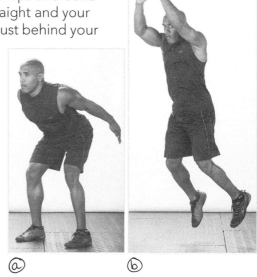

ⓐ ⓑ

Bench Scissor Jump

Setup

Facing a weight bench, stand with your feet hip-width apart and your arms at your sides. Place your right foot on top of the bench, with your rear heel off the ground, thus putting most of your weight on your front leg (see figure a).

Action and Coaching Tips

Lean forward by hinging at your hips and step up onto the bench by explosively extending your right knee (see figure b) and jumping into the air as high as possible while scissoring your legs (see figures c and d) so that you land in the same position but with the opposite leg on top of the bench.

Land as quietly and lightly as possible, using each landing to load the next jump. Each time you land, hinge at your hips and lean forward slightly. Keep your knees in the same line as your toes; your knees should not come toward your body's midline at any time. Jump again, repeating the action. Swing your arms up as you explode to help propel you on each jump.

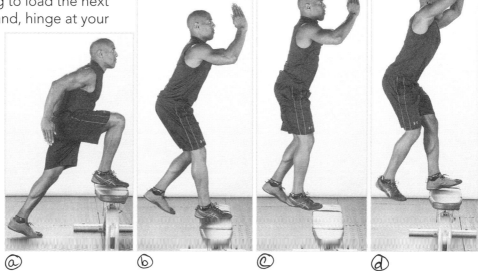

ⓐ ⓑ ⓒ ⓓ

Lateral Bench Scissor Jump

Setup

Stand with a weight bench on your left side, your feet hip-width apart, and your arms at your sides. Place your left foot on top of the bench and place most of your weight on your left leg (see figure a). From the side view, your right foot, that's on the floor, will be behind your left foot, that's on the bench.

Action and Coaching Tips

Step up onto the bench by explosively extending your left knee (see figure b) and jumping into the air as high as possible while you move across the bench

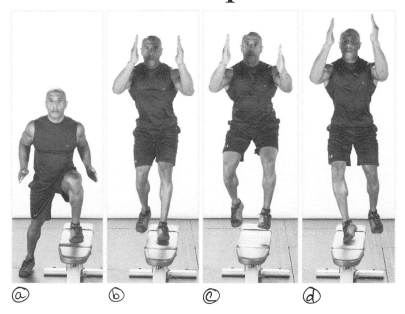

and scissor your legs (see figures c and d) so that you land in the same position on the other side, with the opposite leg on top of the bench.

Land as quietly and lightly as possible, using each landing to load the next jump. Each time you land, hinge at your hips, leaning forward slightly, and keep your knees in the same line as your toes; your knees should not come toward your body's midline at any time. Jump again, repeating the action. Swing your arms up as you explode to help propel you on each jump.

Lateral Bound

Setup

Balance on your right leg. Hold your left leg off the ground by bending your knee and lifting your heel behind you (see figure a). Squat and reach across your body with your left arm.

Action and Coaching Tips

Explode toward your left side, jumping as far you can at a 45-degree angle (see figure b). Land softly on your left leg in a single-leg squat position, reaching across your body with your right arm (see figure c). Each time you land, keep your knees in the same line as your toes; your knees should not come toward your body's midline at any time.

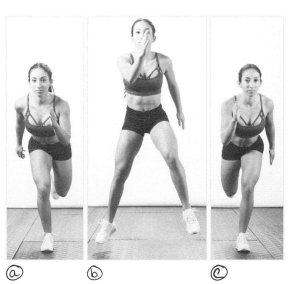

Land with a soft knee into a squat position to ensure maximal force absorption and maximal power production on the next jump. Repeat by jumping back to the right side at a 45-degree angle and make an all-out effort on each repetition.

Trap Bar Squat

Setup

Although some people refer to this exercise as a deadlift rather than a squat, the torso and hip positions in this exercise more closely resembles that of a barbell squat than that of a barbell deadlift.

For this exercise, you need the trap bar. Stand inside the bar, holding on to the handles and with your feet roughly shoulder-width apart (see figure a).

Action and Coaching Tips

Slowly lower yourself down so the weight plates you have loaded on the bar touch the floor. As you lower your body, keep your feet flat and your knees in line with your toes (see figure b). Maintain a strong inward arch in your lower back while lowering into a squatting position. Stand up tall so that your hands end up directly outside of your hips. Slowly lower back into the squat until the weight plates on the bar touch the floor.

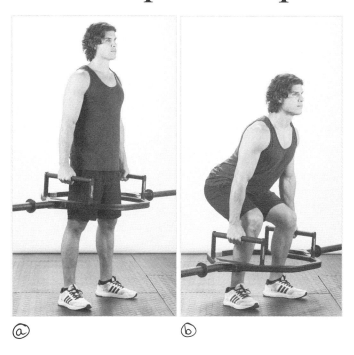

ⓐ   ⓑ

Barbell Romanian Deadlift

Setup

Standing tall with your feet hip-width apart, hold a barbell in front of your thighs with your arms straight; grip the bar just outside your hips (see figure a).

Action and Coaching Tips

Keeping your back straight, hinge at your hips and bend forward toward the floor; keep your knees bent at a 15- to 20-degree angle (see figure b). As you hinge forward, drive your hips backward and do not allow your back to round out. Once your torso is roughly parallel to the floor, drive your hips forward toward the barbell, reversing the motion to stand tall again without overextending at your lower back. Keep the barbell close to you throughout; it should touch your shins at the bottom and track against the fronts of your legs as you perform each repetition.

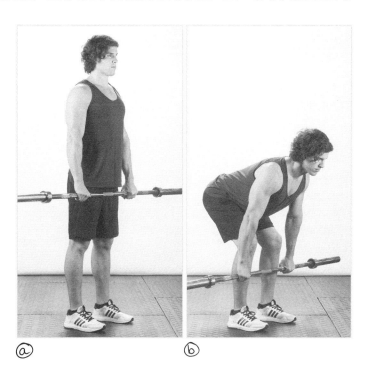

ⓐ   ⓑ

Barbell Rack Pull

Setup

Stand inside a gym rack, with your feet hip-width apart and your knees up against a barbell that's resting at knee height. Keeping your back straight, hinge at your hips and bend forward toward the floor; keep your knees bent at a 15- to 20-degree angle (see figure a). As you hinge forward, drive your hips backward and do not allow your back to round out. Grip the bar just outside your hips.

Action and Coaching Tips

Keeping your back straight, drive your hips toward the barbell as you lift the barbell off the rack (see figure b). Stand tall without overextending your lower back. Reverse the motion; slowly lower the barbell down to the rack. Keep the barbell close to you throughout; it should touch your knees at the bottom and track against the fronts of your legs as you perform each repetition.

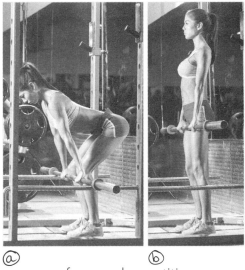

ⓐ ⓑ

One-Leg Angled Barbell Romanian Deadlift

Setup

Place one end of a barbell in a corner or inside a landmine device that's on your right side. Stand parallel to the barbell in a split stance, with your right foot behind your left. Keep your right heel off the ground. Position the middle of your left foot so it's underneath the weighted end of the barbell. Keeping your back straight, hinge at your hips and bend forward toward the floor; keep your knees bent at a 15- to 20-degree angle (see figure a). As you hinge forward, keep most of your weight on your left leg and drive your hips backward. Do not allow your back to round out. Grab the end of the barbell with your right hand and keep your thumbs on the top.

Action and Coaching Tips

Keeping your back straight, drive your hips toward the barbell as you lift the barbell up and stand tall without overextending your lower back (see figure b). As you lift the barbell up by pressing your left foot into the ground, simultaneously press yourself toward the anchor point of the barbell by leaning toward your right side so your body is at a slight angle at the top of each rep. Be sure to drive your hips toward the anchor point of the barbell, and don't just lean with your shoulders (see figure c). Reverse the motion and slowly lower the barbell back down to the starting position. Keep the barbell close to you throughout. Perform all the reps on the same side before switching sides.

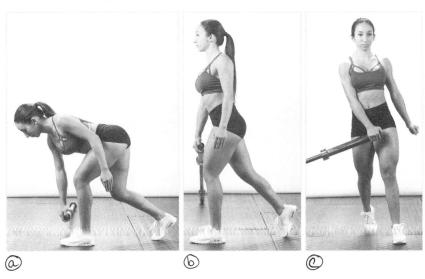

ⓐ ⓑ ⓒ

Dumbbell Goblet Squat

Setup

Stand with your feet just farther than shoulder-width apart and your toes turned out 10 to 15 degrees. Grab one end of a dumbbell with both hands. Place the dumbbell against the top of your chest, with your elbows clamped down on the bottom end of the dumbbell (see figure a).

Action and Coaching Tips

Bend at your knees and hips and lower your body toward the floor as low as you can without losing the arch in your lower back or allowing your heels to lift off the ground (see figure b). Once you've gone as deep as you can control in the squat, reverse the motion by extending your legs and returning to the standing position to complete the rep. Keep your knees tracking in the same direction as your toes; do not allow your knees to drop in toward the midline of your body.

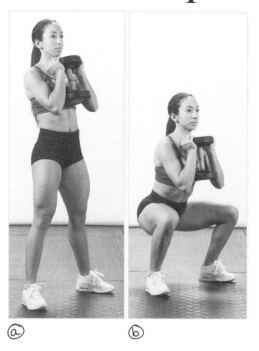

ⓐ   ⓑ

Stability Ball Wall Squat

Setup

Stand with your feet shoulder-width apart and your toes pointed straight as you lean against a 22- to 26-inch (55-65 cm) stability ball that's on the wall at your lower back (see figure a). Your feet should be about 12 to 20 (30-50 cm) inches in front of your hips, and your knees should be slightly bent. Hold a dumbbell in each hand by your hips. You can also do this exercise using only body weight by allowing your hands to hang down at your sides or by interlacing your fingers behind your head.

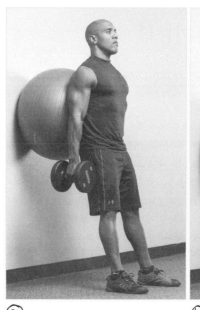 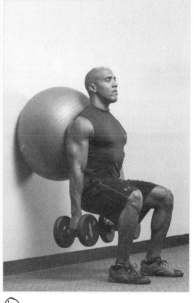

ⓐ   ⓑ

Action and Coaching Tips

Keeping your torso upright, bend at your knees and hips and lower your body toward the floor as much as you can without losing the arch in your lower back (see figure b). Once you've gone as deep as you can control in the squat, reverse the motion by extending your legs and returning to the standing position to complete the rep. Keep your knees tracking in the same direction as your toes; do not allow your knees to drop in toward the midline of your body throughout.

Dumbbell Romanian Deadlift

Setup

Stand tall with your feet hip-width apart (see figure *a*). Hold the dumbbells in front of your thighs.

Action and Coaching Tips

Keeping your back straight, hinge at your hips and bend forward toward the floor, with your knees bent at roughly a 15- to 20-degree angle (see figure *b*). As you hinge forward, drive your hips backward and do not allow your back to round out. Once your torso is roughly parallel to the floor, drive your hips forward toward the dumbbells, reversing the motion to stand tall again without overextending your lower back. Keep the dumbbells close to you throughout; it should touch your shins at the bottom and track against the fronts of your legs as you perform each repetition.

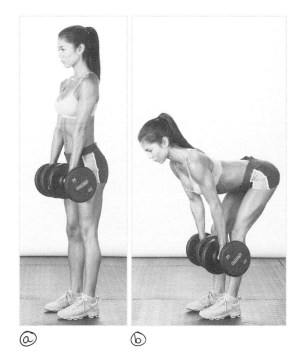

ⓐ   ⓑ

Dumbbell Lateral Romanian Deadlift Lunge

Setup

Stand tall, with your feet hip-width apart (see figure *a*). Hold dumbbells in each hand.

Action and Coaching Tips

Step laterally, with one leg just outside your shoulder width. Keep your front knee bent 15 to 20 degrees and your back knee nearly straight. As your stepping foot hits the ground, shift your weight over your foot and hinge forward at your hips, allowing the dumbbells to track on each side of your leg (see figure *b*). Once your torso becomes parallel to the floor with your back straight, do not allow your back to round out at the bottom of each lunge. Reverse the motion by stepping back to the starting stance and return to an upright position. Then perform the same motion by stepping laterally to the opposite side with the other leg. Use good rhythm and timing; do the step and the hip hinge simultaneously and reverse the motion smoothly and with coordination. Do not let the dumbbells touch the floor at any point during this exercise.

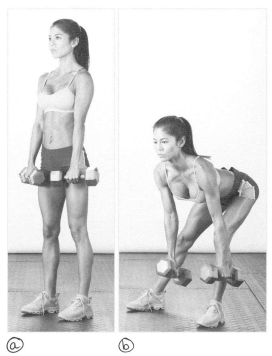

ⓐ   ⓑ

Dumbbell Fighter's Lunge

Setup

This exercise got its name because it resembles the motion of a fighter throwing a knee strike. Stand tall, with your feet hip-width apart (see figure a). Hold a dumbbell in each hand. The dumbbell in your left hand should be outside of your left hip, and the dumbbell in your right hand should be in front of your right thigh.

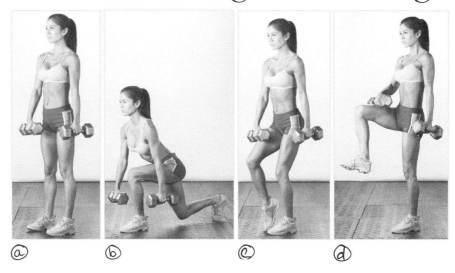

ⓐ ⓑ ⓒ ⓓ

Action and Coaching Tips

Perform a reverse lunge by stepping backward with your right leg, allowing your right knee to gently touch the ground as you lean forward slightly (see figure b). As you return to the standing position, allow your right thigh to meet the center handle of the dumbbell (see figure c). Your thigh should meet the dumbbell gently. Smashing into it makes the exercise uncomfortable to perform.

With the dumbbell against the middle of your right thigh, flex your hip and raise your knee just above a 90-degree angle with the floor. As you flex your hip, lift your knee just above your hip joint (see figure d). Lift the dumbbell with your hip, not your arm. Step backward again with your right leg and repeat. Perform all reps on one side before switching to the other side.

Traveling Dumbbell Lunge

Setup

Stand tall, with your feet hip-width apart (see figure a). Hold a dumbbell in each hand at your sides.

Action and Coaching Tips

Keeping your torso upright, take a large step forward and drop your body so that your back knee lightly touches the floor (see figure b). Stand back up tall while bringing your rear leg forward to meet your front leg and step forward with the opposite leg—the one that was behind you on the last rep. Repeat as you travel down the room.

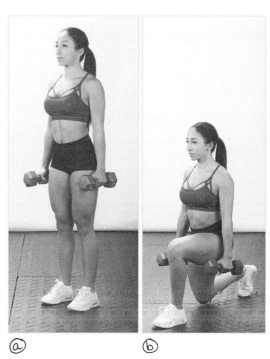

ⓐ ⓑ

Traveling Dumbbell Romanian Deadlift Lunge

Setup

Stand tall, your feet hip-width apart (see figure a).
Hold a dumbbell in each hand at your sides.

Action and Coaching Tips

Step forward with one leg, keeping your front
knee bent 15 to 20 degrees and your back knee
straight or slightly bent. As your front foot hits the
ground, lean forward by hinging at your hips and
allowing your rear heel to come off the ground
(see figure b). Your torso should be no lower than
parallel to the floor and your back should be
straight. Do not allow your back to round out at
the bottom of each lunge. Stand back up tall while
bringing your rear leg forward to meet your front
leg and step forward with the opposite leg—the
one that was behind you on the last rep. Repeat
as you travel down the room.

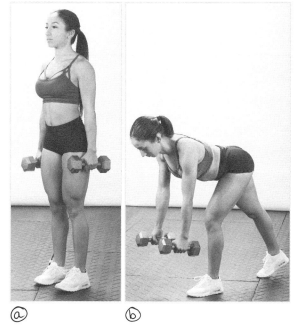

Establish good rhythm and timing by perform-
ing the step and the hip hinge simultaneously and by reversing the motion smoothly. Do not let
the dumbbells touch the floor at any point.

One-Leg One-Arm Dumbbell Romanian Deadlift

Setup

Stand on one leg and hold a dumbbell in
the opposite hand at your hip (see figure
a).

Action and Coaching Tips

Keeping your back and arm straight, hinge
at your hip and bend forward toward the
floor; keep your weight-bearing knee bent
at roughly a 15- to 20-degree angle. As
you hinge, allow your non-weight-bearing leg to elevate so that it remains in a
straight line with your torso and keep your
hips and shoulders flat without allowing
them to rotate (see figure b). Do not allow
your lower back to round out as you hinge
your hips and lower your torso. Once your
torso and non-weight-bearing leg are
roughly parallel to the floor, reverse the

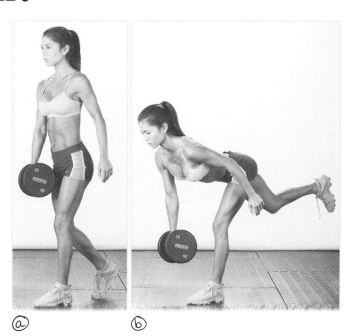

motion by driving your hips forward to stand tall again, thus completing the rep. Perform all repetitions on one side before switching to the other side.

One-Leg Dumbbell Bench Hip Thrust

Setup

Sit on the floor, your shoulders elevated on a weight bench or chair with the shoulders resting on the bench. Position the right arm out to the side across the bench; hold a dumbbell in your left hand in front of your left hip. Position the dumbbell over your hip in a way that feels comfortable to you. Position your legs so that your knees are bent about 90 degrees and your feet are directly below your knees. Keeping your right knee bent 90 degrees, lift your right knee above your hip and lift your hips so that your body makes a straight line from knee to nose (see figure a).

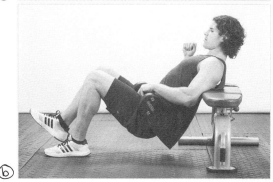

Action and Coaching Tips

Keeping your right leg lifted, lower your hips toward the floor until you either lightly contact the floor or can't go any deeper (see figure b). Drive your hips back up to the top position, making sure to extend from your hips, not your lower back, thus completing the rep. Push through your heel on each repetition; do not lift the heel off the ground at the top. Pause for one or two seconds at the top of each repetition.

One-Leg Bench Hip Thrust

Setup

Sit on the floor with your shoulders elevated on a weight bench or chair and your shoulders resting on the bench. Position your arms out to the sides across the bench. Position your legs so that your knees are bent about 90 degrees and your feet are directly below your knees. Keeping your left knee bent 90 degrees, lift your right knee above your hip and lift your hips so that your body makes a straight line from knee to nose (see figure a).

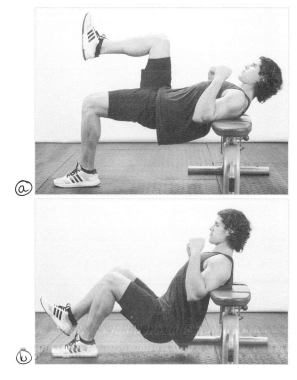

Action and Coaching Tips

Keeping your right leg lifted, lower your hips toward the floor until you either lightly contact the floor or can't go any deeper (see figure b). Drive your hips back up to the top position, making sure to extend from your hips, not your lower back, thus completing the rep. Push through your heel on each repetition; do not lift the heel off of the ground at the top. Pause for one or two seconds at the top of each repetition.

One-Leg Hip Bridge

Setup

Lie on your back (supine) on the floor with your knees bent and heels on the floor. Lift your right knee above your hip so your knee is in front of your rib and chest area (see figure a).

Action and Coaching Tips

Keeping your right leg lifted, drive your hips up as high as you can without overextending your lower back (see figure b). Pause for two or three seconds at the top position before slowly lowering yourself down to the floor. Repeat all the reps on the same side before switching legs.

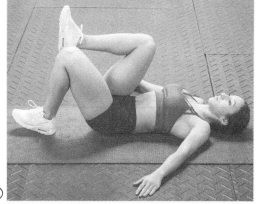

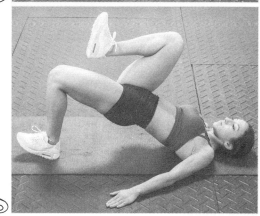

One-Leg Hip Lift with Weight Plate

Setup

Lie on your back with your legs together, your knees bent 15 degrees, and your feet resting on top of a weight bench or chair. Raise one leg off the bench or chair, flexing your hip and knee a little beyond a 90-degree angle (see figure a). Hold a weight plate at your shin of the flexed leg with both hands.

Action and Coaching Tips

With your one leg flexed, raise your hips straight up as high as you can while keeping a slight bend in your knee (see figure b). Do not over-extend your lower back at any time; don't allow your hips to rotate during the exercise. Slowly reverse the motion, allowing your hips to lightly touch the floor. Complete all repetitions on one side before switching to the other leg.

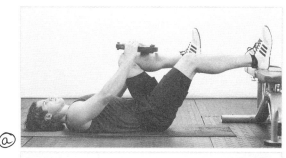

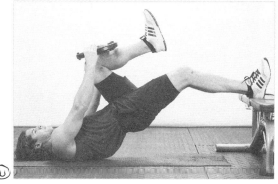

One-Leg Hip Lift

Setup

Lie on your back with your legs together, your knees bent 15 degrees, and your feet resting on top of a weight bench or chair. Raise one leg off the bench or chair, flexing your hip and knee a little beyond a 90-degree angle (see figure *a*). Place your arms on the floor or in a position that is comfortable.

Action and Coaching Tips

With your one leg flexed, raise your hips straight up as high as you can while keeping a slight bend in your knee (see figure *b*). Do not overextend your lower back, and don't allow your hips to rotate during the exercise. Slowly reverse the motion, allowing your hips to lightly touch the floor. Complete all repetitions on one side before switching to the other leg.

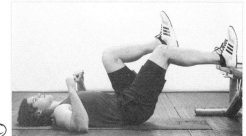

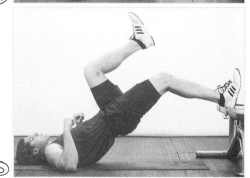

One-Leg 45-Degree Cable Romanian Deadlift

Setup

This exercise is performed exactly like the one-leg one-arm Romanian deadlift with a dumbbell, except that it uses a cable column on the low setting to change the vector of resistance to a 45-degree angle. Stand tall on one leg, holding the cable handle in your opposite hand (see figure *a*). You can also perform this exercise with a resistance band that is anchored low, no higher than your ankle level.

Action and Coaching Tips

Keeping your back and arm straight, hinge at your hip and bend forward toward the floor; keep your weight-bearing knee bent at a 15- to 20-degree angle

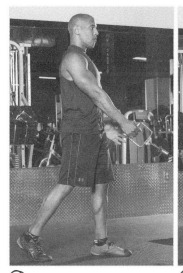
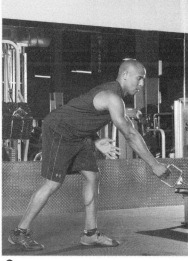

(see figure *b*). Do not allow your lower back to round out as you hinge your hips and lower your torso. As you hinge forward, lift the heel of your non-weight-bearing leg so that it remains in a straight line with your torso. At the bottom position, keep your hips and shoulders flat and do not allow them to rotate; the foot of your non-weight-bearing leg should point at the floor. Once your torso and non-weight-bearing leg are at about a 45-degree angle to the floor, reverse the motion by driving your hips forward toward the cable to stand tall again, thus completing the rep. Perform all repetitions on one side before switching sides.

The range of motion is shorter when using the cable than when using the dumbbell because the force you're working against is at a higher point. The dumbbell pulls you toward the floor; the cable pulls you toward its anchor point at a 45-degree angle.

One-Leg Cable Hip Adduction

Setup

Stand tall, a few feet away from a cable column on the low setting. The column should be at your left side, and the ankle cuff attachment should be around your left ankle (see figure a). Hold on to a dowel rod against the ground or the cable column with your left hand for balance. You can also perform this exercise with a resistance band that is anchored low, no higher than your ankle level.

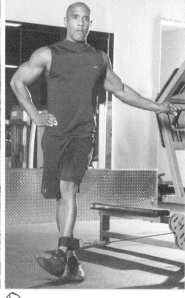

@   b

Action and Coaching Tips

Keeping your knees slightly bent, lift your left foot off the ground and drive your left leg across the front of your body as far as you can without losing your balance or your tall standing position (see figure b). Slowly reverse the motion, allowing your left leg to go as far toward the cable's origin as possible, again keeping your balance and your tall standing position. Perform all reps on one side before switching sides.

Resistance Band Loop Hybrid Deadlift

Setup

First, put your left foot inside one end of the resistance band loop and your right foot on top of the band (see figure a). Stand with your feet just outside of shoulder-width apart and turned out 15 degrees. Grab the end of the band that's on the outside of your right foot, pull it over your right foot, and loop the end around your left foot the way you did in the first step (see figure b). Lower your torso to about a 45-degree angle and grab the middle of the band, keeping your hands roughly shoulder-width apart. Hinge at your hips and bend your knees while keeping your back straight and maintaining an arch in your lower back (see figure c).

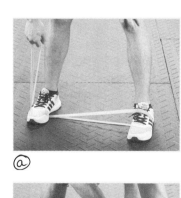

@

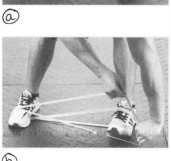

b

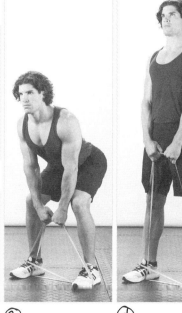

©   d

Action and Coaching Tips

Keeping your back straight, do this exercise fast by driving your hips forward while straightening your legs and standing tall (see figure d). Be sure to extend at your hips, not by overextending your lower back. Reverse the motion and slowly lower yourself back down to the starting position to complete one rep.

Resistance Band Mini Loop Low Lateral Shuffle

Setup

Place a resistance band mini loop around your legs just above your knees. With your hands on your hips and your feet hip-width apart, squat down until your thighs are almost parallel with the floor (see figure a).

Action and Coaching Tips

Take small steps laterally to your left, always maintaining tension on the band (see figure b). Then sidestep back to your right. Do not allow your knees to give into the band and drop toward the midline. Don't allow your torso to wobble from side to side. Keep your knees in line with your feet throughout.

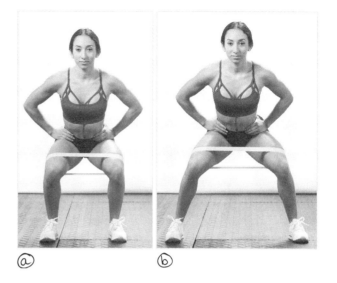

ⓐ　　　　ⓑ

Mid-Platform Machine Leg Press

Setup

For this exercise, you'll need to use the machine that's commonly known as the leg press machine. Sit with a tall torso and place your feet flat roughly shoulder-width apart on the middle of the platform (see figure a).

Action and Coaching Tips

Bend at your knees and hips as far as you can while keeping your feet flat on the platform and maintaining your starting alignment (see figure b). Once you've gone as deep as you can control, reverse the motion by extending your legs and finishing each rep without locking out your knees.

Keep your knees tracking in the same direction as your toes, and do not allow your knees to drop in toward the midline of your body as you perform the action.

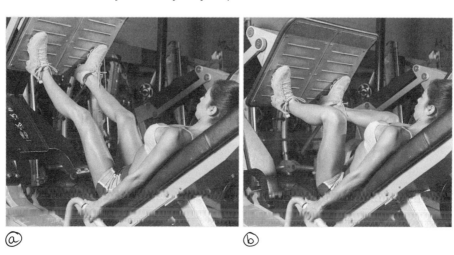

ⓐ　　　　　　　ⓑ

High-Platform Machine Leg Press

Setup

This version of the leg press changes the muscular focus of this exercise by adjusting your foot placement on the platform. A higher foot placement stresses the glutes and hamstrings more, whereas a lower foot placement (as described in the previous version of the leg press) tends to place more stress on the quadriceps.

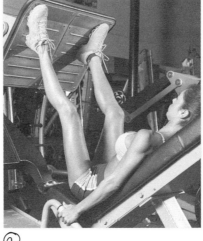 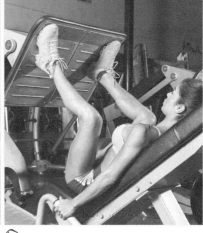

For this exercise, you'll need to use the machine that's commonly known as the leg press machine. Sit with a tall torso and place your feet roughly shoulder-width apart and near the top of the platform (see figure a).

Action and Coaching Tips

Bend at your knees and hips as far as you can while keeping your feet flat on the platform and maintaining your starting alignment (see figure b). Once you've gone as deep as you can control, reverse the motion by extending your legs and finishing each rep without locking your knees.

Keep your knees tracking in the same direction as your toes, and do not allow your knees to drop in toward the midline of your body as you perform the action.

Machine Seated Hamstring Curl

Setup

For this exercise, use a seated hamstring curl (leg curl) machine. Sit tall and position the pad you'll be pushing at the bottom of your calves. Position your legs hip-width apart and straight out, keeping the backs of your knees in contact with the seat pad (see figure a).

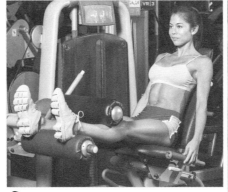 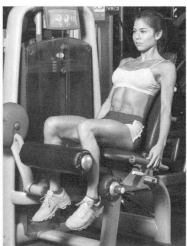

Action and Coaching Tips

Holding on to the handles, pull your calves against the pad by bending your knees to curl your legs underneath you as far as the machine will allow (see figure b). Slowly reverse the motion under control to complete the rep. Do not allow the portion of the weight stack that you're moving to rest on the other portion of the stack; rather, allow it to just gently touch the rest of the stack at the end of each rep.

Machine Lying Hamstring Curl

Setup

For this exercise, you'll need to use the machine that's commonly known as the lying hamstring curl or lying leg curl machine. Lie face down with your legs straight and your hip joint on top of the apex of the pads (see figure a). Adjust the pad you'll be pushing against so it's at the bottom of your calves.

Action and Coaching Tips

Hold on to the handles, and with your legs hip-width apart, pull your heels toward your glutes as far as possible (see figure b). Slowly reverse the motion, under control. Do not allow the portion of the weight stack that you're moving to rest on the other portion of the stack; rather, allow it to just gently touch the rest of the stack at the end of each rep.

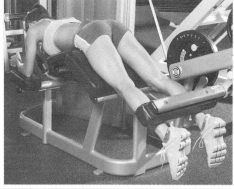

(a)

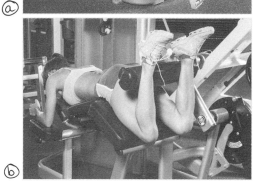

(b)

Machine Leg Extension

Setup

For this exercise, you'll need to use the machine that's commonly known as the leg extension machine. Sit tall, with the pad you'll use to extend your legs roughly low-shin level, your legs hip-width apart, and the backs of your knees in contact with the seat pad (see figure a).

Action and Coaching Tips

Holding on to the handles, push your shins into the pad and extend your legs, keeping your ankles dorsiflexed until just before your knees are fully straight (see figure b). Slowly reverse the motion to complete one rep. Do not allow the weight stack to rest back on the stack. Just allow it to gently touch at the end of each rep.

It's important to note that the machine leg extension exercise often gets bad rap, as many trainers and coaches believe it to be "nonfunctional" (i.e., not beneficial) and even universally dangerous. However, when looked at more scientifically and skeptically, these beliefs are based more on conjecture (10).

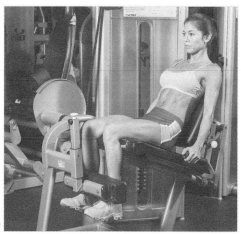

(a)

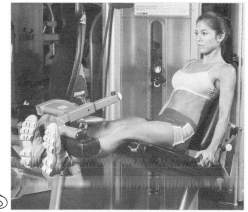

(b)

Machine Hip Adduction

Setup

For this exercise, you'll need to use the machine that's commonly known as the (seated) hip adduction machine. Sit tall, with the pad you'll be pressing the insides of your legs against set as wide as you're able to manage without discomfort (see figure a).

Action and Coaching Tips

Holding on to the handles, push the insides of your thighs into the pads and drive your legs together until the outsides of the pads touch or until your thighs are roughly parallel with each other (see figure b). Slowly reverse the motion to complete one rep. Do not allow the weight stack

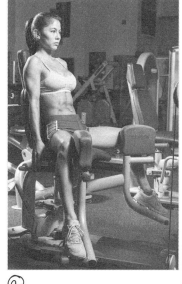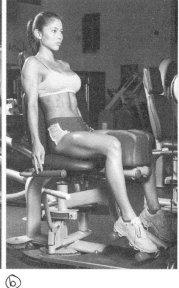

you're moving to rest back on the stack. Just allow it to gently touch at the end of each rep.

This exercise, like the machine leg extension, often gets an unjustified bad rap. The misconceptions about using exercises like the machine hip adduction were addressed in chapter 2, Function and Performance.

Zombie Squat

Setup

Stand tall, with your feet shoulder-width apart and your toes turned out about 10 degrees (see figure a). Extend your arms in front of you at shoulder height. Keeping your arms extended in front of you at shoulder height serves as a counterbalance to help keep your torso upright as you lower yourself down on each rep.

Action and Coaching Tips

Squat by bending your knees and sitting back at your hips. Go down so your thighs are almost parallel to the floor without allowing your lower back to round out (see figure b). As you squat, do not allow your heels to come off the ground or your knees to come together toward the midline of your body. Your knees should track in the same direction as your toes. Reverse and stand back up to complete one rep.

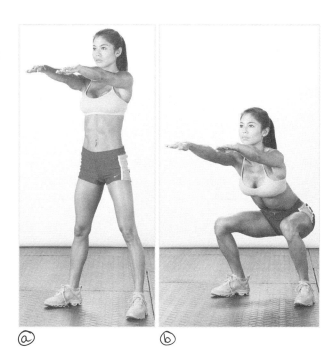

Side-Lying Hip Adduction

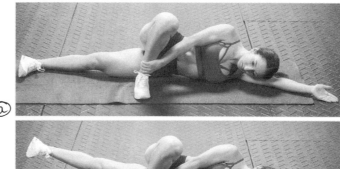

Setup

Lie on your left side, with your head resting on your left arm (your bottom arm), which is extended across the floor at roughly a 45-degree angle above you. Keep your left leg (your bottom leg) straight and in line with your torso. Bend your right leg (your top leg) and bring it up until your foot is flat on the floor in front of your bottom knee (see figure a). Grab your right ankle with your right (top) hand.

Action and Coaching Tips

Keeping your knee straight and your ankle flexed, lift your left leg off the ground as a high as you can without allowing your hip to flex (see figure b). Your bottom leg should stay in line with your torso, and do not allow your torso to roll at any point; keep your shoulders and hips perpendicular to the floor. Pause for two to three seconds at the top. Slowly reverse the motion, allowing your leg to return to the floor. Perform all reps on one side before switching sides.

Nordic Hamstring Curl

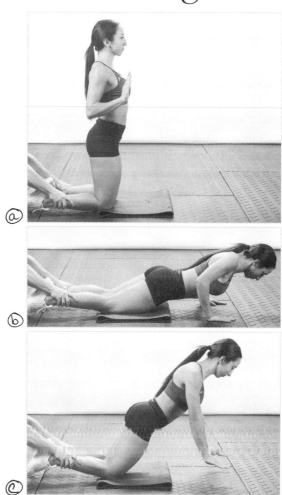

Setup

This exercise requires either a partner or suitable gym equipment to securely lock your lower legs in place. Kneel tall, with your legs hip-width apart and your calves anchored (see figure a).

Action and Coaching Tips

Keeping your hips and back straight, slowly lower yourself toward the floor by extending at your knees. At the point where you can no longer lower yourself with control, allow your body to fall to the floor, using your hands to control your descent and landing in a position that resembles a kneeling push-up (see figure b). Use your hands to push back off the floor (see figure c) and help you reverse the motion so that you return to the tall kneeling position, thus completing the rep.

Do not allow your hips to drift more than a few degrees behind you. Maintain a nearly straight line from your knees to your shoulders throughout.

Stability Ball Leg Curl

Setup

Lie on your back on the floor, with your legs hip-width apart, your heels resting on top of a 22- to 26-inch (55-65 cm) stability ball, and your arms out to the sides for balance. Raise your hips off the floor until your body forms a straight line (see figure a).

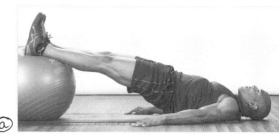

Action and Coaching Tips

Pull your heels toward your body while raising your hips toward the sky until your feet are underneath you (see figure b). Your body should form a straight line from your shoulders to your knees at the top of each rep. Slowly reverse the motion and repeat without allowing your hips to rest on the floor.

Do not overextend your lower back at any time. If your feet drift lower on the ball while performing a set, adjust the foot position as needed.

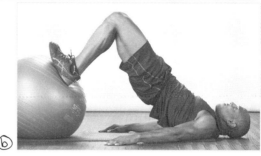

One-Leg Stability Ball Leg Curl

Setup

Lie on your back on the floor, with your legs hip-width apart, your heels resting on top of 18- to 22-inch (45-55 cm) stability ball, and your arms out to the sides for balance. Raise your hips off the floor until your body forms a straight line, then raise one leg off the ball, flexing your hip and knee slightly above a 90-degree angle (see figure a).

Action and Coaching Tips

With your one leg flexed, pull the ball toward your body with the heel that's on the ball while raising your hips toward the sky until your foot is underneath you (see figure b). Your body should form a straight line from your shoulders to your knee at the top of each rep. Slowly reverse the motion and repeat without allowing your hips to rest on the floor. Complete all repetitions on one side before switching to the other leg. Do not overextend your lower back at any time. If your feet drift lower on the ball while performing a set, adjust foot position as needed.

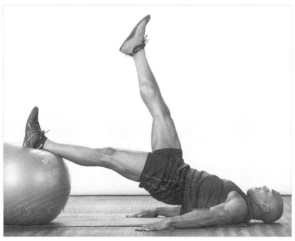

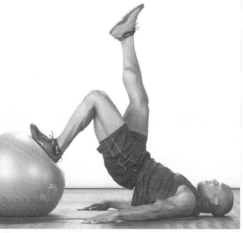

{ Core Exercises

8

Core training is always a hot topic. There are hundreds of different exercises to choose from, and it can be difficult to know which ones give you the best value. In this chapter, we'll clarify the confusion by showing you a variety of scientifically supported exercises that help you maximize your training time.

Let's kick things off in the next two sections by first covering some of the popular beliefs about core training that even advanced trainers and coaches think are true. From there, we'll finish this chapter by showing how to perform a variety exercises for the core.

Core Confusion: The Truth About Squats and Deadlifts

A few studies have taken the position that multijoint, free-weight exercises such as barbell squats and deadlifts activate core muscles better than more targeted core exercises like the ones later in this chapter, including stability ball crunches, dumbbell plank rows, etc. These studies have led many trainers, coaches, athletes, and exercise enthusiasts to mistakenly think that you don't need to do exercises that focus on strengthening your abs and obliques, because squats and deadlifts do the job more effectively. The truth is, when you look at the scientific evidence, the claim that (heavy) barbell squats and deadlifts are all you need to strengthen your abs and obliques doesn't make sense. Let's review the science so you can see for yourself.

One of the two studies most commonly quoted as scientific "evidence" that squats and deadlifts work better for strengthening your abs and obliques is entitled "Systematic Review of Core Muscle Activity During Physical Fitness Exercises." The purpose of this article was to "systematically review the literature on the electromyographic (EMG) activity of three core muscles (lumbar multifidus, transverse abdominis, and quadratus lumborum) during physical fitness exercises in healthy adults." (1) (You scientific detective types will notice that when the authors say "core muscles," they're not referring to the rectus abdominis and the obliques.)

The major findings of this research review were as follows:

- No studies were uncovered for quadratus lumborum EMG activity during physical fitness exercises.
- Moderate levels of evidence indicate that lumbar multifidus EMG activity is greater during free-weight exercises compared with stability ball/device exercises and is similar during core stability and stability ball/device exercises.
- Transverse abdominis EMG activity is similar during core stability and stability ball/device exercises.

It's clear that the results of this research review certainly don't demonstrate that squats and deadlifts create more activation of the rectus abdominis and oblique musculature than exercises that focus on those core muscles. However, these findings do tell us that if you're doing exercises like squats and deadlifts, you're not neglecting the deep (local) core stabilizing muscles like the transverse abdominis and the lumbar multifidus.

The researchers concluded that, "the available evidence suggests that strength and conditioning specialists should focus on implementing multijoint free-weight exercises, rather than core-specific exercises, to adequately train the core muscles in their athletes and clients" (1). Now, if you only read that conclusion and failed to ask which core muscles the researchers of this study looked at, you can clearly see how the study was misrepresented as demonstrating that squats and deadlifts create more abdominal activation than core-focused exercises directed at those specific muscles.

Core Strength Training Is Overrated for Athletic Performance

Core training has reached almost mythic status, and many people would be gravely concerned if a potential function and performance training program didn't emphasize it.

A 2015 systematic review and meta-analysis (i.e., a study or studies) concluded that trunk muscle strength plays only a minor role for physical fitness and athletic performance in trained individuals. The authors of the paper stated that "core muscle strength was associated with only limited gains in physical fitness and athletic performance measures when compared with no or only regular training." (2)

Now, this certainly doesn't mean that the trunk (i.e., core) musculature is not an important area to train. If it wasn't, it would not be included in the list of exercises in this chapter. It simply means the benefit that trunk muscle strengthening has on performance is often misunderstood and is overstated by many trainers and coaches. So although core training exercises should still be included as a component of your training, there is no need to view the core as exclusive to function and performance training or treat core exercises as something that requires special emphasis over strengthening the upper and lower body.

Another study often misrepresented is entitled "Trunk Muscle Activity During Stability Ball and Free-Weight Exercises." In it, barbell squats and deadlifts were done with loads of approximately 50, 70, 90, and 100 percent of the subject's 1RM (i.e., one repetition max). Subjects also completed three stability ball exercises: birddog (lying prone over the stability ball while extending one arm and the opposite leg), hip bridge (lying supine with your heels on the stability ball and raising your hips off the ground), and ball back extension (lying prone over the stability ball while extending your torso toward the sky) (3).

The major findings of this study were as follows:

- No significant differences were observed in the rectus abdominis and external oblique muscles during any of the exercises.
- Activity of the trunk muscles during squats and deadlifts is greater or equal to that which is produced during the stability ball exercises.
- Squats and deadlifts are recommended for increasing strength and hypertrophy of the back extensors.

Once again, if you stopped reading at the second bullet point, you'd mistakenly think that this study demonstrates that you don't need to do targeted abdominal exercises if you're dong squats and deadlifts. However, this study showed that squats and deadlifts elicit high levels of activation in the posterior core muscles (i.e., the back extensors, as highlighted in the third bullet point) when compared to other exercises that target the posterior core muscles. But they didn't compare squats and deadlifts to exercises like those featured in this chapter that activate the anterior core (abdominals and obliques) musculature.

In summary, the research to date demonstrates that exercises like barbell squats and deadlifts effectively activate the posterior core muscles (i.e., back extensors, lumbar stabilizers). However, it does not show that they activate the anterior core muscles (i.e., abdominals, obliques) better than exercises focused on the anterior aspect of the core. Indeed, this reality should be obvious because squats and deadlifts try to drive the torso forward into flexion, which makes the back extensors work constantly to resist that force and maintain spinal alignment.

So, squats and deadlifts likely *don't* provide sufficient stimulus to train the anterior core aspects. The question is, What move or moves offer the most benefit for working these anterior core muscles (i.e., abdominals, obliques)? The answer is, the exercises highlighted in this chapter! And the next few paragraphs tell you why.

With all the available abdominal exercise variations out there, along with all the varying opinions and conflicting information, it can be confusing for even the most experienced exerciser or fitness professional to decide which abs moves may offer the most benefit. Research can help us see through the confusion and find which abdominal exercise options are the most effective in activating muscles.

A study that looked at the muscle activity of a variety of traditional and nontraditional abdominal exercises found that the stability ball rollout and stability ball pike were the most effective exercises in activating the abdominal muscles (rectus abdominis and internal and external obliques) while also creating the lowest EMG activity in the lower back and hip flexors muscles (4).

It's important to note that both the stability ball rollout and stability ball pike exercises involve the shoulders and hips because another study found that the

How Useful Are Abdominal Elbow Planks?

The abdominal elbow plank is a static hold, where you hover over the floor on your forearms. The abdominal elbow plank makes sense in the early stages injury rehabilitation and when trainers use it to help entry-level clients build awareness of optimal body alignment in a static position. However, the problem is when the abdominal elbow plank is always used without moving past it to more dynamic and challenging exercises.

If you can do a basic abdominal plank for around 30 seconds, it's time to stop boring yourself with them and move on to using more interesting plank versions and challenging abdominal exercises (that also involve the shoulders or hips to a greater degree), like the ones featured in this chapter.

greatest activation of abdominal muscles is during abdominal exercises that also require recruitment of shoulder or hip musculature (5). This provides a guiding principle in judging the potential effectiveness for any abdominal-focused exercise. As you'll see, all the exercises highlighted in the chapter involve the shoulders or hips.

Basic Core Exercises: PERFECTED

The following section provides basic core exercises that create or resist torso bending and twisting while also showing you how to do them better than the way they are commonly performed. This will help you train smarter, more safely, and efficiently. All it takes is a couple of small tweaks.

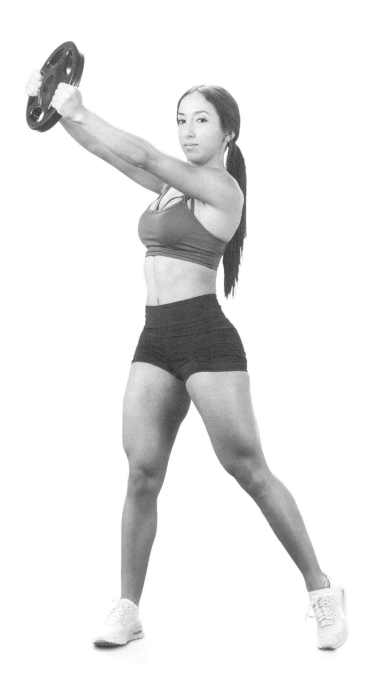

Reverse Crunch

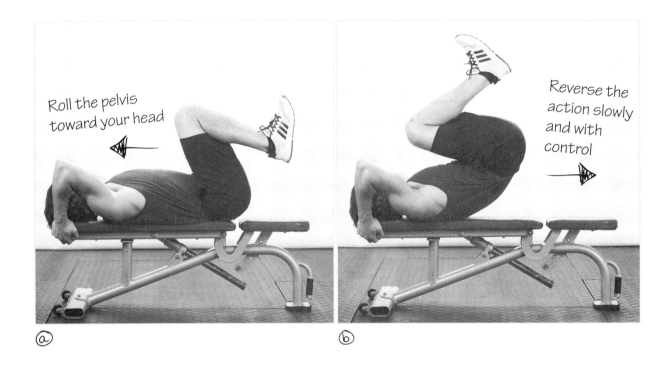

Roll the pelvis toward your head

Reverse the action slowly and with control

ⓐ ⓑ

Setup

Lie on your back on a weight bench, with your knees bent and your hips flexed into your belly (see figure a). With your elbows bent, hold on to the bench just behind and above your head. This exercise can be made more difficult if you lie on an incline bench with your head higher than your legs.

Action and Coaching Tips

Smoothly and with control, do a reverse crunch by rolling your lower back up off the bench and bringing your knees toward your chin (see figure b). Do not use momentum or jerk your body. Slowly reverse this motion, lowering your spine back down toward the bench, one vertebra at a time. Do not allow your legs to extend or your head to lift off the ground at any point.

WHY IT'S BETTER

You eliminate using momentum and avoid jerking your body up. This is done by rolling the pelvis toward your head and reversing the action slowly and with control. When performing this exercise, most people use momentum and jerk their bodies up and down by kicking their legs to create the movement. Eliminating that momentum forces the abdominal musculature to perform the action, which is the main purpose of this exercise.

Benefits

- Reduces cheating
- More focused on using abdominal muscles to perform the action

Hanging Leg Raise

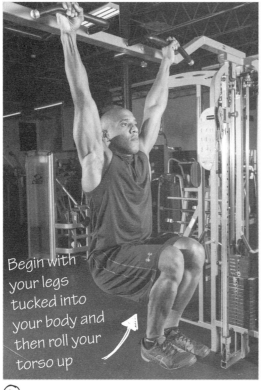

Begin with your legs tucked into your body and then roll your torso up

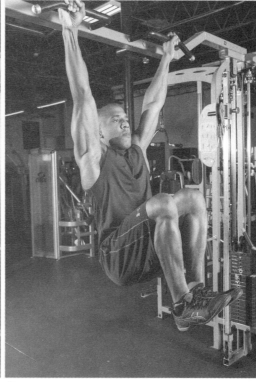

Setup

This is essentially a more advanced version of the reverse crunch. If you're unable to perform reverse crunches as described previously on a bench, it's unlikely you'll possess the strength to perform hanging leg raises in the manner described here.

Hang from a pull-up bar, using an overhand grip and with your hands roughly shoulder-width apart. Flex your hips and bend your knees, holding them above your hips in and in front of your torso (see figure a).

Action and Coaching Tips

Smoothly and with control, roll your torso upward, bringing your knees toward your chin (see figure b). Slowly reverse this motion without allowing your knees to become untucked from your body. Do not use momentum or jerk your body at any point during this exercise.

WHY IT'S BETTER

You begin with your legs tucked into your body and then roll your torso up. The way this exercise is usually performed, with your legs hanging down and by flexing at your hips, is primarily a hip flexion exercises. Although this certainly involves the abdominals, it's to a much less degree than when doing this version. This is because tucking the pelvis better targets the abdominal musculature.

Benefits

- Less cheating by eliminating the use of momentum
- Increases the challenge on the abdominal muscles

Cable Side Bend

Setup

Grab the handle of a cable (or resistance band) that's attached at roughly ankle level with your left hand. Stand tall, with your feet roughly shoulder-width apart and the cable at your left side (see figure a). Stand far enough away from the cable or band so that it's at roughly a 45-degree angle to the floor.

Action and Coaching Tips

Without rotating your body, bend your torso sideways to the left until you feel a mild stretch in the right side of your torso (see figure b). Reverse the action and finish the rep by slightly flexing your torso to the right against the resistance. Perform all reps on the same side before switching sides.

WHY IT'S BETTER

You use a single cable that's at roughly a 45-dgree angle to your body instead of holding two dumbbells. When performing this exercise, most people hold a dumbbell on each side of the body. A great example of a commonly done exercise that doesn't make biomechanical sense is doing side bends while holding a dumbbell on each side. Of course, the weight of the dumbbell offsets the weight on the other side, making this exercise ineffective at loading the lateral flexors of the torso sufficiently compared to performing this exercise while holding a single dumbbell on one side. Even performing side bends while holding a single dumbbell on one side of the body isn't as effective at targeting the lateral core muscles that resist and create lateral trunk flexion as this version because of the angle of force involved. There's not much resistance when using a dumbbell, unlike when using a cable. The dumbbell is very close to your body, giving you a mechanical advantage over the weight. You'd have to hold a very heavy weight, which may exceed your grip strength, to create the same training effect the cable provides with much lower loads.

Benefits

- More consistent resistance through the range of motion
- More effective at targeting the lateral core muscles

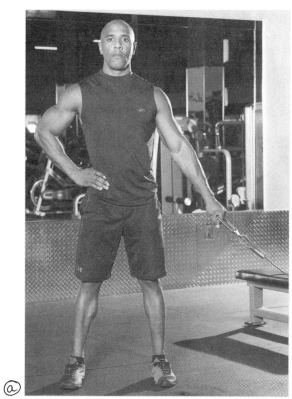

 Use a single cable that's at roughly a 45-dgree angle to your body

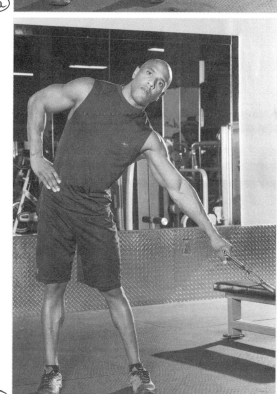

Side Elbow Plank with External Shoulder Rotation

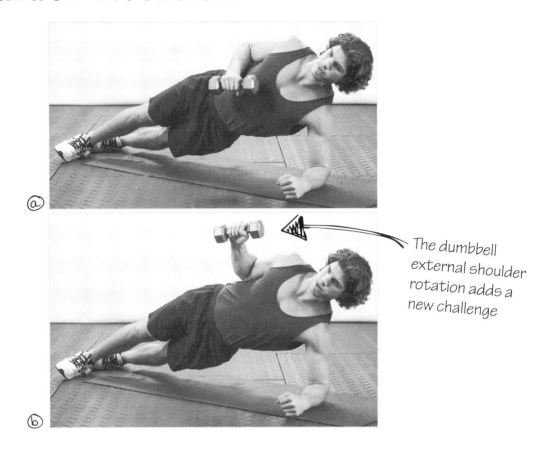

The dumbbell external shoulder rotation adds a new challenge

Setup

Place your left forearm on the floor with your elbow directly underneath your shoulder. Place your right foot in front of your left foot, keeping your hips and knees off the ground and your body in a straight line. Use a pad or a rolled towel underneath your elbow for comfort if necessary. Hold a dumbbell with your top hand, keeping your elbow at your side bent at 90-degrees so the dumbbell is in front of your belly (see figure a).

Action and Coaching Tips

While maintaining the side plank position and keeping your elbow bent at 90 degrees, activate the external shoulder rotators by elevating the dumbbell toward the ceiling as far as possible without raising your elbow off your side (see figure b). Slowly reverse the motion to complete one rep.

WHY IT'S BETTER

Front and side planks are boring exercises to perform. Adding the dumbbell external shoulder rotation adds a new challenge for maintaining the plank position while you move the dumbbell and makes this exercise more interesting to perform. Plus, a lot of what you do in the gym involves using the internal shoulder rotators. Nearly all pushing exercises, as well as a surprising number of pulls, put you in an internally rotated position. However, most programs don't target the external shoulder rotators to balance it out.

Benefits

- Adds a new challenge to the side plank exercise
- Get two things done at once by training the often-neglected shoulder external rotators along with the lateral core muscles

164

Low-to-High Cable Chop

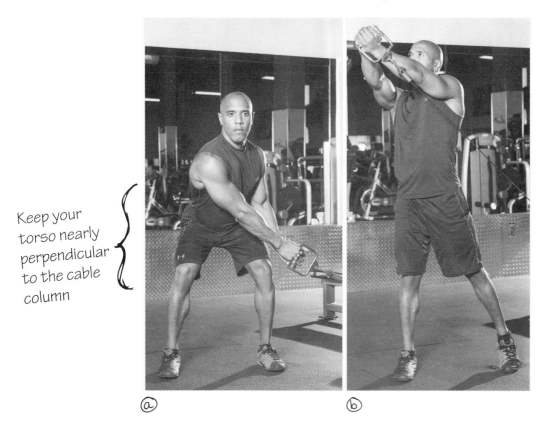

Keep your torso nearly perpendicular to the cable column

ⓐ　　ⓑ

Setup

Stand perpendicular to a cable column (or resistance band) on your left side. With both hands on the handle, which is attached to the lowest position, extend your arms toward the cable's origin. Position your feet slightly farther than shoulder-width apart. Squat and shift most of your weight to your left leg while your arms reach at a downward angle toward the origin of the cable (see figure a).

Action and Coaching Tips

Stand up while shifting your weight toward your right leg and driving the cable diagonally, upward across your body. Finish at the top, with your arms above your head on your right side when the rope gently touches your forearm (see figure b). Reverse the motion to return to the starting position, then repeat. Perform all reps on the same side before switching sides.

WHY IT'S BETTER

You keep your torso nearly perpendicular to the cable column; you do not rotate your torso away from the cable column more than a few degrees as you reach the top of the range of motion. Fully rotating your torso in each direction, as is commonly done when performing this exercise, greatly reduces the rotational tension on your torso muscles. In other words, this modification keeps more constant tension on the torso muscles to create and resist rotation, helping you make the best use of your training time.

Benefits

- More consistent tension of the torso muscles
- Improves the ability of the torso muscles to control rotation while you create rotation from your hips

Cable Tight Torso Rotation with Hip Shift

Setup

Attach the cable to the highest position and stand perpendicular to a cable column on your left side. Hold the handle with both hands and extend your arms toward the cable's origin. Position your feet slightly farther than shoulder-width apart and shift your weight toward your left leg, with your shoulders directly over your hips (see figure a).

Action and Coaching Tips

Keeping your hips moving with your shoulders, shift your weight to your right leg as you move your arms horizontally, pulling the handle across your body to the right until both arms are just outside your right shoulder (see figure b). Stop rotating your hips and shoulders when the cable or band gently touches your forearm. Slowly reverse the motion to return to the starting position and complete one rep. Perform all reps on one side before switching to the other side.

WHY IT'S BETTER

This variation has four adjustments: a wider stance, a weight shift as you rotate, reduced rotational range of motion, and the rotation involves both the hip and shoulders instead of just the shoulders. The wider stance gives you a larger base of support, which allows you to move heavier loads and provide a greater strength challenge to your torso muscles to perform the exercise. Keeping your torso nearly perpendicular to the cable maintains high levels of rotational tension on your torso muscles, helping you make better use of your time. And moving the hips in the same direction and at the same speed as your shoulders is similar to how we produce high levels of power and strength in athletics.

Benefits

- Increased involvement of your core muscles
- Better positioning to perform the movement with more strength

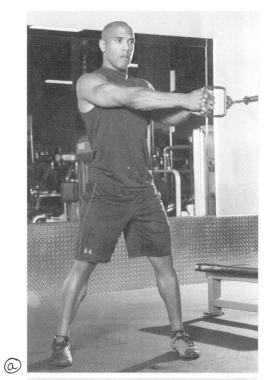

Wider stance gives you a larger base of support

Move the hips in the same direction and at the same speed as your shoulders

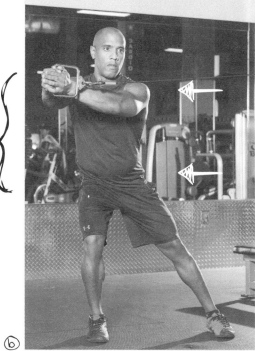

High-to-Low Cable Chop

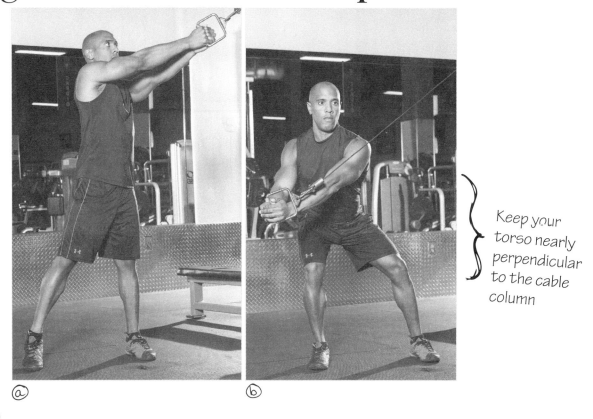

(a)   (b)

Keep your torso nearly perpendicular to the cable column

Setup

Stand perpendicular to a cable column on your left side with the cable attached in the highest position. Hold the handle with both hands and extend your arms toward the cable's origin (see figure a). Position your feet slightly farther than shoulder-width apart.

Action and Coaching Tips

With your arms above your head on your left side and most of your weight shifted onto your left leg, drive the cable diagonally downward across your body as you set your hips back slightly and shift your weight to your right leg (see figure b). Once the cable touches your arm, slowly reverse the motion to complete the rep. Perform all reps on the same side before switching sides. Throughout this exercise, keep your spine in a neutral position and keep your torso nearly perpendicular to the cable column; do not rotate your torso away from the cable column more than a few degrees as you reach the bottom of the range of motion (doing so greatly reduces the rotational tension on your torso muscles).

WHY IT'S BETTER

As with an earlier exercise, the low-to-high cable chop, this exercise also involves keeping your torso nearly perpendicular to the cable column; you do not rotate your torso away from the cable column more than a few degrees as you reach the top of the range of motion. Fully rotating your torso in each direction, as is commonly done when performing this exercise, greatly reduces the rotational tension on your torso muscles. In other words, this modification keeps more constant tension on the torso muscles to create and resist rotation, helping you make the best use of your training time.

Benefits

- More consistent tension of the torso muscles
- Improves the ability of the torso muscles to control rotation while you create rotation from your hips

Ab Wheel Rollout
with Resistance Band

Move through a smaller range of motion instead of extending your arms overhead

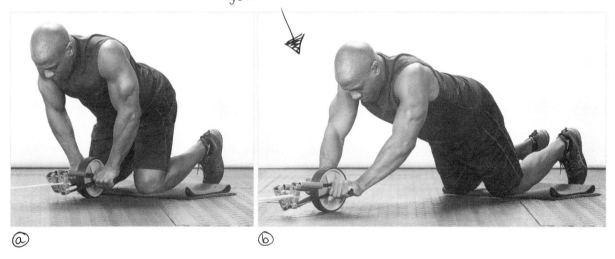

ⓐ   ⓑ

Setup

Anchor a resistance band around something stable (like a weight bench) near the floor. Hook each end of the band around the handles of the ab wheel. Kneel with your hands on the handles of the ab wheel, your wrists just underneath your shoulders, and your arms straight (see figure a). You may also need to place a pad, pillow, or folded towel under your knees for comfort.

Action and Coaching Tips

Drive the ab wheel away from you by extending your hips and arms overhead as if diving into a pool (see figure b). Push the wheel just above your head without allowing your lower back to sag toward the floor and without feeling any pressure in your lower back. Once you've gone as far as you can with control, reverse the motion and pull the wheel back to the starting position, finishing with the wheel under the middle of your torso.

WHY IT'S BETTER

You attach a resistance band to the ab wheel and move through a smaller range of motion instead of extending your arms completely up overhead in a straight line with your torso while rolling the ab wheel away from you. Many people have had difficulty using the ab wheel, or even hurt their backs doing it, simply because they went out too far beyond what they could control. Using a band with the ab wheel makes your abs work harder from the start, so you don't need to go out nearly as far to get the same or more of an effective resistance challenge on your abdominals.

Benefits

- Creates more tension on the abdominals
- Less risk of straining your back due to the reduced range of motion

Stability Ball Plate Crunch

Setup

Lie face up with a 22- to 26-inch (55-65 cm) stability ball in the arch of your lower back and hold a weight plate directly above your chest, your arms outstretched (see figure a).

Action and Coaching Tips

Perform a crunch, keeping the weight plate toward the sky (see figure b). Pause for one or two seconds at the top of each rep, and do not sit all the way up (with your torso perpendicular to the floor); doing so removes the tension from the abs. Slowly reverse the motion, allowing your abdominal muscles to stretch over the ball. Do not allow your neck to hyperextend in the bottom position; keep your neck in a neutral position throughout.

WHY IT'S BETTER

To focus on your abs when doing ball crunches (i.e., to do them properly), the ball doesn't move under you at all. Instead, keep your knees bent at roughly a 90-degree angle throughout, and flex and extend your spine with control over the ball. Be sure to hold the weight plate straight above your shoulders and reach your arm straight up toward the sky as you perform each crunch rep. It's common for the ball to roll back and forth as you perform the crunches. It's primarily your knees (bending and extending) driving the motion, not your abs.

It's important to note that, although some trainers and coaches claim that spinal flexion exercises, like stability ball crunches, are inherently dangerous or less effective than isometric abdominal exercises, research has shown that spinal flexion exercises can not only help promote nutrient delivery to the intervertebral discs but also may provide superior muscle and performance gains versus isomeric abdominal exercises (6).

That said, as with any other type of exercise, some exercises, like stability ball crunches, may be contraindicated for some people who have pain when performing it and for those with existing spinal conditions, such as disc prolapse or herniation (6). However, for those with otherwise healthy spines, the winning combination is to use both isometric and dynamic abdominal exercises because each offers a unique benefit the other may miss. In other words, spinal flexion exercises are no different than any other resistance training exercise. All exercises can induce stress, which causes tissue adaptation. For your back, loading enhances tissue resiliency in general, but there's a tipping point where you exceed your capacity. That's the individual nature of training, and exactly what's meant by training smart!

Benefits

- Allows for greater abdominal muscle stretch than floor crunches
- Not allowing the ball to shift as you crunch keeps consistent tension on the abdominals

Keep your knees bent at roughly a 90-degree angle, not allowing the ball to move

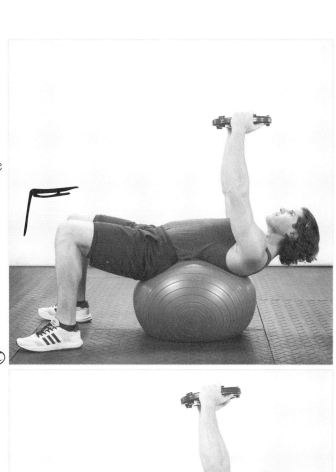

(a)

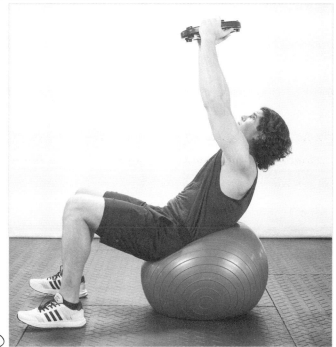

(b)

Stability Ball Arc

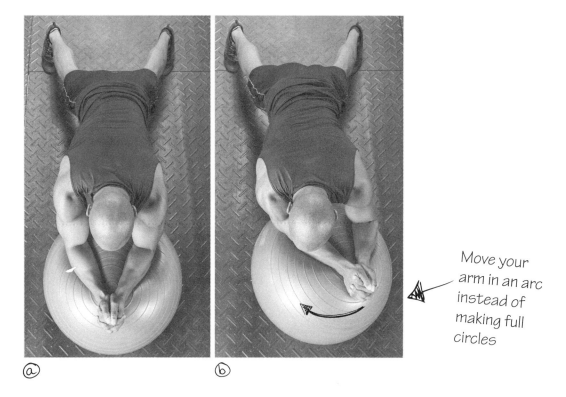

Move your arm in an arc instead of making full circles

(a)   (b)

Setup

Place both forearms on top of a 22- to 26-inch (55-65 cm) stability ball and get into a plank position, with your body in a straight line and your feet just farther than shoulder-width apart (see figure *a*). Contract your glutes and posteriorly rotate your pelvis by bringing your front hip bones toward your head and your tailbone toward your feet. In other words, if you imagine your pelvis as a bucket of water, the posterior pelvic tilt would tip the bucket so that water would spill out of your back, whereas an anterior pelvic tilt would make water spill out from the front.

Action and Coaching Tips

Move your arms in small arcs, from where your elbows are underneath the left side of your torso, to straightening your arms as you reach out above your head, to bringing your arms back underneath the right side of your torso (see figure *b*). Alternate between left-to-right arcs and right-to-left arcs without allowing your head or hips to sag toward the floor. On each arc, squeeze your glutes tightly each time that you reach your arms out. Reach your arms as far as you can without feeling discomfort in your lower back.

WHY IT'S BETTER

You move your arm in an arc instead of making full circles, as if you're stirring a big pot. Making full circles is unnecessary and awkward when your arms are close. Eliminating the bottom end of the circle takes away the part of the exercise when your arms are fully underneath you, which is easiest on your abs but hardest on your shoulders.

Benefits

- More constant tension on the abdominals
- Less awkward to perform

Leg Lowering with Resistance Band

Bend your knees instead of keeping them straight

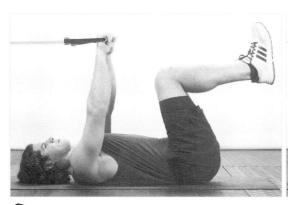
ⓐ

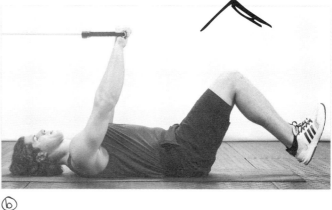
ⓑ

Setup

Lie on your back on the floor, with your knees bent, your hips flexed more than 90 degrees, and your arms outstretched above your torso just below shoulder level (see figure *a*). In each hand, hold the handle of a resistance band that's attached about 12 inches (about 30 cm) off the floor to a stable structure or inside a doorjamb behind you.

Action and Coaching Tips

Maintaining tension against the band with your arms, slowly lower your legs toward the floor (see figure *b*). Keep your knees bent and do not allow your lower back to come off the floor. Once your heels lightly touch the floor, reverse the motion and bring your knees back above your hips.

To make this exercise more challenging, simply extend your legs farther as you lower them toward the floor—the farther you straighten your legs, the harder the exercise; the closer your heels are to your hips, the easier the exercise.

WHY IT'S BETTER

Instead of keeping your legs almost straight and arbitrarily lowering them to or just above the floor while allowing your lower back to arch off the floor, this version forces you to better use your abdominal muscles to resist the weight of your legs pulling your spine into extension (arching your lower back off the floor). Plus, this version is more individualized to your strength level by allowing you to manipulate how much you extend your legs and how much you lower them without allowing your lower back to arch. The addition of the band further enhances abdominal muscle activation.

Allowing your lower back to arch off the floor reduces the involvement of your abdominal musculature to resist spinal extension and places more stress on the lower back, which may end up extending to the point of discomfort and increase the risk of injury.

Benefits

- Potentially safer on the lower back
- More constant tension on the abs

Angled Barbell Rainbow

Face the barbell's anchor point as your arms move

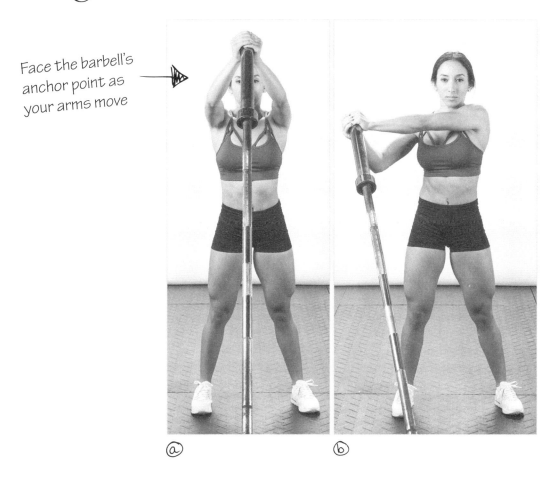

ⓐ ⓑ

Setup

Place one end of a barbell in a corner or into a landmine device. Hold the other end with both hands while standing tall, your feet roughly shoulder-width apart (see figure a).

Action and Coaching Tips

Move the barbell from side to side in a rainbow-like arc from one shoulder to the other while maintaining a straight spine and keeping a slight bend in your elbows throughout (see figure b). The movement of the barbell should come from your shoulders, not your elbows. Avoid any rotation at your torso; as you move the barbell from side to side, your torso should face the barbell's anchored end.

WHY IT'S BETTER

Instead of rotating your hips and shoulders, which is perfectly fine to do as a different exercise, this involves avoiding any torso movement by working to remain facing the barbell's anchor point as your arms move. Maintaining a stiff and stable torso position forces your torso musculature to resist the lateral side-bending forces that are being placed on them as your move the barbell out to the side of your body.

Benefits

- Increased focus on resisting the lateral movement of your torso to maintain your posture and position
- Easily modifiable by reducing the range of motion to best fit your ability

Weight Plate Speed Chop

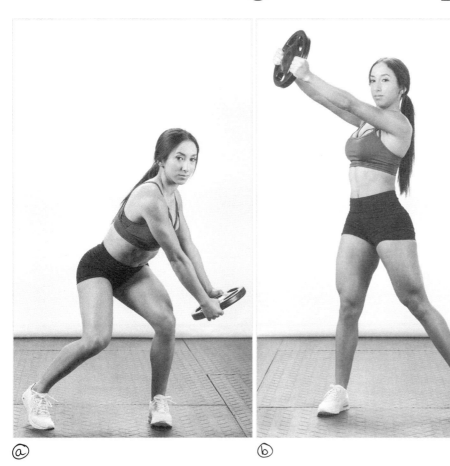

Perform a shorter range of motion at a faster speed

(a)   (b)

Setup
Squat and rotate your hips and torso while holding a weight plate weighing 10 to 45 pounds (4.5-20 kg) outside your left knee (see figure a).

Action and Coaching Tips
Stand up as you quickly rotate to your right side and drive the plate across your body in a diagonal pattern, finishing with it just above your head (see figure b). Without pausing, quickly reverse the motion by driving the plate back down across your body on the same diagonal path you used to lift it. Perform all reps to one side, then repeat the exercise to the other side.

Do this exercise fast, but smoothly and with a consistent rhythm, coordinating your upper body and lower body during both the lifting and the lowering phase of each repetition.

WHY IT'S BETTER

A shorter range of motion is performed at a faster speed. Increasing the speed of the action doesn't just require you to lift the weight up with more intensity but also forces you to decelerate the weight plate and pull the weight back down, increasing the demand on your muscles.

Benefits
- More athletic
- Increased muscular activation

Stability Ball Rollout

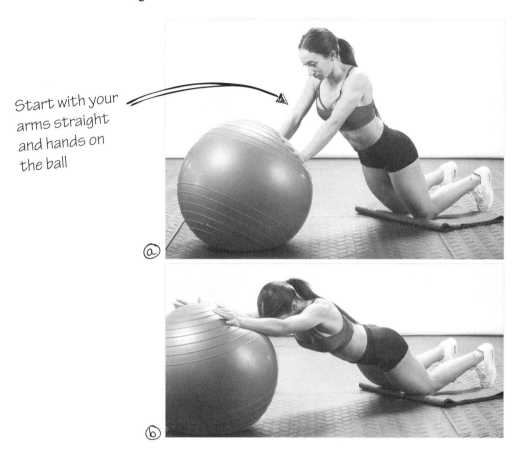

Start with your arms straight and hands on the ball

ⓐ

ⓑ

Setup
Kneel on the floor on a 22- to 26-inch (55-65 cm) stability ball, with your knees hip-width apart, your arms straight, and your palms shoulder-width apart (see figure a).

Action and Coaching Tips
Drive the ball away from you by reaching your arms overhead as if diving into a pool (see figure b). Roll the ball out as far as you can without allowing your head or lower back to sag toward the floor. Once you've gone as far as you can, or your arms are completely overhead in a straight line with your torso, reverse the motion by driving your arms downward into the ball and pull it back to the starting position without allowing your hips to flex.

To make this exercise more difficult, use a smaller ball. Use a larger ball to make this exercise easier.

WHY IT'S BETTER
You perform this exercise with your arms straight and hands starting on the ball instead of with your elbows bent and forearms starting on the ball. Keeping the arms straight allows you to better incorporate the shoulders by driving into the ball as you pull it back toward you, which increases both the shoulder and abdominal muscle involvement.

Benefits
- Better incorporates the shoulders
- Increased abdominal muscle involvement

Stability Ball Pike

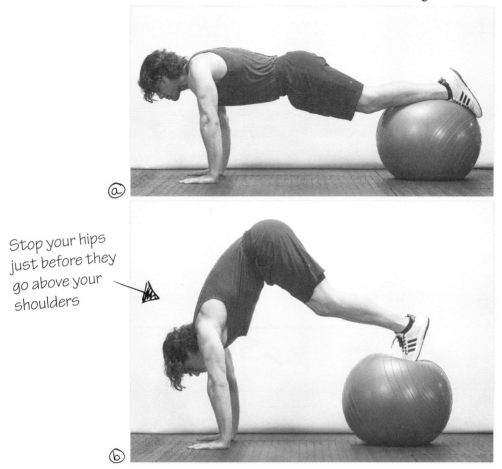

Stop your hips just before they go above your shoulders

Setup

Begin in a push-up position, with your hands directly underneath your shoulders and your feet and shins hip-width apart on top of a 22- to 26-inch (55-65 cm) stability ball (see figure *a*).

Action and Coaching Tips

Use your abs to raise your hips toward the sky while keeping your legs almost straight. Raise your hips until just before they reach above your shoulders (see figure *b*). Slowly lower to the starting position with your body straight. Do not allow your hips or head to sag toward the floor as you extend your hips back into the starting position.

To make the exercise easier, start with the ball closer to your belly button.

WHY IT'S BETTER

In this exercise, you stop your hips until just before they reach above your shoulders, instead of stacking your hips directly above your shoulders at the top of the pike motion. Stopping your hips until just before they reach above your shoulders keeps more constant tension on your abdominal musculature than if you stack your hips directly over your shoulders. Once your hips are directly above your shoulders, the tension gets placed mostly on your shoulders, instead of your abs, to maintain the position.

Benefits

- Constant tension on the abdominal muscles
- More concentrated on the abs

Stability Ball Pike Rollout

Setup

This exercise combines the ball pike and the ball rollout into one abdominal exercise. Hold yourself in a push-up position, with your hands directly underneath your shoulders and your feet hip-width apart on top of a 22- to 26-inch (55-65 cm) ball (see figure *a*).

Action and Coaching Tips

Keep your legs straight and perform the pike portion by pushing your hips toward the ceiling while keeping your back nearly flat (see figure *b*). During the pike portion of the exercise, raise your hips until just before they reach above your shoulders.

After straightening your hips and coming back to the starting position, perform the rollback portion by pushing your body backward on the ball until your arms are fully extended in front of you and your legs are fully extended behind you (see figure *c*). Do not allow your hips or head to sag toward the floor as you extend your arms into the rollback portion of the exercise. Reverse the motion, then repeat.

To make the exercise easier, start with the ball closer to your belly button.

WHY IT'S BETTER

You add a rollback to the end of the movement by pushing your body backward on the ball until your arms are fully extended in front of you. The rollback portion of the exercise adds another dynamic to the movement by increasing the range of motion, which then increases the challenge on the abdominals and shoulders.

Benefits

- Incorporates effective abdominal exercises into one comprehensive exercise
- Increases demand on the abdominal muscles

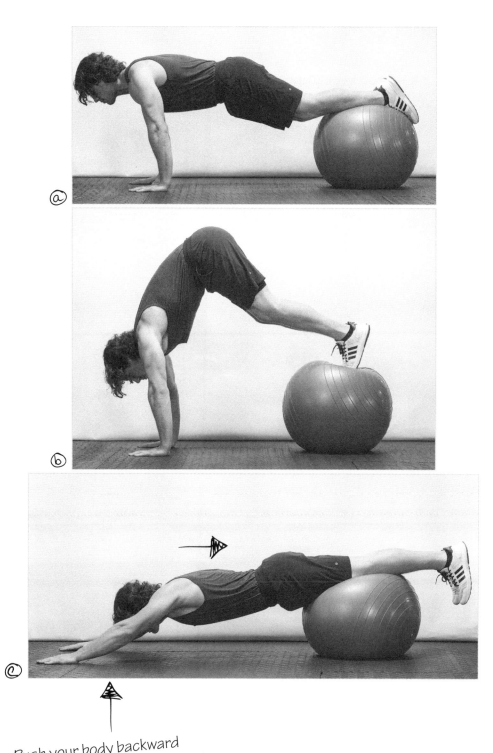

Push your body backward
until your arms are extended

Additional Core Exercises

The exercises in this section also focus on helping you maximize the strength and development of your abdominal muscles, but there aren't unique adjustments for doing them, so they don't warrant the same level of description as the exercises in the previous section. You also may find some not-so-common core exercises here to help you incorporate some variety into your workouts.

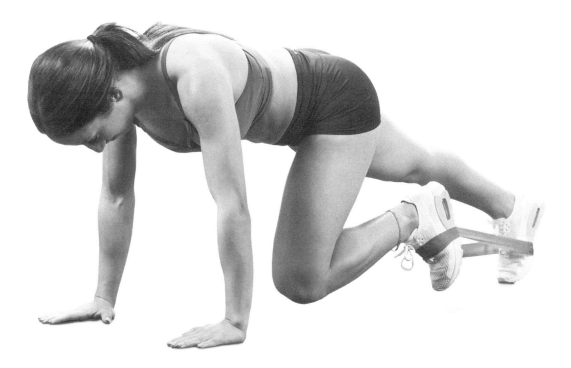

Stability Ball Knee Tuck

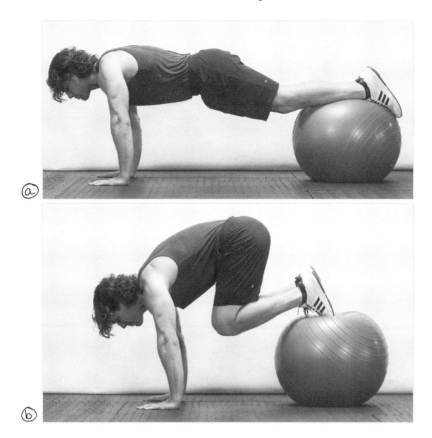

Setup

Hold yourself in a push-up position with your hands directly underneath your shoulders and your feet and shins resting on top of a 22- to 26-inch (55-65 cm) stability ball (see figure a). Keep your legs hip-width apart.

Action and Coaching Tips

Pull your knees in to your chest (see figure b). Reverse the motion and repeat, performing the exercise smoothly with deliberate control. Do not allow your head or lower back to sag toward the floor.

Weight Plate Around the World

Setup

Stand tall, with your feet about six-inches more than shoulder-width. Hold a weight plate weighing 2.5 to 25 pounds (1-12 kg) in both hands above your head (see figure a). Extend your arms and bend your elbows a little.

Action and Coaching Tips

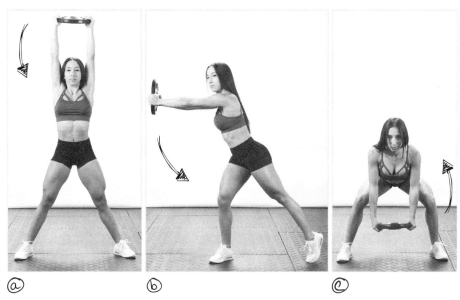

While keeping your arms extended and elbows slightly bent, use your entire body to make the biggest circles (more like horizontal ovals) that you can make around your body (see figures b and c). Move from the outside of your body, to just above the floor, to outside your body, to above your head to complete one rep. As you make circles, bend your knees and hips at the bottom aspects of the movement and shift your weight to the same side the plate is on while you reach your arms out and way from you as far as possible while maintaining a neutral spine. Also, reach high to the sky at the top aspects of this exercise. Perform all reps in the same direction before reversing the circular motion and repeating the exercise in the opposite direction.

Do this exercise fast, but smoothly and with a consistent rhythm, coordinating your upper body and lower body during both the lifting and the lowering phase of each repetition.

Dumbbell Plank Row

Setup

Begin in a push-up position with each of your hands gripping a dumbbell placed on the floor (see figure a). Your feet are shoulder-width apart and your wrists directly below your shoulders. To ensure that the dumbbells do not roll, place your hands directly underneath your shoulders.

Action and Coaching Tips

From the push-up position, pick up the dumbbell in your left hand and row it into your body (see figure b). Slowly lower it to the floor and repeat the action with your right hand. Continue to alternate hands.

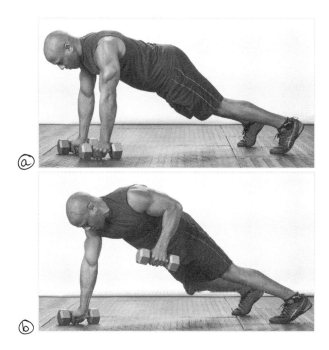

One-Arm Plank

Setup

Begin in a push-up position, with your hands shoulder-width apart and your feet a few inches farther than shoulder-width apart (see figure a).

Action and Coaching Tips

Lift one arm off the ground without allowing your shoulders or hips to rotate or your head or belly to sag toward the floor (see figure b). Pause for several seconds before switching hands. To make this exercise more difficult, you can perform it from your elbows; if you do so, place a pad, pillow, or folded towel under your elbow for protection. You can also increase the challenge of both the straight-arm and elbow-supported version of this exercise by extending your free arm out to your side so your arm is parallel with the floor.

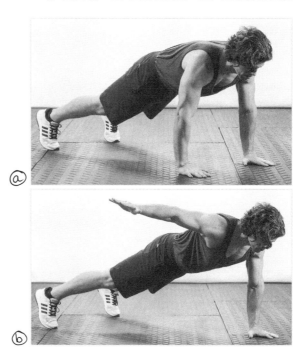

Arm Walkout

Setup

Kneel, keeping your hands flat on the floor just above your shoulders and your arms straight under your shoulders (see figure a). Your torso should form a nearly straight line from your head to your knees. You may also need to place a pad, pillow, or folded towel under your knees for comfort.

Action and Coaching Tips

Walk your arms out in front of you as far as possible without feeling discomfort in your lower back and while keeping your body in a straight line (see figure b); do not allow your hips or head to sag toward the floor. Squeeze your glutes tightly each time that you walk your hands out to the long position. Reverse the motion, walking your hands back so that they end up just in front of your shoulders.

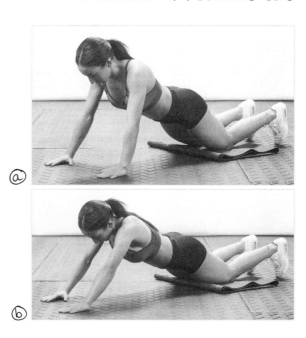

Medicine Ball Arm Walkout

Setup

Kneel, putting your hands on the top of a rubber or sand-filled 2 kg or 4.4 lb medicine ball that is on the ground just above your shoulders, and keep your arms straight (see figure a). Your torso should form a nearly straight line from your head to your knees. You may also need to place a pad, pillow, or folded towel under your knees for comfort.

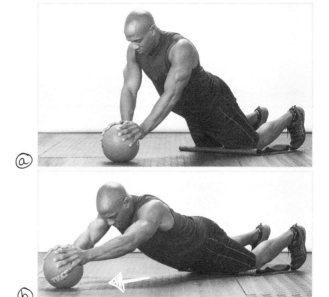

Action and Coaching Tips

Roll the ball out in front of you by walking with your arms, hand-over-hand, as far as you can without feeling discomfort in your lower back and while keeping your body in a straight line (see figure b); do not allow your hips or head to sag toward the floor. Squeeze your glutes tightly each time that you walk your hands out to the long position. Reverse the motion, rolling the ball back toward you by walking your hands back so that they end up just in front of your shoulders.

If using a rubber medicine ball (the kind found at most gyms), choose one that is fully inflated and large enough—at least 8 pounds (3.5 kg)—to accommodate both of your hands. If using a sand-filled ball, you can make the exercise harder by using a heavier ball.

Off-Bench Side Lean Hold

Setup

Sit in the center of a weight bench with one leg on each side. Turn your body to the right so your torso is now in-line with the bench. With your knee bent to roughly 90-degrees, lean slightly over to your right side while hooking your right heel and left toes underneath the padded part the bench (see figure a). Your left leg will be your top leg.

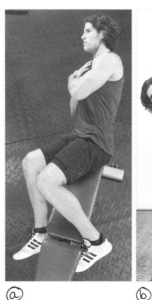
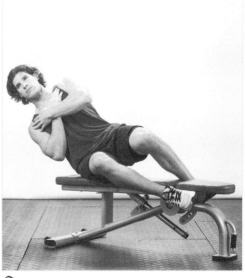

Action and Coaching Tips

Once both your feet are securely and comfortably hooked underneath the padded platform of the bench, lower your torso as far as you can without resting the weight of your torso on the bench. Once you've gone as low as you're able to go while keeping your spine straight, hold this position (see figure b). Then perform the same action on the other side by turning your torso to the left—your right leg will be your top leg—while hooking your right toes and left heel underneath the padded platform of the bench.

Plank March with Resistance Band Mini Loop

Setup

Begin in a push-up position, with a mini band around your feet, your legs hip-width apart, and your wrists directly underneath your shoulders (see figure a).

Action and Coaching Tips

Keeping your body in a nearly straight line and your ankles flexed by pulling your toes toward your nose, flex one hip and bring your knee toward your head until your hip is bent a little more than 90 degrees without allowing your toes to touch the floor (see figure b). Reverse the motion by a placing your foot back to the start position, then repeat the same motion on the other leg.

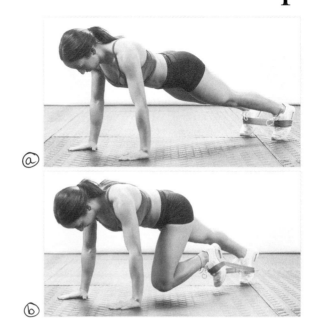

Cross-Body Plank

Setup

Begin in a push-up position, your wrists underneath your shoulders and your feet shoulder-width apart (see figure a).

Action and Coaching Tips

Without allowing your head or hips to sag, simultaneously raise your right foot and left hand off the ground. Bring your right knee to your left elbow while keeping your left hand in contact with your chin (see figure b). Pause for two or three seconds, then reverse this motion on the opposite side, touching your left knee to your right elbow. Do not allow your hips or shoulders to rotate at any time.

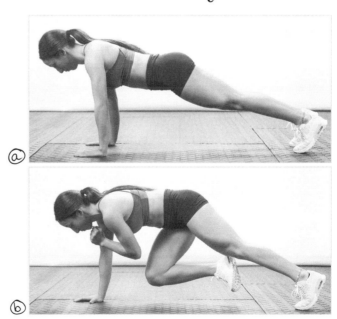

Shoulder Tap Plank

Setup

Begin in a push-up position. Keep your wrists underneath your shoulders and your feet shoulder-width apart (see figure a).

Action and Coaching Tips

Without allowing your head or hips to sag, raise your left hand off the ground and touch your right shoulder. Pause for one or two seconds, then reverse this motion on the opposite side, touching your right hand to your left shoulder. Do not allow your hips or shoulders to rotate.

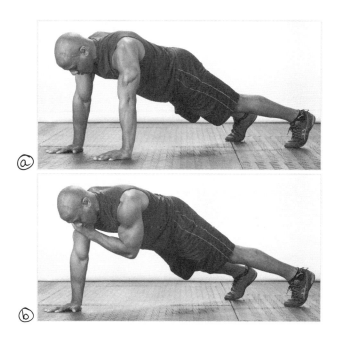

Fast-Hands Plank

Setup

Begin in a push-up position, with your hands a few inches outside shoulder-width apart and your feet a few inches farther than shoulder-width apart (see figure a).

Action and Coaching Tips

Without allowing your shoulders or hips to rotate or your head or belly to sag toward the floor, as fast as you can, lift one hand off the ground and tap the top of your opposite hand (see figure b). Then, place that hand back on the ground and repeat the action with the other hand. Perform each rep as fast as possible but with control.

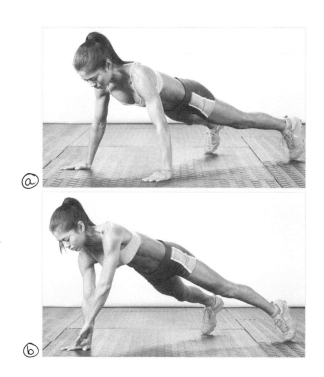

9 Conditioning Exercises

The conditioning exercises featured in this chapter increase your endurance and help you get into great shape. They complement your strength training and are utilized in the workout programming chapters later in this book to finish the resistance training portion of the workouts. These conditioning exercises and complexes provide a metabolically demanding challenge to your workouts that'll have your heart pounding and muscles burning.

Basic Conditioning Exercises: PERFECTED

The following basic conditioning exercises have been revised so you can do them better than the way they are commonly performed. This will help you train smarter, more safely, and efficiently. All it takes is a couple of small tweaks.

25-Yard Dash

Setup
Place two cones roughly 25 yards (23 m) apart.

Action and Coaching Tips
Jog up to the first cone, then sprint as fast as you can to the other cone. Do not take short, choppy steps; take powerful strides. While sprinting, keep your elbows bent at roughly a 90-degree angle and drive with your arms. Once you pass the second cone, jog several steps before you stop. Walk back to the start cone and repeat.

WHY IT'S BETTER

Instead of going from a still position and exploding off the line into a sprint, you jog to the line and begin sprinting once the starting line is reached. Many strength and conditioning professionals and sports therapists have found that it's quite common for athletes to injure their hamstrings while doing a "quick start" when beginning to sprint. With this in mind, a jog up to the starting point is a precautionary measure that reduces the potential risk of injury from quick starts.

It's important to note that if an athlete training for a specific (combine type) event that demands beginning a sprint from the still position, the athlete would certainly need to train for that event by using quick starts. In cases like this, there's no reason you can't also integrate some jogging starts to work on sprinting speed while making efforts to minimize any potential injury that quick starts may present.

Benefits
- Potentially safer
- More applicable to a wider population

300-Yard Shuttle Run

Setup
Place two cones 25 yards (23 m) apart.

Action and Coaching Tips
Jog up to the start cone, then sprint as fast as you can back and forth between the cones for six round trips, which equals a total of 300 yards (274 m). On each reversal of direction, stay upright as you turn around (with control) and run back toward the other cone.

WHY IT'S BETTER

In addition to jogging up to the starting point to reduce the risk of injury that was discussed in the previous exercise, staying upright as you turn around on each reversal of direction, instead of reaching down to touch the cone, can also help reduce the chance of an injury when changing direction.

As with the 25-yard dash, if one is training for a specific (combine type) event, where one has to touch each cone in transition, the athlete would certainly need to train for that.

Benefits
- Potentially safer
- More applicable to a wider population

Gorilla Burpee

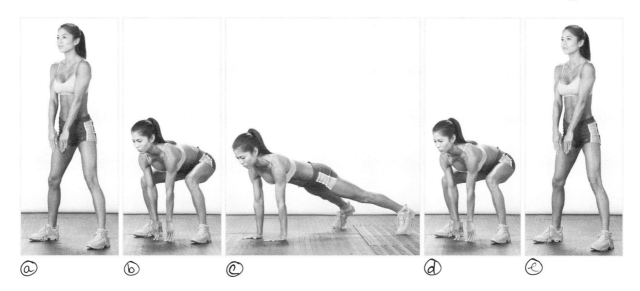

ⓐ   ⓑ   ⓒ   ⓓ   ⓔ

Setup

With your feet slightly farther than shoulder-width apart, hold your arms straight in front of your body (see figure a).

Action and Coaching Tips

Bend your knees and hinge forward at your hips so that your torso leans forward. Place your hands on the ground, with your wrists directly below your shoulders (see figure b), and jump backward to move into a push-up position (see figure c). Make sure that your body forms a straight line and that you do not allow your hips to sag toward the floor in the push-up position. Jump back up so your feet are outside your hands (see figure d), then return to a tall standing position to complete the rep (see figure e).

WHY IT'S BETTER

You start with your feet slightly farther than shoulder-width apart, instead of the way the burpee is commonly done, which has them closer together. Then, in this version, you're lowering and raising your torso by mainly bending and extending from your knees and your hips, which places more emphasis on the lower body. Burpees are commonly performed by bending over mostly from your lower back and placing your hands on the floor in front of your feet, involving less contribution from the lower body and placing more stress on the lower back.

Benefits
- More involvement from the lower body
- Less unwanted stress on the lower body

Additional Conditioning Exercises

The exercises in this section also focus on helping you maximize your conditioning levels, but there aren't unique adjustments for doing them, so they don't warrant the same level of description as the exercises in the previous section. You also may find some not-so-common conditioning exercises and sequences here to help you incorporate some variety into your workouts.

One-Mile Run for Time

Setup

You can perform this either outside or on a treadmill. If running outside, you want to begin running on flat terrain such on a street or track with minimal to no hills. If using a treadmill, there shouldn't be any incline.

Action and Coaching Tips

This is not "jog" a mile. *Run* a mile in as little time as possible—just like back in your school days. This drill can be called "the one-mile race" instead of the "mile run" because it helps people better understand that it's about how fast you finish, not just finishing by putting yourself on cruise-control the whole time. As you run, drive your legs and arms to run as fast as you can to complete the mile distance. Do not take short, choppy steps; take a full stride on each step.

High-Resistance Upright Bike Sprints

Setup

The upright or Airdyne bike provides a fantastic option for interval training because it creates a low-impact but very challenging conditioning workout. Adjust the seat so that when you stand next to it, it aligns with your hip joint. On a scale of one to ten, with ten being the heaviest resistance you can manage, set the bike's resistance at a level that puts you around a six or seven.

Action and Coaching Tips

Pedal as hard and as fast and as you can for the time indicated in the workout programs in this book. Rest fully between intervals by not pedaling the bike or getting off the bike completely.

Weight Plate Push

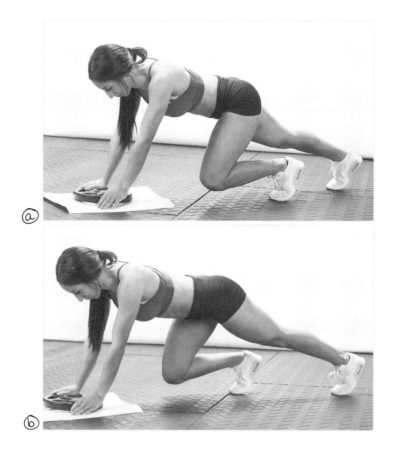

Setup

Place a heavy weight plate—try 35 to 45 pounds (about 15-20 kg)—on top of a towel so that it glides or on a turf surface. For an additional challenge, you can also place a set of dumbbells (25-35 pounds or 11-15 kg) inside the weight plate. Get into push-up position, with your hands on top of the weight plate.

Action and Coaching Tips

Drive with your legs by bringing your knees up toward your chest, first one knee (see figure a) and then the other (see figure b). Push the plate quickly across the floor for 20 to 25 yards (18-23 m) up and back, for a total of 40 to 50 yards (37-46 m). Be sure to take long strides and keep your hips no higher than your shoulders throughout.

Dumbbell Farmer's Walk Complex

A farmer's walk complex consists of a series of dumbbell exercises interspersed with several sets of dumbbell (farmer's) carries. The exercises in this complex are performed back-to-back (circuit style) without rest until all exercises in each complex have been completed.

To begin, use a heavier set of dumbbells for the farmer's portions and a lighter set for the other exercises. The lighter set of dumbbells should be roughly 35 to 40 percent of the weight used for the heavier set. For example, if your heavier set is 80 pounds (about 35 kg) each, then your lighter set should be around 30 pounds (13 kg) each.

To set up for this complex, designate two ends of a room about 20 to 25 yards (18-23 m) apart. Place both pairs of dumbbells at one end of the room. If you don't have much free space in your weight room, just bring the dumbbells into the group fitness room or go outside if the weather is suitable. Perform all the following exercises back-to-back for the reps indicated to complete one round of this complex.

 ## Dumbbell Farmer's Walk

Setup

Stand at one end of the room and hold two heavy dumbbells in each hand, your palms facing your body by your hips (or at your shoulders).

Action and Coaching Tips

Walk to the other end of the room (see figure), then return to your starting point, completing one full lap of 40 to 50 total yards (37-46 m). Take normal strides and move as fast as you can without losing control and maintaining a tall, upright posture as you carry the weight.

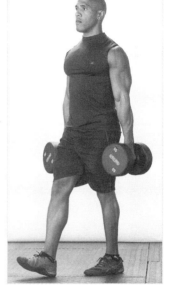

 ## Dumbbell Rotational Shoulder Press

Setup

Stand tall, with your feet roughly shoulder-width apart. Hold a dumbbell in front of each shoulder (see figure a).

Action and Coaching Tips

Press one dumbbell into the air directly over your same-side shoulder as you rotate to the opposite side (see figure b). To better allow your hips to rotate, raise your heel off the ground as you turn. Lower the dumbbell in a smooth, controlled manner as you bring your torso back to facing straight ahead. Then turn to the opposite side to perform the rep with the other arm. Perform 6 to 8 reps on each side.

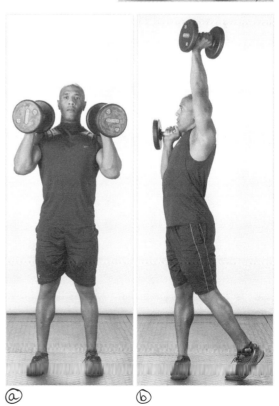

a   b

Dumbbell Farmer's Walk

As described for exercise 1, stand at one end of the room and hold two heavy dumbbells in each hand, with your palms facing your body by your hips (or at your shoulders). Walk to the other end of the room, then return to your starting point, completing one full lap, covering 40 to 50 total yards (37-46 m). Take normal strides, moving as fast as you can without losing control and maintaining a tall, upright posture.

Dumbbell Front Squat

Setup

Stand with your feet shoulder-width apart. Hold lighter dumbbells in each hand at your shoulders—the back ends of the dumbbells will rest on the tops of your shoulders—with your elbows directly underneath the handles of the dumbbells (see figure *a*).

Action and Coaching Tips

Squat as low as you can by bending your knees and sitting your hips back (see figure *b*). Do not allow your heels to rise off the floor or your lower back to round out. Also, do not allow your knees to drop in toward the midline of your body; keep your knees tracking in the same direction as your toes. Reverse the motion and return to the tall standing position to complete a rep. Perform 10 to 14 reps.

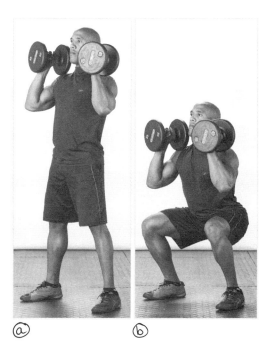

@   b

Dumbbell Farmer's Walk

As described previously, stand at one end of the room and hold two heavy dumbbells in each hand, with your palms facing your body by your hips (or at your shoulders). Walk to the other end of the room, then return to your starting point, completing one full lap, covering 40 to 50 total yards (37-46 m). Take normal strides, moving as fast as you can without losing control and maintaining a tall, upright posture.

Break-Dancer Push-Up

Setup

Begin in a push-up position, with your hands and feet shoulder-width apart (see figure *a*).

Action and Coaching Tips

Perform a push-up; at the top, rotate your entire body toward your left side, driving your right knee to your left elbow while keeping your left hand at your chin (see figures *b* and *c*). Reverse this motion to perform another push-up and repeat this action on the opposite side, touching your left knee to your right elbow. Be sure to rotate your hips and shoulders together at the same rate, and do not allow your head and hips to sag toward the floor. Perform 10 to 16 reps total.

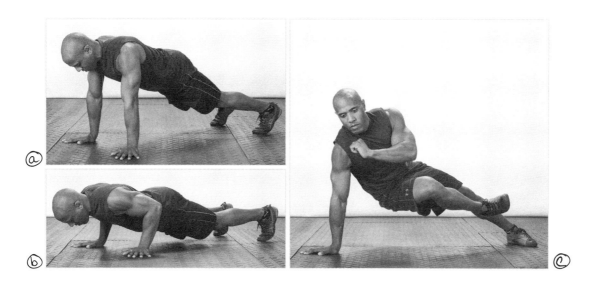

⑦ Dumbbell Farmer's Walk

As described previously, stand at one end of the room and hold two heavy dumbbells in each hand, with your palms facing your body by your hips (or at your shoulders). Walk to the other end of the room, then return to your starting point, completing one full lap, covering 40 to 50 total yards (37-46 m). Take normal strides, moving as fast as you can without losing control and maintain a tall, upright posture.

⑧ Deadlift Jump

Setup

Stand with your feet roughly shoulder-width apart and with your arms at your thighs.

Action and Coaching Tips

With your feet roughly shoulder-width apart, hinge at your hips and bend forward toward the floor (see figure a). Keep your back straight and your knees bent at a 15- to 20-degree angle. Let your arms hang in front of your body, keeping your elbows slightly bent. Jump straight up by simultaneously extending your hips and knees (see figure b). Land as lightly and quietly as possible, thus returning to the starting position. Do not allow your back to round out at the bottom of each repetition.

Each time you set up for the next jump, keep your knees in the same line as your toes; your knees should not come toward one another at any time. Jump as high as you can on each repetition. Perform 10 to 14 reps.

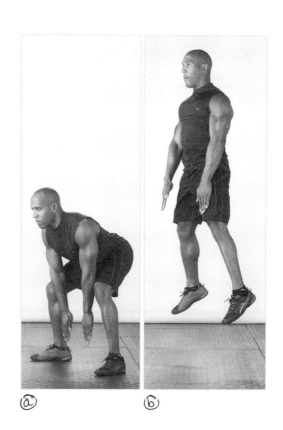

Unilateral Farmer's Walk Complex

This complex is performed in the same way as the previous dumbbell farmer's walk complex, except that here, you do two laps of each farmer's walk: one lap carrying a dumbbell in your right hand and one more lap carrying it in your left hand.

To perform this complex, use a heavier dumbbell for the farmer's-walk portions and a lighter dumbbell for the other exercises. The lighter dumbbell should be roughly 35 to 40 percent of the weight used for the heavier dumbbell. For example, if your heavier dumbbell is 80 pounds (about 35 kg), then your lighter dumbbell should be around 30 pounds (13 kg).

To set up for this complex, designate two ends of a room about 20 to 25 yards (18-23 m) apart. Place both dumbbells at one end of the room. If you don't have much free space in your weight room, just bring the dumbbells into the group fitness room or go outside if the weather is suitable. Perform all the following exercises back-to-back for the reps indicated to complete one round of this complex.

 One-Arm Dumbbell Rotational Shoulder Press

Setup

Stand tall, with your feet roughly shoulder-width apart. Hold a dumbbell in front of one shoulder (see figure a).

Action and Coaching Tips

Press the dumbbell into the air directly over your same-side shoulder as you rotate to the opposite side (see figure b). To better allow your hips to rotate, raise your heel off the ground as you turn. Lower the dumbbell smoothly and with control as you bring your torso back to facing straight ahead before you begin the next rep. Perform 6 to 8 reps on each side.

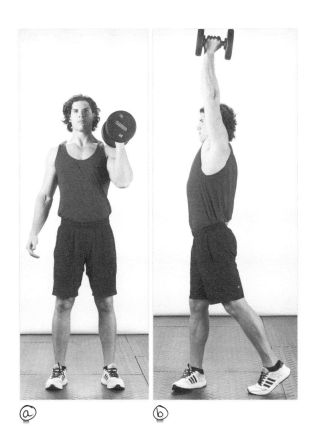

a   b

One-Arm Dumbbell Farmer's Walk

Setup

Stand tall at one end of the room while holding a heavy dumbbell on the left side of your body and your palm facing your body by your hip (or at your shoulder).

Action and Coaching Tips

Walk to the other end of the room (see figure), then return to your starting point and complete one full lap, covering 40 to 50 total yards (37-46 m). Switch hands and do another lap. Take normal strides and move as fast as you can without losing control. Maintain a tall, upright posture as you carry the weight.

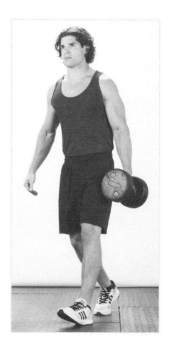

 ## One-Leg Reverse Lunge with Dumbbell at Shoulder

Setup

Stand tall, with your feet about hip-width apart. Hold a lighter dumbbell in your left hand at your left shoulder (see figure a). The back of the dumbbell should rest on top of your shoulder throughout.

Action and Coaching Tips

Step backward with your left foot, as you simultaneously drop your body so that your knee lightly touches the floor (see figure b). Keep your back straight and your torso centered. Do not lean to one side. Reverse the movement by coming out of the lunge and bringing your foot forward so that you are back in the starting position. Perform a series of reverse lunges by stepping back with only this one leg. Perform 10 to 12 reps on each side.

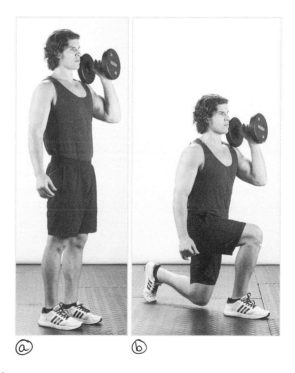

ⓐ   ⓑ

 ## One-Arm Dumbbell Farmer's Walk

As described for exercise 2, stand at one end of the room and hold a heavy dumbbell on the left side of your body, with your palm facing your body by your hip (or at your shoulder). Walk to the other end of the room, then return to your starting point and complete one full lap, covering 40 to 50 total yards (37-46 m). Switch hands and perform another lap. Take normal strides and move as fast as you can without losing control. Maintain a tall, upright posture as you carry the weight.

⑤ One-Arm Plank

Setup
Begin in a push-up position, with your hands shoulder-width apart and your feet a few inches farther than shoulder-width apart (see figure *a*).

Action and Coaching Tips
Lift one arm off the ground without allowing your shoulders or hips to rotate or your head or belly to sag toward the floor (see figure *b*). Pause for several seconds before switching hands. To make this exercise more difficult, you can perform it from your elbows; if you do so, place a pad, pillow, or folded towel under your elbow for protection. You can also increase the challenge of both the straight-arm and elbow-supported version of this exercise by extending your free arm out to your side so your arm is parallel with the floor. Hold for 12 to 20 seconds on each side.

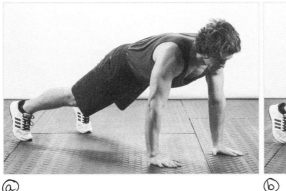 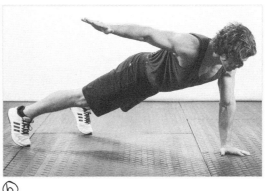

ⓐ   ⓑ

⑥ One-Arm Dumbbell Farmer's Walk

As described previously, stand at one end of the room and hold a heavy dumbbell on the left side of your body, with your palm facing your body by your hip (or at your shoulder). Walk to the other end of the room, then return to your starting point and complete one full lap, covering 40 to 50 total yards (37-46 m). Switch hands and do another lap. Take normal strides and move as fast as you can without losing control. Maintain a tall, upright posture as you carry the weight.

⑦ Leaning Split Squat Scissor Jump

Setup
Assume a split stance, with your legs hip-width apart and your rear heel off the ground, thus putting most of your weight on your front leg (see figure *a*).

Action and Coaching Tips
Lean forward by hinging at your hips and reach your arms down, keeping them just in front of your toes. Jump as high as possible while scissoring your legs (see figures *b* and *c*) so that you land in the same position but with the opposite leg forward (see figure *d*). Jump again, repeating the action. Land as quietly and lightly as possible, using each landing to load the next jump. Each time you land, hinge forward at your hips, keeping your spine straight. Each time you explode back up, raise your torso. Perform 16 to 20 total reps (8 to 10 reps per leg).

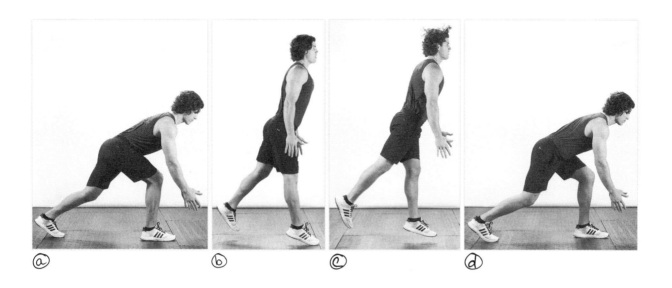

@ ⓑ ⓒ ⓓ

⑧ One-Arm Dumbbell Farmer's Walk

As described previously, stand at one end of the room and hold a heavy dumbbell on the left side of your body, with your palm facing your body by your hip (or at your shoulder). Walk to the other end of the room, then return to your starting point and complete one full lap, covering 40 to 50 total yards (37-46 m). Switch hands and do another lap. Take normal strides and move as fast as you can without losing control. Maintain a tall, upright posture as you carry the weight.

Dumbbell Complex

This complex uses two dumbbells, one in each hand. After you've finished performing 2 reps of the two-arm dumbbell swing and 1 rep of each of the remaining exercises in this complex, which is 1 rep of the complex, position your body properly to start the first exercise and repeat the sequence. You'll do 15 to 20 total reps of the exercises in this combination.

Two-Arm Dumbbell Swing

Setup

With your feet roughly shoulder-width apart, hold a dumbbell in each hand in front of your hips.

Action and Coaching Tips

Keeping your back and arms straight, drive the dumbbells between your legs as if hiking a football and hinge forward at your hips, keeping your knees bent at roughly a 15- to 20-degree angle (see figure *a*). Once your forearms contact your thighs, explosively reverse the motion by simultaneously driving your hips forward and swinging the dumbbells upward to roughly eye level to complete 1 rep (see figure *b*). Perform 2 reps.

As you hinge forward, be sure that you drive your hips backward and do not allow your back to round out. Also, allow your forearms to touch the insides of your thighs at the bottom

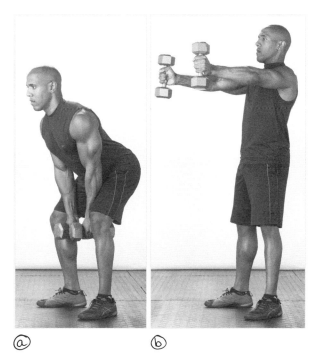

Ⓐ   Ⓑ

of each swing. Use your hips to powerfully drive your arms forward off your thighs to swing the dumbbells up on each rep. This ensures that you're doing the exercise properly by emphasizing the involvement of your leg and hip musculature instead of just lifting the dumbbell with your arms.

Down Gorilla Burpee

Setup

Stand with your feet wider than shoulder-width apart and hold dumbbells in front of your hips, with your arms straight so they are hanging between your feet.

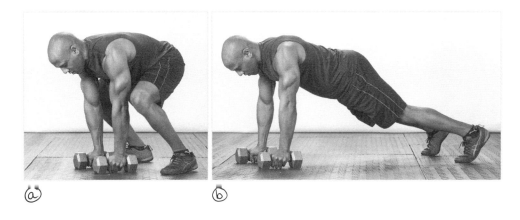

Ⓐ   Ⓑ

Action and Coaching Tips

Bend your knees and hinge forward at your hips to place the dumbbells on the floor between your feet directly under each shoulder (see figure a). Jump backward so you end up in push-up position, with your body forming a straight line, and do not allow your hips to sag toward the floor (see figure b). Remain in this position and move to the next exercise. Perform 1 rep.

 ## Dumbbell Push-Up

Setup

With dumbbells directly under your shoulders, place one hand on the handle of each dumbbell.

Action and Coaching Tips

Do a push-up by lowering your body to the floor while keeping your elbows directly above your wrists the entire time (see figure a). Once your ribs touch the dumbbells, reverse the motion by pushing your body up (see figure b). Be sure you do not allow your head or hips to sag toward the floor at any time. Perform 1 rep.

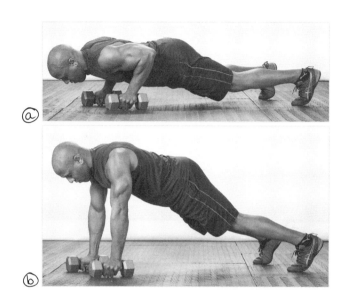

 ## Dumbbell Plank Row

Setup

Begin in a push-up position with each of your hands gripping a dumbbell placed on the floor (see figure a). Your feet are shoulder-width apart and your wrists are directly below your shoulders. To ensure that the dumbbells do not roll, place your hands directly underneath your shoulders.

Action and Coaching Tips

Pick up the dumbbell and perform a row by pulling it into your body without allowing your head or hips to sag or your torso to rotate (see figure b). Slowly lower it and repeat on the other side. Perform 1 rep on each side.

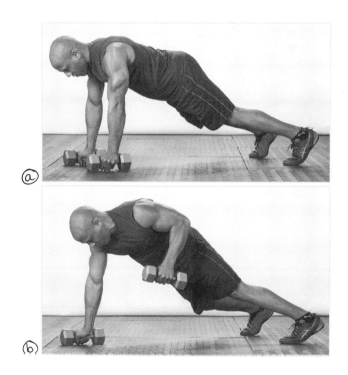

⑤ Up Gorilla Burpee

Setup

Remain in the push-up plank position from the previous exercise (see figure *a*).

Action and Coaching Tips

Jump up to your feet (see figure *b*) and simply stand up tall. Perform 1 rep.

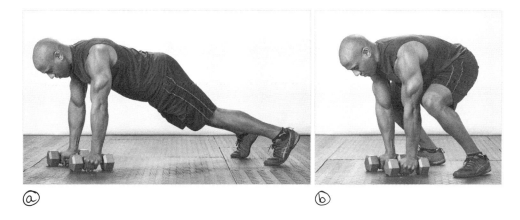

ⓐ   ⓑ

⑥ Dumbbell Squat and Shoulder Press

Setup

Stand tall, with your feet shoulder-width apart. Hold a dumbbell in each hand at your shoulders, your elbows directly underneath the handles (see figure *a*).

Action and Coaching Tips

Squat as low as you can by bending your knees and sitting your hips back without allowing your heels to rise off the floor or your lower back to round out (see figure *b*). Reverse the motion by simultaneously standing up and pressing the dumbbells overhead so that your knees and arms straighten at roughly the same time (see figure *c*). Perform 1 rep. Then repeat the sequence beginning with the two-arm dumbbell swing.

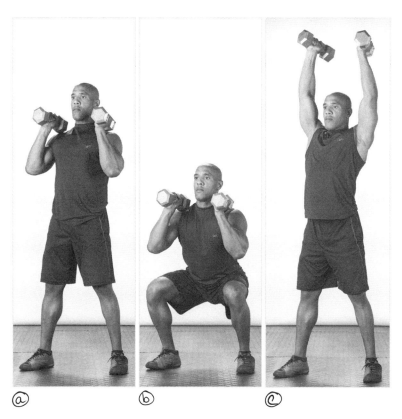

ⓐ   ⓑ   ⓒ

Weight Plate Complex

The following complex requires you to hold each end of a 25-, 35-, or 45-pound Olympic weight plate, which is the traditional type of weight plate found most gyms. The following complex is dynamic and requires good amount of coordination and athleticism. Perform all three exercises back-to-back for the reps indicated to complete one round of this complex.

Weight Plate Speed Chop

Setup

Squat and rotate your hips and torso while holding a weight plate weighing 10 to 45 pounds (4.5-20 kg) near the outside your left knee (see figure a).

Action and Coaching Tips

Stand up as you quickly rotate to your right side and drive the plate across your body in a diagonal pattern, finishing with it just above your head (see figure b). Without pausing, quickly reverse the motion by driving the plate back down across your body on the same diagonal path you used to lift it. Perform all reps to one side, then repeat the exercise to the other side. Do 14 to 16 reps on each side.

Do this exercise fast but smoothly and with a consistent rhythm, coordinating

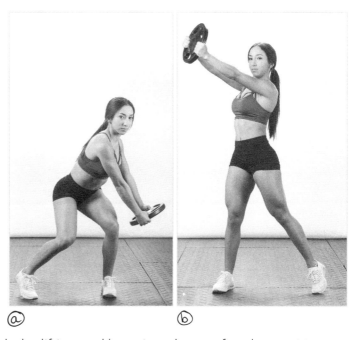

your upper body and lower body during both the lifting and lowering phases of each repetition.

Weight Plate Middle Speed Chop

Setup

Stand with your feet wider than shoulder-width apart (see figure a). Hold a weight plate with both hands.

Action and Coaching Tips

Keeping your back and arms straight, drive the weight plate between your legs as if hiking a football and hinge forward at your hips (see figure b). Keep your knees bent at roughly a 15- to 20-degree angle. As you hinge forward, drive your hips backward; do not allow your back to round out. Once your forearms contact your thighs, explosively reverse the motion by simultaneously driving your hips forward and swinging the weight plate up to eye level. Perform 14 to 16 reps on each side.

Do this exercise fast, but smoothly and with a consistent rhythm, coordinating your upper body and lower body during both the lifting and the lowering phase of each repetition.

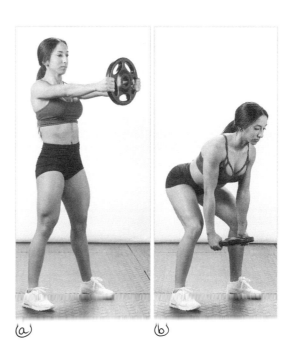

③ Weight Plate Push

Setup

Place a heavy weight plate—try 35 to 45 pounds (about 15-20 kg)—on top of a towel so that it glides or on a turf surface. For an additional challenge, you can also place a set of dumbbells (25-35 pounds or 11-15 kg) inside the weight plate. Get into push-up position, with your hands on top of the weight plate.

Action and Coaching Tips

Drive with your legs by bringing your knees up toward your chest, first one knee (see figure *a*) and then the other (see figure *b*). Push the plate quickly across the floor for 20 to 25 yards (18-23 m) up and back for a total of 40 to 50 yards (37-46 m; see figures a-c). Perform 1 lap.

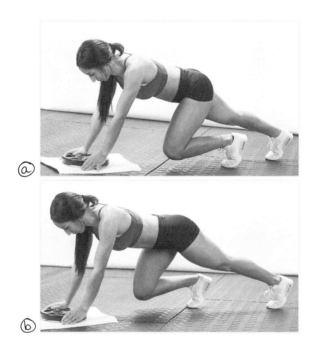

Bodyweight Leg Complex

Do the following exercises back-to-back, fast but with control. Perform all the reps indicated to complete one round of this complex.

Squat Jump with Arm Drive

Setup

Stand with your feet roughly shoulder-width apart.

Action and Coaching Tips

Squat by bending at your knees and hips so that your thighs are just above parallel to the ground while making sure to keep your knees in the same line as your toes (see figure a); your knees should not come toward one another at any time. Reach your arms just behind your hips, keeping your elbows slightly bent. Jump straight up by simultaneously extending your legs and swinging your arms above you (see figure b). Land as lightly and quietly as possible, thus returning to the starting position. Jump as high as you can on each repetition. Perform 10 to 12 reps.

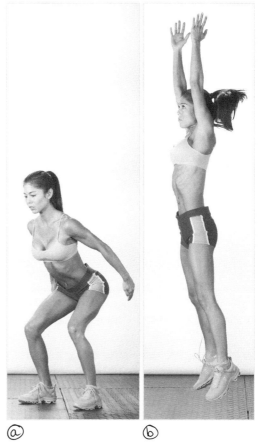

ⓐ   ⓑ

Leaning Split Squat Scissor Jump

Setup

Assume a split stance with your legs hip-width apart and your rear heel off the ground, thus putting most of your weight on your front leg (see figure a).

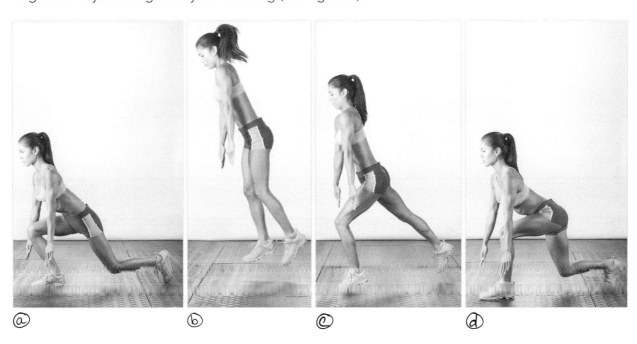

ⓐ   ⓑ   ⓒ   ⓓ

Action and Coaching Tips

Lean forward by hinging at your hips and reach your arms down, keeping them just behind your toes. Jump as high as possible while scissoring your legs (see figures *b* and *c*) so that you land in the same position but with the opposite leg forward (see figure *d*). Jump again, repeating the action. Land as quietly and lightly as possible, using each landing to load the next jump. Each time you land, hinge forward at your hips, keeping your spine straight. Each time you explode back up, raise your torso. Perform 20 to 24 total reps (10 to 12 reps per leg).

Reverse Lunge

Setup

Stand tall, with your feet hip-width apart and your fingers interlaced behind your head (see figure *a*).

Action and Coaching Tips

Step backward on your left leg, placing the ball of your foot on the floor while bending both knees, and lower your body into a lunge (see figure *b*). Once your back knee lightly touches the floor, reverse the motion by stepping back up into the starting position. Do the same motion by stepping back with your other leg. Alternate legs on each rep. Perform each rep as fast as possible but with control. Do 20 to 24 total reps (10-12 reps per leg).

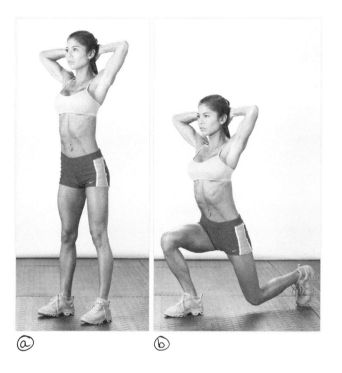

@   ⓑ

Zombie Squat

Setup

Stand tall, with your feet shoulder-width apart and your toes turned out about 10 degrees. Extend your arms in front of you at shoulder height (see figure *a*).

Action and Coaching Tips

Squat by bending your knees and sitting back at your hips (see figure *b*). Your knees should track in the same direction as your toes. Go down so your thighs are almost parallel to the floor without allowing your lower back to round out. Perform each rep as fast as possible but with control. Do 20 to 24 reps.

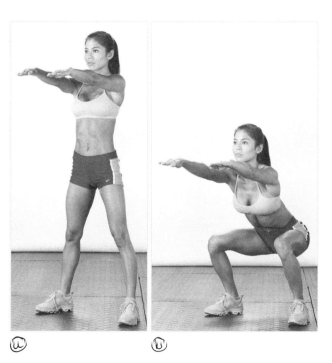

ⓐ   ⓑ

Two-Minute Bodyweight Complex

Perform the following four exercises back-to-back to complete one round of the complex. Do each exercise for 30 seconds each, with no rest between each exercise

 ## Fast-Hands Plank

Setup

Begin in a push-up position, with your hands a few inches outside shoulder-width apart and your feet a few inches farther than shoulder-width apart (see figure a).

Action and Coaching Tips

Without allowing your shoulders or hips to rotate or your head or belly to sag toward the floor, as fast as you can, lift one hand off the ground and tap the top of your opposite hand (see figure b). Then, place that hand back on the ground and repeat the action with the other hand. Perform each rep as fast as possible but with control in 30 seconds.

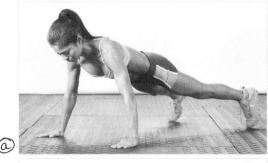

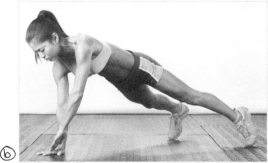

 ## Gorilla Burpee

Setup

With your feet slightly farther than shoulder-width apart, hold your arms straight in front of your body (see figure a).

Action and Coaching Tips

Bend your knees and hinge forward at your hips so that your torso leans forward. Place your hands on the ground, with your wrists directly below your shoulders (see figure b), and jump backward to move into a push-up position (see figure c). Make sure that your body forms a straight line and that you do not allow your hips to sag toward the floor in the push-up position. Jump back up so your feet are outside your hands (see figure d), then return to a tall standing position to complete the rep (see figure e).

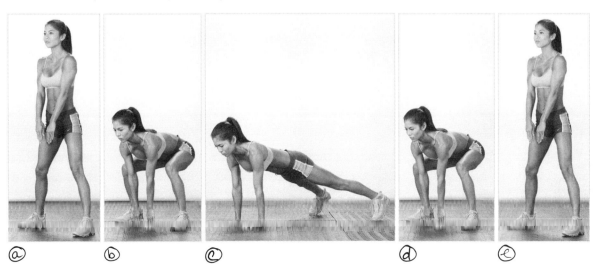

③ Squat Jump with Arm Drive

Setup
Stand with your feet roughly shoulder-width apart.

Action and Coaching Tips
Squat by bending at your knees and hips so that your thighs are just above parallel to the ground (see figure a). Make sure to keep your knees in the same line as your toes; your knees should not come toward one another at any time. Reach your arms just behind your hips, keeping your elbows slightly bent. Jump straight up by simultaneously extending your legs and swinging your arms above you (see figure b). Land as lightly and quietly as possible, thus returning to the starting position. Jump as high as you can on each repetition. Perform as many reps as possible but with control in 30 seconds.

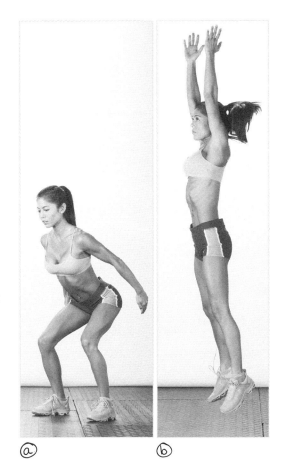

a   b

④ Seal Jack

Setup
Stand with your feet together and your arms extended in front of you at shoulder level, your hands together (see figure a).

Action and Coaching Tips
As you open your arms horizontally to the side, jump up just enough to spread your feet wide (see figure b). Without pausing, quickly reverse the movement. Do the exercise smoothly, opening and closing your legs and arms simultaneously. Be as light on your feet as possible. Minimize the time that your feet are in contact with the ground. Perform each rep as fast as possible but with control.

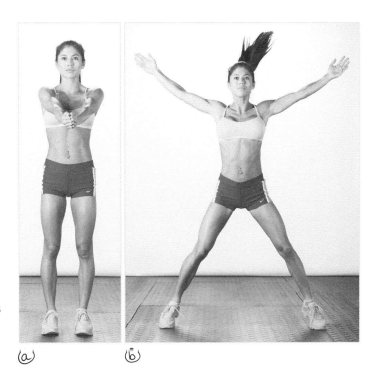

a   b

Bodyweight and Resistance Band Complex

This complex involves using a resistance band that's attached at roughly shoulder height to a stable structure or inside a doorjamb (many resistance bands come with an attachment for this). Perform the following exercises back-to-back, fast but with control, to complete one round of this complex.

Resistance Band Alternate-Arm Row

Setup

Stand tall in a split stance, with your right foot forward and your knees slightly bent. Face a band that's attached at roughly chest height. Hold one handle in each hand.

Action and Coaching Tips

As you pull the band toward your body with one arm, let the other arm straighten without allowing your torso or hips to rotate more than a few degrees (see figure a). Alternate your arms in a quick motion, making sure that the elbow on the arm that you're rowing with goes past your torso (see figure b). Perform each rep as fast as possible but with control. Do 20 to 25 total reps per stance. Once you you've completed all the reps with your right foot in front, switch your stance and perform the same amount of reps with your left foot in front.

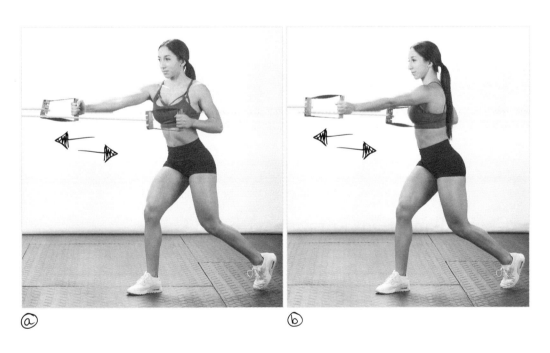

ⓐ   ⓑ

Resistance Band Alternate-Arm Chest Press

Setup

Face away from a band that's attached at roughly shoulder height. Hold one handle in each hand, with your elbows out to your sides and your forearms parallel to the floor. Stand in a split stance, with your left foot forward and your knees slightly bent.

Action and Coaching Tips

As you press the band horizontally away your body with one arm, let the other arm straighten without allowing your torso or hips to rotate more than a few degrees (see figure a). Alternate your arms in a quick motion, making sure that the elbow on the arm that you're getting ready to press with goes past your torso (see figure b). Perform each rep as fast as possible but with control. Perform 20 to 25 total reps per stance. Once you have completed all the reps with your left foot in front, switch your stance and perform the same number of reps with your right foot in front.

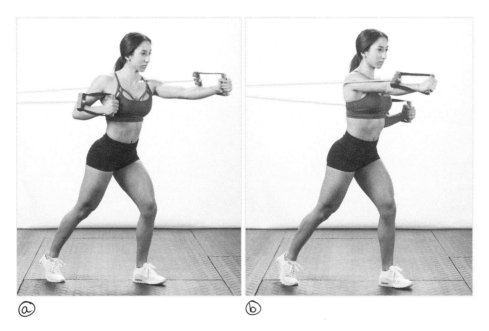

@   ⓑ

Resistance Band Tight Rotation with Hip Shift

Setup

Stand with your feet shoulder-width apart, your knees slightly bent, and the handles of a resistance band on your right side at shoulder level. Hold the handles on your right side, with your elbows slightly bent. Position your feet slightly father than shoulder-width apart and your weight shifted towards your right leg with your shoulders directly over your hips (see figure a).

Action and Coaching Tips

Keeping your hips moving with your shoulders, shift your weight to your left leg as you simultaneously move your arms horizontally, pulling the handles across your body to the left until both arms are just outside your left shoulder. Stop rotating your hips and shoulders when the bands gently touches your forearm (see figure b). The range of motion in this exercise is small—roughly the same as the width of your shoulders. Allow minimal rotation at your hips, which should move in the same direction and at the same speed as your shoulders. Perform each rep as fast as possible but with control for 10 to 15 reps per side. Perform all reps on one side before switching to the other side.

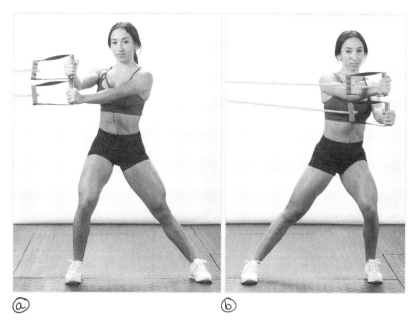

@   ⓑ

④ Gorilla Burpee

Setup

With your feet slightly wider than shoulder-width apart, hold your arms straight down in front of your body (see figure a).

Action and Coaching Tips

Bend your knees and hinge forward at your hips so that your torso leans forward (see figure b). Place your hands on the ground, with your wrists directly underneath your shoulders, and quickly move your legs backward so that you move into a push-up position (see figure c). Make sure that your body forms one straight line and that you do not allow your hips to sag toward the floor in the push-up position. Keeping your hands on the ground, jump up to the outside of your hands and drop your hips into a squat-type position (see figure d) before you return to the tall standing position (see figure e), thus completing the rep. Perform each rep as fast as possible but with control. Perform 15 to 20 reps.

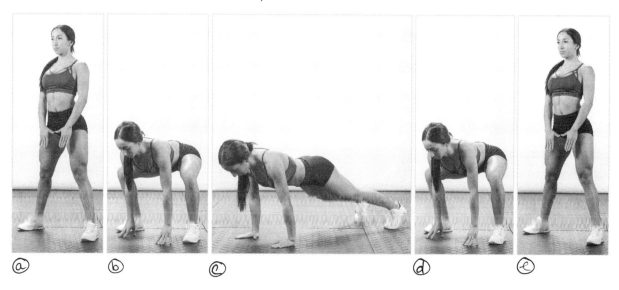

ⓐ   ⓑ   ⓒ   ⓓ   ⓔ

PART III

Programming

10 { General Beginner Programs

This chapter provides beginner workout programs for those who are just starting out or for those who haven't done any regular strength training in a while. Once you've been through these beginner workouts or if you've been regularly performing moderate levels of strength training, you can start with using the fitness programs in chapter 11. Do those exercises for at least six to eight weeks before trying any of the programs found in chapters 12 to 14.

The Basics of General Beginner Programs

This chapter focuses on gym-based programs, but since you can't always make it to the gym and your primary training should be done using equipment, it also provides two home and hotel gym workouts along with two workouts using only bodyweight and resistance band exercises that you can use on the days when you're traveling or don't have access to any kind of gym equipment.

There are guidelines for using the programs in this chapter. Some of these guidelines will be the same for all the program chapters featured in this book, but others differ depending on the type of program you're doing. Let's look at the key points to remember for your beginner programs:

- Perform exercises *a* and *b* as paired sets. Do all the indicated sets and reps in a paired set before moving on to the next set. Once all exercises within a paired set are complete, you can rest a bit longer than indicated between sets (if necessary) to complete the designated number of reps with good control. Completing one round of the exercises in a paired set is considered one set.

- The rep range (i.e., 10-15 reps) is next to each exercise in the programs in the next two sections. If you're using the same weight for each set, you may be able to do 15 reps on the first set, 12 reps on the next set, and 10 reps on the third set due to accumulated fatigue. Or, you can reduce the weight you're using with each consecutive set to achieve the higher end of the given rep range on each consecutive set. Both methods are effective at helping you progress.

- When a program indicates to take rest days, this doesn't mean you have to do nothing. During your days off, you can do some low-impact activities, such as going for long walks, hikes, bike rides, or swims. Also, yoga can be a great option for your active rest periods.

- The main goal of the programs in this chapter is to familiarize your body with the demands of performing basic exercises. Your primary focus when using these programs, especially in phase 1, is not to reach full exercise fatigue but to improve your exercise technique and your muscle awareness when performing the exercises.
- Maintain strict form, without cheating by using additional movements or momentum.
- Mentally focus on the working muscles in each exercise.
- Do the concentric (lifting) portion of each rep at a normal tempo and maintain control during the eccentric (lowering) portion.
- Use a weight load that leaves you unable to perform any more reps than indicated while maintaining proper control and technique.
- If an exercise causes pain or discomfort beyond the sensation associated with muscle fatigue, do an alternative exercise that doesn't hurt. There are plenty of movements in the exercise chapters of this book to choose from.
- Remember, before you begin a workout in the following programs, be sure to perform one of the dynamic warm-up sequences in chapter 5.

Beginner Gym-Based Workout Program

The beginner gym-based workout program is broken down into two phases (see tables 10.1-10.3). Phase 1 consists of a single program, which you'll repeat four times, either two, three, or four times a week on nonconsecutive days. If you're exercising four times per week, you'll complete phase 1 in one week's time. Once you've completed phase 1, you'll move on to phase 2. Phase 2 consists of Program

Your Gym Bag

There are a couple pieces of portable equipment that I recommend you always have in your gym bag—resistance bands with handles and resistance band loops. These bands allow you to group exercises requiring immobile equipment (e.g., squat rack or machine) with bands, which are mobile equipment. This enables you to use band exercises within a paired set or triset while you remain at the immobile equipment and don't have to walk all over the gym, thus potentially losing your equipment to another member.

There are two places online that I recommend you go to purchase high-quality resistance bands: Power-Systems.com and Sorinex.com. At Power Systems, the resistance bands with handles to get are the *Double Cords*; the resistance band loops are called *strength bands*, and resistance band mini loops are called *Versa Loops*. At Sorinex Exercise Equipment, resistance band loops are called *strength bands*, and resistance band mini loops are called *short bands*.

B, which you'll alternate on nonconsecutive days. You'll repeat each program in phase 2 three times, either twice, three times, or four times within a week on nonconsecutive days.

Once you've finished both phases of the beginner programs that follow, you're ready to move on to the Fitness Programs chapter for at least six to eight weeks before trying any of the other programs in part III.

Table 10.1 Beginner Gym-Based Workout Program: Phase 1

		Workout 1	Workout 2	Workout 3	Workout 4	Page
1a.	Dumbbell goblet squat	1× 12-15 (−3)*	1× 12-15 (−2)*	1× 12-15 (−1)*	1× 12-15	141
1b.	Lat pull-down with neutral grip	1× 12-15 (−3)* with 90 seconds rest between paired sets	1× 12-15 (−2)* with 90 seconds rest between paired sets	1× 12-15 (−1)* with 90 seconds rest between paired sets	1× 12-15 with 90 seconds rest between paired sets	91
2a.	Push-up	1× max reps (−3)*	1× max reps (−2)*	1× max reps (−1)*	1× max reps	62
2b.	Dumbbell Romanian deadlift	1× 12-15 (−3)* with 90 seconds rest between paired sets	1× 12-15 (−2)* with 90 seconds rest between paired sets	1× 12-15 (−1)* with 90 seconds rest between paired sets	1× 12-15 with 90 seconds rest between paired sets	142
3a.	One-arm cable row	1× 12-14	1×15-16	1× 17-18	1× 19-20	93
3b.	One-arm cable press	1× 12-15 (−3)* with 90 seconds rest between paired sets	1× 12-15 (−2)* with 90 seconds rest between paired sets	1× 12-15 (−1)* with 90 seconds rest between paired sets	1× 12-15 with 90 seconds rest between paired sets	92
4a.	Machine lying hamstring curl	1× 12-15 (−3)*	1× 12-15 (−2)*	1× 12-15 (−1)*	1× 12-15	151
4b.	Dumbbell shoulder T	1× 12 with 90 seconds rest between paired sets	1× 13 with 90 seconds rest between paired sets	1× 14 with 90 seconds rest between paired sets	1× 15 with 90 seconds rest between paired sets	90
5a.	Machine hip adduction	1× 12-15 (−3)*	1× 12-15 (−2)*	1× 12-15 (−1)*	1× 12-15	152
5b.	Dumbbell side shoulder raise	1× 12-15 (−3)* with 90 seconds rest between paired sets	1× 12-15 (−2)* with 90 seconds rest between paired sets	1× 12-15 (−1)* with 90 seconds rest between paired sets	1× 12-15 with 90 seconds rest between paired sets	71
6a.	Cable triceps rope extension	1× 12-14	1x 15-16	1× 17-18	1× 19-20	98
6b.	Dumbbell biceps curl	1× 12-15 (−3)* with 90 seconds rest between paired sets	1× 12-15 (−2)* with 90 seconds rest between paired sets	1× 12-15 (−1)* with 90 seconds rest between paired sets	1× 12-15 with 90 seconds rest between paired sets	68
7a.	One-leg hip bridge	1× 30 seconds each side	1× 35 seconds each side	1× 40 seconds each side	1× 45 seconds each side	146
7b.	Shoulder tap plank	1× 20 seconds each side	1× 24 seconds each side	1× 28 seconds each side	1× 30 seconds each side	186

*(-1) indicates to stop the set 1 rep before muscle failure. (-2) indicates to stop the set 2 reps before muscle failure, and (-3) indicates to stop the set 3 reps before failure.

Table 10.2 Beginner Gym-Based Workout Program: Phase 2, Program A

		Workout 1	Workout 2	Workout 3	Page
1a.	Mid-platform machine leg press	2× 10-12	2× 13-14	2× 14-16	149
1b.	Stability ball rollout	2× 10-12 with 90 seconds rest between paired sets	2× 13-14 with 90 seconds rest between paired sets	2× 14-16 with 90 seconds rest between paired sets	176
2a.	Machine chest press	2× 10-12	2× 13-14	2× 14-16	102
2b.	One-arm dumbbell off-bench row	2× 10-12 each side with 90 seconds rest between paired sets	2× 13-14 each side with 90 seconds rest between paired sets	2× 14-16 each side with 90 seconds rest between paired sets	83
3a.	Dumbbell incline bench press	2× 10-12	2×13-14	2× 14-16	82
3b.	Dumbbell lateral Romanian deadlift lunge	2× 8 each side with 90 seconds rest between paired sets	2× 9 each side with 90 seconds rest between paired sets	2× 10 each side with 90 seconds rest between paired sets	142
4a.	One-arm half-kneeling angled cable row	2× 10-12 each side	2× 13-14 each side	2× 14-16 each side	95
4b.	Dumbbell side shoulder raise	2× 10-12 with 90 seconds rest between paired sets	2× 13-14 with 90 seconds rest between paired sets	2× 14-16 with 90 seconds rest between paired sets	71
5a.	One-leg cable hip adduction	2× 10-12 each side	2× 13-14 each side	2× 14-16 each side	148
5b.	Dumbbell biceps curl	2× 9-10 with 90 seconds rest between paired sets	2× 11-12 with 90 seconds rest between paired sets	2× 13-15 with 90 seconds rest between paired sets	68
6a.	One-leg dumbbell bench hip thrust	2× 10-12 each side	2× 13-14 each side	2× 14-16 each side	145
6b.	Reverse crunch	2× 8-9 with 90 seconds rest between paired sets	2× 10-11 with 90 seconds rest between paired sets	2× 12-14 with 90 seconds rest between paired sets	160

Table 10.3 Beginner Gym-Based Workout Program: Phase 2, Program B

		Workout 1	Workout 2	Workout 3	Page
1a.	Dumbbell leaning Bulgarian split squat	2× 9-10 each side	2× 11-12 each side	2× 13-15 each side	128
1b.	Push-up	2× max reps (−2)* with 90 seconds rest between paired sets	2× max reps (−1)* with 90 seconds rest between paired sets	2× max reps with 90 seconds rest between paired sets	62
2a.	Lat pull-down	2× 10-12	2× 13-14	2× 14-16	58
2b.	Dumbbell Romanian deadlift	2× 10-12 with 90 seconds rest between paired sets	2× 13-14 with 90 seconds rest between paired sets	2× 14-16 with 90 seconds rest between paired sets	142
3a.	One-arm angled barbell press	2× 10-12 each side	2× 13-14 each side	2× 14-16 each side	77
3b.	Stability ball leg curl	2× 12-13 with 90 seconds rest between paired sets	2× 14-15 with 90 seconds rest between paired sets	2× 16-18 with 90 seconds rest between paired sets	154
4a.	E-Z bar biceps curl	2× 10-12	2× 13-14	2× 14-16	87
4b.	One-arm dumbbell overhead triceps extension	2× 10-12 each side with 90 seconds rest between paired sets	2× 13-14 each side with 90 seconds rest between paired sets	2× 14-16 each side with 90 seconds rest between paired sets	86

	Workout 1	Workout 2	Workout 3	Page
5a. Machine hip adduction	2× 10-12	2× 13-14	2× 14-16	152
5b. Dumbbell plank row	2× 6 each side with 90 seconds rest between paired sets	2× 7 each side with 90 seconds rest between paired sets	2× 8 each side with 90 seconds rest between paired sets	182
6a. Stability ball plate crunch	2× 9-10	2× 11-12	2× 13-15	170
6b. Resistance band mini loop low lateral shuffle	2× 16-18 each side with 90 seconds rest between paired sets	2× 20-22 each side with 90 seconds rest between paired sets	2× 24-25 each side with 90 seconds rest between paired sets	149

*(-1) indicates to stop the set 1 rep before muscle failure and (-2) indicates to stop the set 2 reps before muscle failure.

You'll perform the beginner program at least twice per week but no more than four times per week until you've completed all the workouts in each phase. The sample weekly programs that could be created if you're training two, three, or even four times a week as shown in tables 10.4 through 10.6.

Table 10.4   Sample Beginner Gym-Based Training Setup: Two Times per Week

Week 1	Week 2
Monday: Phase 1, workout 1	*Monday:* Phase 1, workout 3
Tuesday: Rest	*Tuesday:* Rest
Wednesday: Rest	*Wednesday:* Rest
Thursday: Phase 1, workout 2	*Thursday:* Phase 1, workout 4
Friday: Rest	*Friday:* Rest
Saturday: Rest	*Saturday:* Rest
Sunday: Rest	*Sunday:* Rest
Week 3	**Week 4**
Monday: Phase 2, program A, workout 1	*Monday:* Phase 2, program A, workout 2
Tuesday: Rest	*Tuesday:* Rest
Wednesday: Rest	*Wednesday:* Rest
Thursday: Phase 2, program B, workout 1	*Thursday:* Phase 2, program B, workout 2
Friday: Rest	*Friday:* Rest
Saturday: Rest	*Saturday:* Rest
Sunday: Rest	*Sunday:* Rest

Week 5*
Monday: Phase 2, program A, workout 3
Tuesday: Rest
Wednesday: Rest
Thursday: Phase 2, program B, workout 3
Friday: Rest
Saturday: Rest
Sunday: Rest

*After you've competed week five, continue to the fitness programs featured in the next chapter.

Table 10.5   Sample Beginner Gym-Based Training Setup: Three Times per Week

Week 1	Week 2
Monday: Phase 1, workout 1	*Monday:* Phase 1, workout 3
Tuesday: Rest	*Tuesday:* Rest
Wednesday: Phase 2, program B, workout 1	*Wednesday:* Phase 2, program A, workout 3
Thursday: Rest	*Thursday:* Rest
Friday: Phase 1, workout 2	*Friday:* Phase 1, workout 4
Saturday: Rest	*Saturday:* Rest
Sunday: Rest	*Sunday:* Rest
Week 3	**Week 4***
Monday: Phase 2, program A, workout 1	*Monday:* Phase 2, program B, workout 2
Tuesday: Rest	*Tuesday:* Rest
Wednesday: Phase 2, program B, workout 1	*Wednesday:* Phase 2, program A, workout 3
Thursday: Rest	*Thursday:* Rest
Friday: Phase 2, program A, workout 2	*Friday:* Phase 2, program B, workout 3
Saturday: Rest	*Saturday:* Rest
Sunday: Rest	*Sunday:* Rest

*After you've competed week four, continue to the fitness programs featured in the next chapter.

Table 10.6   Sample Beginner Gym-Based Training Setup: Four Times per Week

Week 1	Week 2
Monday: Phase 1, workout 1	*Monday:* Phase 2, program A, workout 1
Tuesday: Phase 1, workout 2	*Tuesday:* Phase 2, program B, workout 1
Wednesday: Rest	*Wednesday:* Rest
Thursday: Phase 1, workout 3	*Thursday:* Phase 2, program A, workout 2
Friday: Rest	*Friday:* Rest
Saturday: Phase 1, workout 4	*Saturday:* Phase 2, program B, workout 2
Sunday: Rest	*Sunday:* Rest
Week 3*	
Monday: Phase 2, program A, workout 3	
Tuesday: Phase 2, program B, workout 3	
Wednesday: Rest	

*After you've competed week three, which only lasts until Wednesday in the above weekly training set-up, continue to the fitness programs featured in the next chapter.

Beginner Home or Hotel Gym Workouts

On days that you're traveling, can't make it to the gym, or don't have access to a gym, you can use the beginner home or hotel gym workouts or the beginner bodyweight and band workouts here. The two workouts in tables 10.7 and 10.8

involve equipment that's either recommended for your home gym or that's commonly found in most hotel gyms. That equipment is as follows:

- A set of dumbbells (up to 50 lb or 20 kg)
- An adjustable weight bench that can be made flat or set at an incline
- A high-quality stability ball that's 55 to 65 centimeters
- A chin-up bar (many are designed to be easily placed inside the top of a doorway)
- A set of resistance bands with handles of varying strengths, from light to very heavy
- Resistance band loops of varying strength, from light to medium
- Resistance band mini loops of varying strength, from light to medium

Resistance bands, resistance band loops, and resistance band mini loops are affordable and available at most sporting goods stores or online, but they are not often found at hotel gyms. We recommend traveling with at least one set of each type of band. They're portable and easy to pack in your luggage. It's also important to note that since the following workouts are designed to be done with limited equipment, some of the exercises included will require small modifications from how they're featured in the exercise descriptions. For example, for a cable-based exercise such as the One-Arm Cable Row, you'd perform it with a resistance band instead of cable if your training environment doesn't feature a cable column. Or, for a dumbbell exercise such as the Dumbbell Shoulder W, you'd simply perform the same movement as shown in the exercise description without holding dumbbells. These modifications are indicated within each of the workouts.

Also, these workouts are intended to be used *only* as an addition to your regular weekly gym-based workouts on the days you can't make it to the gym or when you're traveling. They are not designed to replace your gym-based workouts; your primary training should revolve around using the beginner workout programs in the previous section. Remember, before you begin any of the following workouts, be sure to perform one of the dynamic warm-up sequences in chapter 5.

The two workouts in tables 10.9 and 10.10 have bodyweight exercises and resistance band exercises utilizing three types of bands: resistance bands with handles (these can be attached to any doorway or stable object in matter of seconds), resistance band loops, and resistance mini band loops. A set of high-quality resistance bands with handles and both types of resistance band loops—they come in multiple resistances from light to very heavy—for home use and to take with you when you travel are a must. They are portable and add a number of effective exercise options to your bodyweight training workouts, delivering a value that far exceeds their cost.

Again, the following workouts are *not* intended to be done exclusively and are not designed to replace the gym-based beginner workout program earlier in this chapter. They are intended to be used only as an addition to your regular weekly gym-based workouts on the days you don't have access to any kind of gym.

Table 10.7 Beginner Home or Hotel Gym Workout: Phase 1

Exercise		Sets and reps	Page
1a.	Dumbbell goblet squat	1× 12-15	141
1b.	One-arm motorcycle cable row (with resistance band)*	1× 15-20 each side with 90 seconds rest between paired sets	94
2a.	Push-up	1× max reps	62
2b.	Dumbbell Romanian deadlift	1× 15-20 with 90 seconds rest between paired sets	142
3a.	One-arm cable row (with resistance band)*	1× 15-20 each side	93
3b.	Cable tight torso rotation with hip shift (with resistance band)*	1× 15-20 each side with 90 seconds rest between paired sets	166
4a.	Stability ball leg curl	1× max reps	154
4b.	Dumbbell shoulder T	1× 15-20 with 90 seconds rest between paired sets	90
5a.	Side-lying hip adduction	1× 15-20 each side	153
5b.	Dumbbell side shoulder raise	1× 15-20 with 90 seconds rest between paired sets	71
6a.	Dumbbell triceps skull crusher	1× 15-20	73
6b.	Dumbbell biceps curl	1× 15-20 with 90 seconds rest between paired sets	68
7a.	One-leg hip bridge	1× 20-30 each side	146
7b.	Shoulder tap plank	1× 20-30 seconds	186

*Use a resistance band instead of a cable to perform this exercise in the manner provided in the exercise description.

Table 10.8 Beginner Home or Hotel Gym Workout: Phase 2

Exercise		Sets and reps	Page
1a.	Elevated dumbbell leaning reverse lunge	2× 8-12 each side	125
1b.	Plank march with resistance band mini loop	2× 8-10 each side with 90 seconds rest between paired sets	185
2a.	Dumbbell bench press	2× 14-16	81
2b.	One-arm dumbbell off-bench row	2× 14-16 each side with 90 seconds rest between paired sets	83
3a.	Dumbbell incline bench press	2× 14-16	82
3b.	Dumbbell Romanian deadlift	2× 10-12 with 90 seconds rest between paired sets	142
4a.	One-arm motorcycle cable row (with resistance band)*	2× 15-18 each side	94
4b.	Resistance band overhead triceps extension	2× 14-16 with 90 seconds rest between paired sets	106
5a.	Side-lying hip adduction	2× 15-20 each side	153
5b.	Dumbbell biceps curl	2× 12-15 with 90 seconds rest between paired sets	68
6a.	One-leg dumbbell bench hip thrust	2× 15-20 each side	145
6b.	Low-to-high cable chop (with resistance band)*	2× 12-15 each side	165

*Use a resistance band instead of a cable to perform this exercise in the manner provided in the exercise description.

Table 10.9   Beginner Bodyweight and Band Workout 1

Exercise		Sets and reps	Page
1a.	Zombie squat	1X 15-20	152
1b.	One-arm motorcycle cable row (with resistance band)*	1X 15-20 each side with 90 seconds rest between paired sets	94
2a.	Push-up	1X max reps	62
2b.	Resistance band loop hybrid deadlift	1X 15-25	148
3a.	One-arm cable row (with resistance band)*	1X 15-20 each side	93
3b.	Cable tight torso rotation with hip shift (with resistance band)*	1X 15-20	166
4a.	Stability ball leg curl	1X max reps	154
4b.	Stability ball rollout	1X 15-20	176
5a.	Side-lying hip adduction	1X 15-20 each side	153
5b.	Dumbbell shoulder Y (without dumbbells)**	1X 15-20	89
6a.	Resistance band overhead triceps extension	1X 15-20	106
6b.	Resistance band biceps curl	1X 15-20 with 90 seconds rest between paired sets	109
7a.	One-leg hip bridge	1X 20-30 each side	146
7b.	Shoulder tap plank	1X 20-30 seconds	186

*Use a resistance band instead of a cable to perform this exercise in the manner provided in the exercise description.

** Perform this movement without using dumbbells in the manner provided in the exercise description. You can also perform this movement without the front foot elevated if needed.

Table 10.10   Beginner Bodyweight and Band Workout 2

Exercise		Sets and reps	Page
1a.	Elevated dumbbell reverse lunge (without dumbbells)**	2× 12-15 each side	126
1b.	One-arm motorcycle cable row (with resistance band)*	2× 25-30 seconds with 90 seconds rest between paired sets	94
2a.	Push-up	2× max reps	62
2b.	One-arm cable row (with resistance band)*	2× 15-20 each side with 90 seconds rest between paired sets	93
3a.	Resistance band one-arm incline press	2× 15-20	106
3b.	One-leg 45-degree cable Romanian deadlift (with resistance band)*	2× 15-20 each side with 90 seconds rest between paired sets	147
4a.	Resistance band overhead triceps extension	2× 15-20	106
4b.	Resistance band biceps curl	2× 15-20 with 90 seconds rest between paired sets	109
5a.	Side-lying hip adduction	2× 15-20 each side	153
5b.	Stability ball rollout	2× 15-20 with 90 seconds rest between paired sets	176
6a.	One-leg hip bridge	2× 15-25 each side	146
6b.	Low to high cable chop (with resistance band)*	2× 12-15 each side with 90 seconds rest between paired sets	165

*Use a resistance band instead of a cable to perform this exercise in the manner provided in the exercise description.

**Perform this movement without using dumbbells in the manner provided in the exercise description. Also, if you don't have an aerobic step platform or weight plate to elevate your front foot, you can use a thick book or a folded towel. Or, you can just perform this exercise without the front foot elevated.

11 { Fitness Programs

This chapter is for those who want to improve and maintain their overall health and fitness levels. If you're not necessarily interested in changing your eating habits, but you're exercising more to manage your weight and offset all the foods you love to eat while staying active and building a stronger body that can get things done (i.e., improve performance), then the programs in this chapter are for you!

The programs in this chapter use elements from the function and performance, fat loss, and physique programs and will help you improve your muscle, strength, and metabolism. But they do more than simply help you improve your overall fitness level and general health. They help set the fitness foundation to ensure that your body is ready to safely and more effectively perform the function and performance, fat loss, and physique workouts provided in the next three chapters. Regardless of which of those three workouts you use, it is smartest and safest to start (for at least six weeks) with the fitness programs in this chapter.

The Basics of Fitness Programs

Gauging exercise success doesn't just come in the form of gaining muscle size, lifting bigger weights, or dropping a waist size. You can also judge your exercise success by how much you've enjoyed each workout, how you feel at the end of the workout, and how many workouts you've completed per week. As explained in chapter 1, in addition to the obvious aesthetic and athletic benefits, there are numerous well-documented physical and mental health benefits of regular exercise.

The programs in this book are more similar than they are different. What makes a program more focused on something like function and performance, fat loss, physique, or more general fitness (and health) isn't the exercises that are included—most of the same exercises appear in each—it's how many sets, how many reps, how long you rest, and the organization and order of the workouts.

Gym-based programs are the focus of this chapter. Since you can't always make it to the gym, and while your primary training should

Your Gym Bag

There are a couple pieces of portable equipment that I recommend you always have in your gym bag—resistance bands with handles and resistance band loops. These bands allow you to group exercises requiring immobile equipment (e.g., squat rack or machine) with bands, which are mobile equipment. This enables you to use band exercises within a paired set or triset while you remain at the immobile equipment and don't have to walk all over the gym, thus potentially losing your equipment to another member.

There are two places online that I recommend you go to purchase high-quality resistance bands: Power-Systems.com and Sorinex.com. At Power Systems, the resistance bands with handles to get are the *Double Cords*; the resistance band loops are called *strength bands*, and resistance band mini loops are called *Versa Loops*. At Sorinex Exercise Equipment, resistance band loops are called *strength bands*, and resistance band mini loops are called *short bands*.

be done using equipment, this chapter also provides two home gym or hotel gym fitness workouts along with two more fitness workouts using only bodyweight and resistance band exercises that you can use on the days when you're traveling or don't have access to any kind of gym equipment.

There are guidelines for using the programs in this chapter. Some of these guidelines will be the same for all the program chapters featured in this book, but others differ depending on which type of program you're doing. Let's look at the key points to remember for your fitness programs:

- Perform the exercises designated with *a* or *b* as paired sets, and perform exercises with *a*, *b*, and *c* as trisets. Perform all reps in each set before moving to the next set. Once all exercises within a set are complete, you can rest a bit longer than indicated between sets (if necessary) to complete the designated number of reps with good control. Completing one round of the exercises in a paired or triset is considered one set.

- The rep range (i.e., 10-15 reps) is next to each exercise in the workout in the next two sections. If you're using the same weight for each set, you may be able to do 15 reps on the first set, 12 reps on the next set, and 10 reps on the third set due to accumulated fatigue. Or, you can reduce the weight you're using with each consecutive set to achieve the higher end or given rep range on each consecutive set. Both methods are effective at helping you to progress.

- When a program indicates to take a break before beginning a new cycle, this doesn't mean you have to do nothing. During your days off, you can do some low-impact activities, such as going for long walks, hikes, bike rides, or swims. Also, yoga can be a great option for your active rest periods. If you're already doing yoga each week, as recommended earlier, you can simply increase your yoga practice in your (active) rest week from the gym. Taking 4 to 7 days to "deload" before repeating a workout cycle can minimize the risk of overtraining and helps you continue to make gains. It also makes you hungry to get back into the gym, which can help you avoid getting in the habit of simply going through the motions.

- Maintain strict form, without cheating by using additional movements or momentum. Mentally focus on the working muscles in each exercise.

- Do the concentric (lifting) portion of each rep at a normal tempo and maintain control during the eccentric (lowering) portion.

- Use a weight load that leaves you unable to perform any more reps than indicated while maintaining proper control and technique.

- If an exercise causes pain or discomfort beyond the sensation associated with muscle fatigue, utilize an alternative exercise that doesn't hurt. There are plenty of movements in the exercise chapters of this book to choose from.

- Remember, before you begin a workout in the following programs, be sure to perform one of the dynamic warm-up sequences in chapter 5.

Fitness Workout Programs

There are two versions of each of the eight total body fitness workouts, for a total of 16 different workouts (see tables 11.1-11.8). The B version of each workout consists of the same exercises, but they're done for a different set and rep range than the A version. On the workout days when you're performing fewer overall sets of the resistance exercises, you'll finish with a conditioning component to the workout.

A good ongoing training program should have enough consistency to allow you to see progress while also having enough variety to prevent staleness and boredom. This means using the same basic exercises but in different ways, which is exactly what you're doing when performing the exercises for different set and rep ranges and alternating which workouts include a conditioning finisher.

It's important to note that how often you regularly workout each week depends on why you're exercising to begin with. Most people who are exercising for general fitness and health purposes—working out is often secondary to them—train less frequently than those who are exercising with a focus on function and performance, physique, or fat loss. With this in mind, the workout programs featured here are total body fitness programs that assume you're going to miss the next workout due to life getting in the way. These workouts are designed to be used at least two or three times per week (preferred over twice per week if your schedule allows) but no more than four times per week and no more than two days in a row to maximize recovery and minimize the risk of overtraining. If you're dedicated to exercising more frequently than that, you're not a recreational exerciser who is satisfied with the types of general fitness programs in this chapter. You are an exercise enthusiast who's better off either doing something like yoga, hiking, taking a long bike ride, swimming, etc. on a few of the days you're not doing the workout programs in this chapter. Or you may be interested in trying the workouts in chapter 14, Physique Programs, which gives you an option to train more frequently than four times per week. Tables 11.9-11.11 show a few ways a weekly setup could be used with the fitness programs for training two, three, or four times per week.

Table 11.1   Gym-Based Fitness Program 1

		Workout A	Workout B	Page
1a.	Trap bar squat	4× 8-10	3× 12-15	139
1b.	Stability ball plate crunch	4× 8-10 with 90 seconds rest between paired sets	3× 12-15 with 90 seconds rest between paired sets	170
2a.	Pull-up (with machine or resistance band loop assistance if needed)	4× 6-8	3× 12-15	118
2b.	Dumbbell rotational shoulder press	4× 6-8 with 90 seconds rest between paired sets	3× 10-14 with 90 seconds rest between paired sets	83
3a.	One-arm cable row	3× 12-15 each side	2× 20-25 each side	93
3b.	One-arm cable press	3× 12-15 each side with 90 seconds rest between paired sets	2× 20-25 each side with 90 seconds rest between paired sets	92
4a.	One-leg 45-degree cable Romanian deadlift	3× 12-15 each side	2× 20-25 each side	147
4b.	Cable triceps rope extension	3× 12-15	2× 20-25	98
4c.	Cable rope face pull	3× 12-15 with 90 seconds rest between tri-sets	2× 20-25 with 90 seconds. rest between tri-sets	74
Conditioning			High-resistance upright bike sprints: 10 seconds on (as fast as you can go) and 50 seconds rest × 4-8 rounds	191

Table 11.2   Gym-Based Fitness Program 2

		Workout A	Workout B	Page
1a.	Barbell bent-over row	3× 12-15	4× 8-10	63
1b.	Elevated dumbbell reverse lunge	3× 12-15 each side with 90 seconds rest between paired sets	4× 8-10 each side with 90 seconds rest between paired sets	126
2a.	Machine chest press	3× 12-15	4× 6-8	102
2b.	Stability ball leg curl variations (exercises noted)	Stability ball leg curl 3× 14-20 with 90 seconds rest between paired sets	One-leg stability ball leg curl 4× 6-8 each side with 90 seconds rest between paired sets	154
3a.	Lat pull-down	2× 20-25	3× 12-15	58
3b.	Weight plate speed chop	2× 20-25 each side with 90 seconds rest between paired sets	3× 12-15 each side with 90 seconds rest between paired sets	175
4a.	E-Z bar preacher biceps curl	2× 20-25	3× 12-15	87
4b.	Dumbbell side shoulder raise	2× 20-25	3× 12-15	71
4c.	Cross-body plank	2× 14-16 each side with 90 seconds rest between trisets	3× 8-10 each side with 90 seconds rest between trisets	185
Conditioning		Unilateral farmer's walk complex: 2-3 sets with 2-3 min rest between sets		196

Table 11.3   Gym-Based Fitness Program 3

		Workout A	Workout B	Page
1a.	Dumbbell leaning Bulgarian split squat	4× 8-12 each side	3× 15-18 each side	128
1b.	Reverse crunch	4× 8-10 with 90 seconds rest between paired sets	3× 12-15 with 90 seconds rest between paired sets	160
2a.	One-arm half-kneeling angled cable row	4× 8-10 each side	3× 14-16 each side	95
2b.	Angled barbell shoulder to shoulder press	4× 6-8 each side with 90 seconds rest between paired sets	3× 10-14 each side with 90 seconds rest between paired sets	77
3a.	One-arm compound cable row	3× 12-15 each side	2× 20-25 each side	94
3b.	Standing cable chest press	3× 12-15 each side with 90 seconds rest between paired sets	2× 20-25 each side with 90 seconds rest between paired sets	93
4a.	Machine lying hamstring curl	3× 12-15	2× 20-25	151
4b.	One-arm dumbbell overhead triceps extension	3× 12-15	2× 20-25	86
4c.	Dumbbell shoulder A	3× 12-15 with 90 seconds rest between trisets	2× 20-25 with 90 seconds rest between trisets	88
Conditioning			Weight plate push: 40-50 yd (37-46 m) total distance × 3-5 sets. Rest 90 sec to 3 min between sets	192

Table 11.4   Gym-Based Fitness Program 4

		Workout A	Workout B	Page
1a.	Barbell bent-over row	3× 12-15	4× 8-10	63
1b.	Stability ball wall squat	3× 16-20 with 90 seconds rest between paired sets	4× 10-14 with 90 seconds rest between paired sets	141
2a.	Push-up variations (exercises noted)	Stability ball push-up 3× max reps	Close-grip push-up 4× max reps	114 and 113
2b.	Traveling dumbbell Romanian deadlift lunge	3× 14-16 each side with 90 seconds rest between paired sets	4× 8-10 each side with 90 seconds rest between paired sets	144
3a.	Fighter's cable lat pull-down	2× 20-25 each side	3× 12-15 each side	96
3b.	Dumbbell upright row	2× 20-25 with 90 seconds rest between paired sets	3× 12-15 with 90 seconds rest between paired sets	69
4a.	Low-to-high cable chop	2× 20-25 each side	3× 12-15 each side	165
4b.	Cable compound straight-arm pull-down	2× 20-25	3× 12-15	99
4c.	Abdominal rollout variations (exercises noted)	Stability ball rollout 2× 20-25 with 90 seconds rest between trisets	Arm walkout 3× 6-8 with 90 seconds rest between trisets	176 and 183
Conditioning		Weight plate complex: 3-4 rounds with 2-3 min rest between rounds		203

Table 11.5 Gym-Based Fitness Program 5

		Workout A	Workout B	Page
1a.	Barbell hybrid deadlift	4× 8-10	3× 12-15	124
1b.	Stability ball plate crunch	4× 8-10 with 90 seconds rest between paired sets	3× 12-15 with 90 seconds rest between paired sets	170
2a.	Chin-up (with machine or resistance band loop assistance if needed)	4× 6-8	3×12-15	117
2b.	Dumbbell rotational shoulder press	4× 6-8 each side with 90 seconds rest between paired sets	3× 10-14 each side with 90 seconds rest between paired sets	83
3a.	Two-arm dumbbell bent-over row	3× 12-15	2× 20-25	66
3b.	Machine chest press	3× 12-15 with 90 seconds rest between paired sets	2× 20-25 with 90 seconds rest between paired sets	102
4a.	One-leg dumbbell bench hip thrust	3× 12-16 each side	2× 20-25 each side	145
4b.	Off-bench side lean hold	3× 15-20 sec each side	2× 25-30 sec each side	184
4c.	Dumbbell triceps skull crusher	3× 12-15 with 90 seconds rest between trisets	2× 20-25 with 90 seconds rest between trisets	73
Conditioning			High-resistance upright bike sprints: 10 sec on (as fast as you can) and 50 sec rest × 4-8 rounds	191

Table 11.6 Gym-Based Fitness Program 6

		Workout A	Workout B	Page
1a.	One-arm dumbbell off-bench row	3× 12-15 each side	4× 8-10 each side	83
1b.	Dumbbell step-up	3× 12-15 each side with 90 seconds rest between paired sets	4× 8-10 each side with 90 seconds rest between paired sets	132
2a.	Push-up variations (exercises noted)	Box crossover push-up 3× max reps	Lockoff push-up 4× 6-10 each side	112 and 111
2b.	45-degree hip extension	3× 14-16 with 90 seconds rest between paired sets	4× 8-12 with 90 seconds rest between paired sets	131
3a.	Lat pull-down (neutral grip)	2× 20-25	3× 12-15	91
3b.	Weight plate around the world	2× 20-25 with 90 seconds rest between paired sets	3× 12-15 with 90 seconds rest between paired sets	182
4a.	Side-lying hip adduction	2× 20-25 each side	3× 12-15 each side	153
4b.	Dumbbell biceps curl	2× 20-25	3× 12-15	68
4c.	Stability ball abdominal variations (exercises noted)	Stability ball knee tuck 2× 16-25 with 90 seconds rest between trisets	Stability ball pike 3× 8-12 with 90 seconds rest between trisets	181 and 177
Conditioning		Unilateral farmer's walk complex: 2-3 sets with 2-3 min rest between sets		196

Table 11.7 Gym-Based Fitness Program 7

		Workout A	Workout B	Page
1a.	Elevated dumbbell leaning reverse lunge	4× 7-10 each side	3× 12-15 each side	125
1b.	Abdominal rollout variations (exercises noted)	Ab wheel rollout with resistance band 4× 5-8 with 90 seconds rest between paired sets	Stability ball rollout 3× 14-16 with 90 seconds rest between paired sets	169 and 176
2a.	Leaning lat pull-down	4× 8-10	3× 14-16	60
2b.	One-arm angled barbell press	4× 6-8 each side with 90 seconds rest between paired sets	3× 10-14 each side with 90 seconds rest between paired sets	77
3a.	Underhand grip Smith bar row	3× 12-15	2× 20-25	115
3b.	Dumbbell bench press	3× 12-15 with 90 seconds rest between paired sets	2× 20-25 with 90 seconds rest between paired sets	81
4a.	Machine seated hamstring curl	3× 12-15	2× 20-25	150
4b.	Dumbbell plank row	3× 7-9 each side	2× 12-15 each side	182
4c.	Dumbbell triceps kickback	3× 12-15 with 90 seconds rest between trisets	2× 20-25 with 90 seconds rest between trisets	86
Conditioning			Weight plate push: 40-50 yd (37-46 m) total distance × 3-5 sets. Rest 90 sec to 3 min between sets	192

Table 11.8 Gym-Based Fitness Program 8

		Workout A	Workout B	Page
1a.	One-arm dumbbell freestanding row	3× 12-15 each side	4× 8-10 each side	84
1b.	Mid-platform machine leg press	3× 14-16 with 90 seconds rest between paired sets	4× 8-12 with 90 seconds rest between paired sets	149
2a.	Barbell bench press	3× 12-15	4× 8-10	79
2b.	One-leg one-arm dumbbell Romanian deadlift	3× 12-15 each side with 90 seconds rest between paired sets	4× 8-10 each side with 90 seconds rest between paired sets	144
3a.	Lat pull-down (underhand grip)	2× 20-25	3× 12-15	58
3b.	Dumbbell front shoulder raise	2× 20-25 with 90 seconds rest between paired sets	3× 12-15 with 90 seconds rest between paired sets	70
4a.	High-to-low cable chop	2× 20-25 each side	3× 12-15 each side	168
4b.	Low-cable one-arm face-away biceps curl	2× 18-25 each side	3× 12-15 each side	101
4c.	Low-cable one-arm rear delt fly	2×18-25 each side with 90 seconds. rest between trisets	3× 12-15 each side with 90 seconds rest between trisets	98
Conditioning		Weight plate complex: 3-4 rounds with 2-3 min rest between rounds		203

Table 11.9 Sample Gym-Based Training Setup: Two Times per Week

Week 1	Week 2
Monday: Program 1, workout A	*Monday:* Program 3, workout A
Tuesday: Rest	*Tuesday:* Rest
Wednesday: Rest	*Wednesday:* Rest
Thursday: Program 2, workout A	*Thursday:* Program 4, workout A
Friday: Rest	*Friday:* Rest
Saturday: Rest	*Saturday:* Rest
Sunday: Rest	*Sunday:* Rest
Week 3	**Week 4**
Monday: Program 5, workout A	*Monday:* Program 7, workout A
Tuesday: Rest	*Tuesday:* Rest
Wednesday: Rest	*Wednesday:* Rest
Thursday: Program 6, workout A	*Thursday:* Program 8, workout A
Friday: Rest	*Friday:* Rest
Saturday: Rest	*Saturday:* Rest
Sunday: Rest	*Sunday:* Rest
Week 5*	
Monday: Program 1, workout B	
Tuesday: Rest	
Wednesday: Rest	
Thursday: Program 2, workout B	
Friday: Rest	
Saturday: Rest	
Sunday: Rest	

*On week six, you'd perform program 3, workout B and program 4, workout B. On week seven, you'd perform program 5, workout B; program 6, workout B; and so on. Once you complete week 8, you'll repeat the cycle again, starting with program 1, workout A.

Table 11.10 Sample Gym-Based Training Setup: Three Times per Week

Week 1	Week 2
Monday: Program 1, workout A	*Monday:* Program 4, workout A
Tuesday: Rest	*Tuesday:* Rest
Wednesday: Program 2, workout A	*Wednesday:* Program 5, workout A
Thursday: Rest	*Thursday:* Rest
Friday: Program 3, workout A	*Friday:* Program 6, workout A
Saturday: Rest	*Saturday:* Rest
Sunday: Rest	*Sunday:* Rest
Week 3	**Week 4**
Monday: Program 7, workout A	*Monday:* Program 2, workout B
Tuesday: Rest	*Tuesday:* Rest
Wednesday: Program 8, workout A	*Wednesday:* Program 3, workout B
Thursday: Rest	*Thursday:* Rest

Week 3	Week 4
Friday: Program 1, workout B	*Friday:* Program 4, workout B
Saturday: Rest	*Saturday:* Rest
Sunday: Rest	*Sunday:* Rest
Week 5	**Week 6***
Monday: Program 5, workout B	*Monday:* Program 8, workout B
Tuesday: Rest	*Tuesday:* Rest
Wednesday: Program 6, workout B	*Wednesday:* Program 1, workout A
Thursday: Rest	*Thursday:* Rest
Friday: Program 7, workout B	*Friday:* Program 2, workout A
Saturday: Rest	*Saturday:* Rest
Sunday: Rest	*Sunday:* Rest

*On week six, you'll repeat the cycle again, starting with program 1, workout A, and so on.

Table 11.11   Sample Gym-Based Training Setup: Four Times per Week

Week 1	Week 2
Monday: Program 1, workout A	*Monday:* Program 5, workout A
Tuesday: Program 2, workout A	*Tuesday:* Program 6, workout A
Wednesday: Rest	*Wednesday:* Rest
Thursday: Program 3, workout A	*Thursday:* Program 7, workout A
Friday: Program 4, workout A	*Friday:* Program 8, workout A
Saturday: Rest	*Saturday:* Rest
Sunday: Rest	*Sunday:* Rest
Week 3	**Week 4***
Monday: Program 1, workout B	*Monday:* Program 5, workout B
Tuesday: Program 2, workout B	*Tuesday:* Program 6, workout B
Wednesday: Rest	*Wednesday:* Rest
Thursday: Program 3, workout B	*Thursday:* Program 7, workout B
Friday: Program 4, workout B	*Friday:* Program 8, workout B
Saturday: Rest	*Saturday:* Rest
Sunday: Rest	*Sunday:* Rest

*In this setup, you've have completed the entire cycle of workouts in four weeks. It will be four weeks until you repeat the same workout by beginning the cycle again with program 1, workout A.

Sample Fitness Home or Hotel Gym Workouts

On days that you're traveling, can't make it to the gym, or don't have access to a gym, you can use these home or hotel gym workouts or the band and bodyweight workouts for function and performance. The two workouts in tables 11.12 and 11.13 use equipment that's either recommended for your home gym or that's commonly found in most hotel gyms. That equipment is as follows:

- A set of dumbbells (up to 50 lb or 20 kg)
- An adjustable weight bench that can be made flat or set at an incline
- A high-quality stability ball that's 55 to 65 centimeters

- A chin-up bar (many are designed to be easily placed inside the top of a doorway)
- A set of resistance bands with handles of varying strengths from light to very heavy
- Resistance band loops of varying strength from light to medium
- Resistance band mini loops of varying strength from light to medium

Resistance bands, resistance band loops, and resistance band mini loops are affordable and available at most sporting goods stores or online, but they are not often found at hotel gyms. I recommend traveling with at least one set of each type of band. They're portable and easy to pack in your luggage. It's also important to note that since the following workouts are designed to be done with limited equipment, some of the exercises included will require small modifications from how they're featured in the exercise descriptions. For example, for a cable-based exercise such as the One-Arm Cable Row, you'd perform it with a resistance band instead of cable if your training environment doesn't feature a cable column. Or, for a dumbbell exercise such as the Dumbbell Shoulder W, you'd simply perform the same movement as shown in the exercise description without holding dumbbells. These modifications are indicated within each of the following workouts.

Also, these workouts are intended to be used *only* as an addition to your regular weekly gym-based workouts on days when you're traveling, can't make it to the gym, or don't have access to a gym. These workouts are *not* intended to replace your gym-based workouts; your primary training should revolve around using the gym-based programs in the previous section. Before you begin any of the following workouts, be sure to perform one of the dynamic warm-up sequences in chapter 5.

The two workouts in tables 11.14 and 11.15 have bodyweight exercises and resistance band exercises utilizing three types of bands: resistance bands with handles (these can be attached to any doorway or stable object in matter of seconds), resistance band loops, and resistance mini band loops. A set of high-quality resistance bands with handles and both types of resistance band loops—they come in multiple resistances from light to very heavy—for home use and to take with you when you travel are a must. They are portable and add a number of effective exercise options to your bodyweight training workouts, delivering a value that far exceeds their cost.

Again, the following workouts are *not* intended to be done exclusively and are not designed to replace the gym-based programs earlier in this chapter. They are only an addition to your regular weekly gym-based workouts on days when you don't have access to any kind of gym.

Table 11.12 Fitness Home or Hotel Gym Workout 1

Exercise	Sets and reps	Page
1a. Elevated dumbbell reverse lunge**	4× 8-10 each side	126
1b. Stability ball plate crunch***	4× 12-15 with 90 seconds rest between paired sets	170
2a. Pull-up (resistance band loop assistance if needed)	4× 6-8	118
2b. Dumbbell rotational shoulder press	4× 6-8 each side with 90 seconds rest between paired sets	83
3a. One-arm cable row (with resistance band)*	3× 14-16 each side	93
3b. One-arm cable press (with resistance band)*	3× 14-16 each side with 90 seconds rest between paired sets	92
4a. Dumbbell lateral Romanian deadlift lunge	3× 10-12 each side	142
4b. Dumbbell triceps skull crusher	3× 12-15 with 90 seconds rest between paired sets	73
5. Low-to-high cable chop (with resistance band)*	2× 12-15 each side with 90 seconds rest between sets	165
Conditioning	Two-minute bodyweight complex: × 2-3 rounds with 2-3 min rest between rounds	207

*Use a resistance band instead of a cable to perform this exercise in the manner provided in the exercise description.

**If you don't have an aerobic step platform or weight plate to elevate your front foot, you can use a thick book or a folded towel. Or, you can just perform this exercise without the front foot elevated.

***If you don't have a weight plate, you can hold each side of a dumbbell instead.

Table 11.13 Fitness Home or Hotel Gym Workout 2

Exercise	Sets and reps	Page
1a. Dumbbell bench press	3× 12-15	81
1b. Dumbbell leaning Bulgarian split squat	3× 10-15 each side with 90 seconds rest between paired sets	128
2a. Two-arm dumbbell bent-over row	3× 12-15	66
2b. Stability ball leg curl	3× 15-25 with 90 seconds rest between paired sets	154
3a. One-arm motorcycle cable row (with resistance band)*	3× 15-20	94
3b. Cable tight torso rotation with hip shift (with resistance band)*	2× 20-25 each side with 90 seconds rest between paired sets	166
4a. Dumbbell biceps curl	2× 20-25	68
4b. Dumbbell side shoulder raise	2× 20-25	71
4c. Cross-body plank	2× 14-16 each side with 90 seconds rest between trisets	185
Conditioning	Bodyweight and resistance band complex: 3 rounds of 15-20 reps each exercise with 2-3 min rest between sets	209

*Use a resistance band instead of a cable to perform this exercise in the manner provided in the exercise description.

Table 11.14　Fitness Bodyweight and Band Workout 1

Exercise	Sets and Reps	Page
1a. Squat jump with arm drive	4× 8-10	136
1b. Reverse crunch	4× 8-12 with 90 seconds rest between paired sets	160
2a. One-arm compound cable row (with resistance band)*	3× 8-10 each side	94
2b. One-arm cable press (with resistance band)*	3× 12-16 each side with 90 seconds rest between paired sets	92
3a. One-arm half-kneeling angled cable row	3× 14-18 each side	95
3b. One-leg hip lift	3× 12-18 each side with 90 seconds rest between paired sets	147
4a. High-to-low cable chop (with resistance band)*	3× 12-15 each side	168
4b. Resistance band triceps extension	3× 12-15	105
4c. Dumbbell shoulder Y (without dumbbells)**	3× 12-15 with 90 seconds rest between tri-sets	89
Conditioning	Bodyweight and resistance band complex: 3 rounds of 15-20 reps each exercise with 2-3 min rest between sets	209

*Use a resistance band instead of a cable to perform this exercise in the manner provided in the exercise description.

**Perform this movement without using dumbbells in the manner provided in the exercise description.

Table 11.15　Fitness Bodyweight and Band Workout 2

Exercise	Sets and reps	Page
1a. Resistance band loop hybrid deadlift	4× 15-20	148
1b. Arm walkout	4× 4-7 with 90 seconds rest between paired sets	183
2a. One-arm motorcycle cable row (with resistance band)*	3× 15-20	94
2b. Cable tight torso rotation with hip shift (with resistance band)*	2× 20-25 each side with 90 seconds rest between paired sets	166
3a. Resistance band bent-over row	3× 15-20	107
3b. Push-up	3× max reps with 90 seconds rest between paired sets	62
4a. Low-to-high cable chop (with resistance band)*	3× 12-15 each side	165
4b. Resistance band biceps curl	3× 12-18 each side	109
4c. One-leg bench hip thrust**	3× 12-18 each side with 90 seconds rest between tri-sets	145
Conditioning	Two-minute bodyweight complex: × 2-3 rounds with 2-3 min rest between rounds	207

*Use a resistance band instead of a cable to perform this exercise in the manner provided in the exercise description.

**If you don't have a weight bench, you can perform this exercise with your shoulders resting on the seat of a padded chair.

12 { Function and Performance Programs

This chapter is for those who aren't necessarily making a career in athletics but are interested in improving overall athleticism. If you're a recreational athlete or weekend warrior and like to gauge success by improvements in your overall strength, explosiveness, and conditioning (ability to resist fatigue), then the workout programs in this chapter are intended for you!

The Basics of Function and Performance Programs

The programs in this chapter focus on improving performance by emphasizing increases in your strength, explosiveness, and conditioning. In each consecutive workout you'll do, you increase strength by adding weight and performing fewer reps for a greater number of sets than in the preceding workout. And, in each consecutive workout, you improve explosiveness by performing more sets of fewer reps than in the preceding workout, adding with a focus on speed. Unlike the programs in the physique, fat loss, or fitness program chapters, which all cycle through different workout sequences frequently, the workouts in this chapter repeat the same exercises for several weeks before switching to different exercises. This ensures progress in the areas these workouts are emphasizing.

Not everyone who is exercising for improved function and performance (i.e., improved strength, power, and conditioning levels) is doing so because they're recreational athletes or weekend warriors looking to improve an ability to play a sport or do a variety of athletic activities outside the gym. Some people are simply interested in improving their performance at the gym by increasing metrics in strength, power, and conditioning during various exercises. Although both types gauge success the same way—making progress in the gym—how often an individual exercises throughout the week is usually (and should be) different. If you're a recreational athlete or weekend warrior, it means you're regularly (one or two times per week) engaging in playing (or practicing) a sport. If so, you should

Your Gym Bag

There are a couple pieces of portable equipment that I recommend you always have in your gym bag—resistance bands with handles and resistance band loops. These bands allow you to group exercises requiring immobile equipment (e.g., squat rack or machine) with bands, which are mobile equipment. This enables you to use band exercises within a paired set or triset while you remain at the immobile equipment and don't have to walk all over the gym, thus potentially losing your equipment to another member.

There are two places online that I recommend you go to purchase high-quality resistance bands: Power-Systems.com and Sorinex.com. At Power Systems, the resistance bands with handles to get are the *Double Cords*; the resistance band loops are called *strength bands*, and resistance band mini loops are called *Versa Loops*. At Sorinex Exercise Equipment, resistance band loops are called *strength bands*, and resistance band mini loops are called *short bands*.

be exercising less often than an exercise enthusiast who is serious about making improvements in strength, power, and conditioning because you do not have to account for recovering from the physical demands of playing and practicing in addition to your training in the gym. Therefore, this chapter provides programs for those who are training two to three times per week and programs for those who are training four to five times per week. Both programs utilize a load–explode theme, which means the workout programs in this chapter incorporate a heavily loaded lift and a lightly loaded explosive movement.

Gym-based programs are the focus of this chapter, but since you can't always make it to the gym or use gym equipment, this chapter also provides two home and hotel gym workouts along with two workouts using only bodyweight and resistance band exercises. You can use them on the days that you're traveling or don't have access to any kind of gym equipment.

There are guidelines for using the programs in this chapter. Some of these guidelines will be the same for all the program chapters featured in this book, but others differ depending on which type of program you're doing. Let's look at the key points to remember for your function and performance programs:

- Perform the exercises designated with *a* or *b* as paired sets, and perform exercises with *a*, *b*, and *c* as trisets. Perform all reps in a given set before moving to the next set. Once all exercises within a set are complete, you can rest a bit longer than indicated between sets (if necessary) to complete the designated number of reps with good control. Completing one round of the exercises in a paired or triset is considered one set.

- The rep range (i.e., 10-15 reps) is next to each exercise in the workout programs in the next two sections. If you're using the same weight for each set, you may be able to do 15 reps on the first set, 12 reps on the next set, and 10 reps on the third set due to accumulated fatigue. Or, you can reduce the weight you're using with each consecutive set to achieve the higher end of given rep range on each consecutive set. Both methods are effective at helping you to progress.

- When a program indicates to take a break before beginning a new cycle, this doesn't mean you have to do nothing. During your days off, you can do some low-impact activities, such as going for long walks, hikes, bike rides, or swims. Also, yoga can be a great option for your active rest periods. If you're already doing yoga each week, as recommended earlier, you can simply increase your yoga practice in your (active) rest week from the gym. Taking 4 to 7 days to "deload" before repeating a workout cycle can minimize the risk of overtraining and helps you continue to make gains. It also makes you hungry to get back into the gym, which can help you avoid getting in the habit of simply going through the motions.

- For the load exercise in each program, use the heaviest weight load that allows you to perform the indicated number of reps while maintaining optimal technique. Perform the concentric lifting portion of each rep as forcefully as you can; during the eccentric (lowering) portion, maintain good control. On the explode exercises, perform each rep as fast and explosively as possible while maintaining optimal technique.

- The rest of the exercises in the programs in this chapter constantly vary sets and reps to make your workouts more comprehensive. Maintain strict form, without cheating by using additional movements or momentum. This involves performing the concentric (lifting) portion of each rep at a normal tempo and maintaining control during the eccentric (lowering) portion. Be sure to use a weight load that leaves you unable to perform any more reps than indicated while maintaining proper control and technique.

- If an exercise causes pain or discomfort beyond the sensation associated with muscle fatigue, utilize an alternative exercise that doesn't hurt. There are plenty of movements in the exercise chapters of this book to choose from.

- Remember, before you begin a workout in the following programs, be sure to perform one of the dynamic warm-up sequences in chapter 5.

Function and Performance Programs

Before you perform these function and performance programs, first complete the beginner programs in chapter 10 if you're just starting out or haven't worked out in a while. If you have been regularly working out or you've completed the beginner programs, it's also recommended that you complete at least six to eight weeks of the fitness programs in chapter 11 before using the following programs.

Gym-Based Function and Performance Programs: Two or Three Times per Week

This section has four different programs with two different total body workouts (see tables 12.1-12.4). You'll alternate between two versions of a workout in each program for four to seven times before switching to another program and repeating those workouts for another four to seven times. The first time you do each workout in a program, it's considered a *reload* workout. A reload workout is simply a lower-intensity version of the workout, which helps you stay active and acclimate yourself to the movements and sequencing of the new program you're doing. Reloading also allows you to use a weight load that doesn't fatigue you so you can recover between programs. It also provides active recovery days between workout programs. See tables 12.5 and 12.6 for sample gym-based function and performance workouts that are appropriate if you work out two to three times per week

The workouts in each program have at least one load exercise where you focus on increasing your strength and at least one explode exercise where you focus on increasing your explosiveness on each consecutive workout. Other exercises are included to vary the set and reps and finish with a conditioning component on the days where you're performing fewer overall sets of the resistance exercises in the mixed set/rep scheme utilized. Explanations for load, explode, and reload are in the previous section, where we discussed key points about these function and performance programs.

The previous total body workouts assume that you're regularly (approximately one to two times per week) engaging in playing (or practicing) in a sport. These workouts are designed to be used at least two or three times per week (three times is preferred over twice per week if your schedule allows). The following tables show how a weekly setup could be used for the two to three times per week program.

Table 12.1 Gym-Based Function and Performance Program 1: Two or Three Times per Week

Program 1A					
	Workout 1: reload*	Workouts 2 and 5	Workouts 3 and 6	Workouts 4 and 7	Page
1. Load: barbell hybrid deadlift	2× 8-10 with 2-3 minutes rest between sets	4× 6-7 with 3-5 minutes rest between sets	5× 4-5 with 3-5 minutes rest between sets	6× 2-3 with 3-5 minutes rest between sets	124
2. Explode: barbell high pull	2× 3-4 with 2-3 minutes rest between sets	6× 3-4 with 2-3 minutes rest between sets	5× 5-6 with 2-3 minutes rest between sets	4× 7-8 with 2-3 minutes rest between sets	76
3a. Dumbbell step-up	2× 6-8 each side	4× 6-8 each side	3× 10-14 each side	2× 17-20 each side	132
3b. Stability ball plate crunch	2× 6-8 with 90 seconds rest between paired sets	4× 6-8 with 90 seconds rest between paired sets	3× 10-12 with 90 seconds rest between paired sets	2× 15-17 with 90 seconds rest between paired sets	170
4a. Standing cable chest press	2× 8-10	4× 8-10	3× 12-14	2× 17-20	93
4b. One-arm compound cable row	2× 6-8 each side with 90 seconds rest between paired sets	4× 6-8 each side with 90 seconds rest between paired sets	3× 10-14 each side with 90 seconds rest between paired sets	2× 17-20 each side with 90 seconds rest between paired sets	94
5a. Cable triceps rope extension	2× 8-10	4× 6-8	3× 10-14	2× 17-20	98
5b. Cable rope face pull	2× 8-10 with 90 seconds rest between paired sets	4× 6-8 with 90 seconds rest between paired sets	3× 10-14 with 90 seconds rest between paired sets	2× 17-20 with 90 seconds rest between paired sets	74

	Program 1A				
	Workout 1: reload*	Workouts 2 and 5	Workouts 3 and 6	Workouts 4 and 7	Page
Conditioning			High-resistance upright bike sprints: 10 sec on and 50 sec off × 4-8 rounds	Unilateral farmer's walk complex: 2-3 sets with 2-3 min rest between sets	191 and 196

	Program 1B				
	Workout 1: reload*	Workouts 2 and 5	Workouts 3 and 6	Workouts 4 and 7	Page
1. Load: chin-up (with machine or resistance band loop assistance if needed)	8-10 with 2-3 minutes rest between sets	4× 6-7 with 3-5 minutes rest between sets	5× 4-5 with 3-5 minutes rest between sets	6× 2-3 with 3-5 minutes rest between sets	117
2. Explode: squat jump with arm drive	2× 3-4 with 2-3 minutes rest between sets	6× 3-4 with 2-3 minutes rest between sets	5× 5-6 with 2-3 minutes rest between sets	4× 7-8 with 2-3 minutes rest between sets	136
3a. Dumbbell rotational shoulder press	2× 6-8 each side	3× 10-14 each side	2× 16-18 each side	4× 6-8 each side	83
3b. One-arm cable row	2× 6-8 each side with 90 seconds rest between paired sets	3× 10-14 each side with 90 seconds rest between paired sets	2× 17-20 each side with 90 seconds rest between paired sets	4× 6-8 each side with 90 seconds rest between paired sets	93
4a. One-leg dumbbell bench hip thrust	2× 6-8 each side	3× 10-14 each side	2× 17-20 each side	4× 6-8 each side	145
4b. Dumbbell plank row	2× 6-8 each side with 90 seconds rest between paired sets	3× 8-9 each side with 90 seconds rest between paired sets	2× 11-12 each side with 90 seconds rest between paired sets	4× 5-6 each side with 90 seconds rest between paired sets	182
5a. Hamstring variations (exercises noted)	Machine lying hamstring curl 2× 8-10	One-leg stability ball leg curl 3× 10-14 each side	Machine seated hamstring curl 2× 17-20	Machine lying hamstring curl 4× 6-8	151, 154, 150, and 151
5b. Dumbbell biceps curl	2× 8-10 with 90 seconds rest between paired sets	3× 10-14 with 90 seconds rest between paired sets	2× 17-20 with 90 seconds rest between paired sets	4× 6-8 with 90 seconds rest between paired sets	68
6. Conditioning		300-yd (274 m) shuttle run: 1-3 sets with 2-4 min rest between sets	Weight plate complex: 3-4 rounds with 2-3 min rest between rounds		188 and 203

*Reload: Perform all exercises at a low intensity. On a scale of 1 to 10, you should be working at about a 3 or 4. Work at 7 to 9 on all other workouts.

Table 12.2 Gym-Based Function and Performance Program 2: Two or Three Times per Week

		Program 2A				
		Workout 1: reload*	Workouts 2 and 5	Workouts 3 and 6	Workouts 4 and 7	Page
1.	Load: trap bar squat or barbell front squat	2× 8-10 with 2-3 minutes rest between sets	4× 6-7 with 3-5 minutes rest between sets	5× 4-5 with 3-5 minutes rest between sets	6× 2-3 with 3-5 minutes rest between sets	139 or 122
2.	Explode: explosive box crossover push-up	2× 3-4 each side with 2-3 minutes rest between sets	6× 3-4 each side with 2-3 minutes rest between sets	5× 5-6 each side with 2-3 minutes rest between sets	4× 7-8 each side with 2-3 minutes rest between sets	113
3a.	Barbell Romanian deadlift	2× 8-10	4× 6-8	3× 10-14	2× 17-20	139
3b.	Reverse crunch	2× 6-8 with 90 seconds rest between paired sets	4× 6-8 with 90 seconds rest between paired sets	3× 10-14 with 90 seconds rest between paired sets	2× 17-20 with 90 seconds rest between paired sets	160
4a.	Fighter's cable lat pull-down	2× 8-10 each side	4× 6-8 each side	3× 10-14 each side	2× 17-20 each side	96
4b.	Dumbbell rotational shoulder press	2× 6-8 each side with 90 seconds rest between paired sets	4× 6-8 each side with 90 seconds rest between paired sets	3× 10-12 each side with 90 seconds rest between paired sets	2× 18-20 each side with 90 seconds rest between paired sets	83
5a.	Dumbbell incline bench biceps curl	2× 8-10	4× 6-8	3× 10-14	2× 17-20	88
5b.	Dumbbell shoulder T	2× 8-10 with 90 seconds rest between paired sets	4× 6-8 with 90 seconds rest between paired sets	3× 10-14 with 90 seconds rest between paired sets	2× 17-20 with 90 seconds rest between paired sets	90
Conditioning				Weight plate push: 40-50 yd (37-46 m) total distance × 3-5 sets. Rest 90 sec -3 min between sets	Dumbbell farmer's walk complex: 3-4 rounds with 2-3 min rest between rounds	192 and 193

		Program 2B				
		Workout 1: reload*	Workouts 2 and 5	Workouts 3 and 6	Workouts 4 and 7	Page
1.	Load: one-arm dumbbell row	2× 8-10 each side with 2-3 minutes rest between sets	4× 6-7 each side with 3-5 minutes rest between sets	5× 4-5 each side with 3-5 minutes rest between sets	6× 2-3 each side with 3-5 minutes rest between sets	64
2.	Explode: lateral bench scissor jump	2× 4-5 each side with 2-3 minutes rest between sets	6× 3-4 each side with 2-3 minutes rest between sets	5× 5-6 each side with 2-3 minutes rest between sets	4× 7-8 each side with 2-3 minutes rest between sets	138

Program 2B					
	Workout 1: reload*	Workouts 2 and 5	Workouts 3 and 6	Workouts 4 and 7	Page
3a. One-arm angled barbell press	2× 8-10 each side	3× 10-14 each side	2× 17-20 each side	4× 6-8 each side	77
3b. Lat pull-down (underhand grip)	2× 8-10 with 90 seconds rest between paired sets	3× 10-14 with 90 seconds rest between paired sets	2× 17-20 with 90 seconds rest between paired sets	4× 6-8 with 90 seconds rest between paired sets	58
4a. 45-degree hip extension	2× 6-8 each side	3× 10-14 each side	2× 17-20 each side	4× 6-8 each side	131
4b. Cross-body plank	2× 5-6 each side with 90 seconds rest between paired sets	3× 10-12 each side with 90 seconds rest between paired sets	2× 14-15 each side with 90 seconds rest between paired sets	4× 6-8 each side with 90 seconds rest between paired sets	185
5a. Hip adduction variations (exercises noted)	Machine hip adduction 2× 8-10	One-leg cable hip adduction 3× 10-14 each side	Side-lying hip adduction 2× 17-20 each side	Machine hip adduction 4× 6-8	152, 148, 153, and 152
5b. One-arm dumbbell overhead triceps extension	2× 8-10 each side with 90 seconds rest between paired sets	3× 10-14 each side with 90 seconds rest between paired sets	2× 17-20 each side with 90 seconds rest between paired sets	4× 6-8 each side with 90 seconds rest between paired sets	86
Conditioning		One-mile (1.6 km) run (outside or on treadmill) for time	Weight plate complex: 3-4 rounds with 2-3 min rest between rounds		191 and 203

*Reload: Perform all exercises at a low intensity. On a scale of 1 to 10, you should be working at about a 3 or 4. Work at 7 to 9 on all other workouts.

Table 12.3 Gym-Based Function and Performance Program 3: Two or Three Times per Week

Program 3A					
	Workout 1: reload*	Workouts 2 and 5	Workouts 3 and 6	Workouts 4 and 7	Page
1. Load: barbell rack pull	2× 8-10 with 2-3 minutes rest between sets	4× 6-7 with 3-5 minutes rest between sets	5× 4-5 with 3-5 minutes rest between sets	6× 2-3 with 3-5 minutes rest between sets	140
2. Explode: angled barbell press and catch	2× 3-4 each side with 2-3 minutes rest between sets	6× 3-4 each side with 2-3 minutes rest between sets	5× 5-6 each side with 2-3 minutes rest between sets	4× 7-8 each side with 2-3 minutes rest between sets	76
3a. Elevated dumbbell reverse lunge	2× 6-8 each side	4× 6-8 each side	3× 10-14 each side	2× 17-20 each side	126
3b. Stability ball plate crunch	2× 8-10 with 90 seconds rest between paired sets	4× 6-8 with 90 seconds rest between paired sets	3× 10-14 with 90 seconds rest between paired sets	2× 17-20 with 90 seconds rest between paired sets	170

> continued

Table 12.3   > *continued*

Program 3A					
	Workout 1: reload*	Workouts 2 and 5	Workouts 3 and 6	Workouts 4 and 7	Page
4a. Barbell bent-over row	2× 8-10	4× 6-8	3× 10-14	2× 17-20	63
4b. Push-up variations (exercises noted)	Push-up 2× 8-10 with 90 seconds rest between paired sets	Resistance band loop push-up 4× 6-8 with 90 seconds rest between paired sets	Push-up or feet-elevated push-up (depending on your strength level) 3× 10-14 with 90 seconds rest between paired sets	Stability ball push-up 2× 17-20 with 90 seconds rest between paired sets	62, 105, 62 or 114, and 114
5a. Machine rear delt fly	2× 8-10	4×6-8	3× 10-14	2× 17-20	103
5b. Dumbbell biceps curl	2× 8-10 with 90 seconds rest between paired sets	4× 6-8 with 90 seconds rest between paired sets	3× 10-14 with 90 seconds rest between paired sets	2× 17-20 with 90 seconds rest between paired sets	68
Conditioning			High-resistance upright bike sprints: 10 sec on and 50 sec off × 4-8 rounds	Unilateral farmer's walk complex: 2-3 sets with 2-3 min rest between sets	191 and 196

Program 3B					
	Workout 1: reload*	Workouts 2 and 5	Workouts 3 and 6	Workouts 4 and 7	Page
1. Load: lat pull-down with neutral grip	2× 8-10 with 2-3 minutes rest between sets	4× 6-7 with 3-5 minutes rest between sets	5× 4-5 with 3-5 minutes rest between sets	6× 2-3 with 3-5 minutes rest between sets	91
2. Explode: broad jump	2× 3-4 with 2-3 minutes rest between sets	6× 3-4 with 2-3 minutes rest between sets	5× 5-6 with 2-3 minutes rest between sets	4× 7-8 with 2-3 minutes rest between sets	137
3a. Dumbbell incline bench press	2× 8-10	4× 6-8	3× 10-14	2× 17-20	82
3b. Two-arm dumbbell bent-over row	2× 8-10 with 90 seconds rest between paired sets	4× 6-8 with 90 seconds rest between paired sets	3× 10-14 with 90 seconds rest between paired sets	2× 17-20 with 90 seconds rest between paired sets	66
4a. Dumbbell lateral Romanian deadlift lunge	2× 6-8 each side	3× 10-14 each side	2× 16-18 each side	4× 6-8 each side	142
4b. One-arm plank	2× 6-8 each side with 90 seconds rest between paired sets	3× 8-9 each side with 90 seconds rest between paired sets	2× 11-12 each side with 90 seconds rest between paired sets	4× 5-6 each side with 90 seconds rest between paired sets	183

		Program 3B				
		Workout 1: reload*	Workouts 2 and 5	Workouts 3 and 6	Workouts 4 and 7	Page
5a.	Hamstring variations (exercises noted)	Machine seated hamstring curl 2× 8-10	One-leg stability ball leg curl 3× 10-14 each side	Machine seated hamstring curl 2× 17-20	Machine lying hamstring curl 4× 6-8	150, 154, 150, and 151
5b.	Dumbbell triceps kickback	2× 8-10 with 90 seconds rest between paired sets	3× 10-14 with 90 seconds rest between paired sets	2× 17-20 with 90 seconds rest between paired sets	4× 6-8 with 90 seconds rest between paired sets	86
	Conditioning		300-yd (274 m) shuttle run: 1-3 sets with 2-4 min rest between sets	Weight plate complex: 3-4 rounds with 2-3 min rest between rounds		188 and 203

*Reload: Perform all exercises at a low intensity. On a scale of 1 to 10, you should be working at about a 3 or 4. Work at 7 to 9 on all other workouts.

Table 12.4 Gym-Based Function and Performance Program 4: Two or Three Times per Week

		Program 4A				
		Workout 1: reload*	Workouts 2 and 5	Workouts 3 and 6	Workouts 4 and 7	Page
1.	Load: one-leg squat or dumbbell leaning Bulgarian split squat	2× 8-10 each side with 2-3 minutes rest between sets	4× 6-7 each side with 3-5 minutes rest between sets	5× 4-5 each side with 3-5 minutes rest between sets	6× 2-3 each side with 3-5 minutes rest between sets	130 and 128
2.	Explode: explosive push-up	2× 3-4 with 2-3 minutes rest between sets	6× 3-4 with 2-3 minutes rest between sets	5× 5-6 with 2-3 minutes rest between sets	4× 7-8 with 2-3 minutes rest between sets	112
3a.	One-leg one-arm dumbbell Romanian deadlift	2× 6-8 each side	4× 6-8 each side	3× 10-14 each side	2× 17-20 each side	144
3b.	Stability ball abdominal variations (exercises noted)	Stability ball knee tuck 2× 8-10 with 90 seconds rest between paired sets	Stability ball pike rollout 4× 6-8 with 90 seconds rest between paired sets	Stability ball pike 3× 10-14 with 90 seconds rest between paired sets	Stability ball knee tuck 2× 17-20 with 90 seconds rest between paired sets	181, 178, 177, and 181
4a.	Leaning lat pull-down	2× 8-10	4× 6-8	3× 10-14	2× 17-20	60
4b.	Angled barbell shoulder to shoulder press	2× 6-8 each side with 90 seconds rest between paired sets	4× 6-8 each side with 90 seconds rest between paired sets	3× 10-14 each side with 90 seconds rest between paired sets	2× 17-20 each side with 90 seconds rest between paired sets	77
5a.	E-Z bar preacher biceps curl	2× 8-10	4× 6-8	3× 10-14	2× 17-20	87
5b.	Dumbbell shoulder A	2× 8-10 with 90 seconds rest between paired sets	4× 6-8 with 90 seconds rest between paired sets	3× 10-14 with 90 seconds rest between paired sets	2× 17-20 with 90 seconds rest between paired sets	88

> continued

Table 12.4 > *continued*

Program 4A					
	Workout 1: reload*	Workouts 2 and 5	Workouts 3 and 6	Workouts 4 and 7	Page
Conditioning			Weight plate push: 40-50 yd (37-46 m) total distance × 3-5 sets. Rest 90 sec-3 min between sets	Dumbbell complex: 3-4 rounds with 2-3 min rest between rounds	192 and 200

Program 4B					
	Workout 1: reload*	Workouts 2 and 5	Workouts 3 and 6	Workouts 4 and 7	Page
1. Load: machine back row	2× 8-10 with 2-3 minutes rest between sets	4× 6-7 with 3-5 minutes rest between sets	5× 4-5 with 3-5 minutes rest between sets	6× 2-3 with 3-5 minutes rest between sets	102
2. Explode: deadlift jump	2× 3-4 with 2-3 minutes rest between sets	6× 3-4 with 2-3 minutes rest between sets	5× 5-6 with 2-3 minutes rest between sets	4× 7-8 with 2-3 minutes rest between sets	136
3a. Dumbbell rotational shoulder press	2× 6-8	3× 10-14	2× 17-20	4× 6-8	83
3b. Fighter's cable lat pull-down	2× 6-8 each side with 90 seconds rest between paired sets	3× 10-14 each side with 90 seconds rest between paired sets	2× 17-20 each side with 90 seconds rest between paired sets	4× 6-8 each side with 90 seconds rest between paired sets	96
4a. Elevated dumbbell leaning reverse lunge	2× 6-8 each side	3× 10-14 each side	2× 17-20 each side	4× 6-8 each side	125
4b. Stability ball arc	2× 5-6 each side with 90 seconds rest between paired sets	3× 10-12 each side with 90 seconds rest between paired sets	2× 14-15 each side with 90 seconds rest between paired sets	4× 6-8 each side with 90 seconds rest between paired sets	172
5a. Hip adduction variations (exercises noted)	One-leg cable hip adduction 2× 8-10 each side	One-leg cable hip adduction 3× 10-14 each side	Side-lying hip adduction 2× 17-20 each side	Machine hip adduction 4× 6-8	148, 148, 153, and 152
5b. Overhead cable triceps rope extension	2× 8-10 with 90 seconds rest between paired sets	3× 10-14 with 90 seconds rest between paired sets	2× 17-20 with 90 seconds rest between paired sets	4× 6-8 with 90 seconds rest between paired sets	97
Conditioning		One-mile (1.6 km) run (outside or on treadmill) for time	Weight plate complex: 3-4 rounds with 2-3 min rest between rounds		191 and 203

*Reload: Perform all exercises at a low intensity. On a scale of 1 to 10, you should be working at about a 3 or 4. Work at 7 to 9 on all other workouts.

Table 12.5   Sample Gym-Based Function and Performance Training Setup: Two Times per Week

Week 1	Week 2*
Monday: Program 1A, workout 1	*Monday:* Program 1A, workout 2
Tuesday: Rest	*Tuesday:* Rest
Wednesday: Rest	*Wednesday:* Rest
Thursday: Program 1B, workout 1	*Thursday:* Program 1B, workout 2
Friday: Rest	*Friday:* Rest
Saturday: Rest	*Saturday:* Rest
Sunday: Rest	*Sunday:* Rest

*Repeat this sequence four to seven times. You can change the days you perform the workouts from what is listed, as long as you allow at least one day between workouts to maximize your performance in your next workout. Once you've completed program 1 four to seven times, you can move on to another program for four to seven times, and so on.

Table 12.6   Sample Gym-Based Function and Performance Training Setup: Three Times per Week

Week 1	Week 2*
Monday: Program 1A, workout 1	*Monday:* Program 1B, workout 2
Tuesday: Rest	*Tuesday:* Rest
Wednesday: Program 1B, workout 1	*Wednesday:* Program 1A, workout 3
Thursday: Rest	*Thursday:* Rest
Friday: Program 1A, workout 2	*Friday:* Program 1B, workout 3
Saturday: Rest	*Saturday:* Rest
Sunday: Rest	*Sunday:* Rest

*Repeat this sequence four to seven times. You can change the days you perform the workouts from what is listed as long as you allow at least one day between workouts to maximize your performance in the following workout. Once you've completed program 1 four to seven times, you can move on to another program for four to seven times, and so on.

Gym-Based Function and Performance Programs: Four or Five Times per Week

Each program in this section has four different workouts (see tables 12.7 to 12.10). These programs feature two workouts focused on the lower body and two for upper body. The first two workouts in each program have a load emphasis, which is increasing at least one heavy lift each consecutive week. The second two workouts in each program emphasize the explode, which is performing at least one explosive exercise progressively (set/rep) each consecutive week. Explanations for what load, explode, and reload are is in the previous section, where we discussed key points about these function and performance programs.

You'll alternate between workouts A, B, C, and D in each program for four to seven times before switching to another program and repeating those workouts for another four to seven times. The first time you do each workout in a program, it's considered a reload workout. A reload workout is simply a lower-intensity version of the workout, which helps you stay active and acclimate yourself to the movements and sequencing of the new program you're starting. Reloading also allows you to use workouts in a way that doesn't fatigue you so you can recover between programs. It also provides active recovery days between workout programs. See tables 12.11 and 12.12 for sample gym-based function and performance workouts that are appropriate if you work out four or five times per week

The workouts in each program also have other exercises to vary set and reps. They finish with a conditioning component on the days you're doing fewer overall sets of the resistance exercises.

These workouts assume that you're not necessarily playing (or practicing) a sport on a regular basis but are interested in improving performance at the gym by increasing metrics in strength, power, and conditioning. These workouts are designed to be used four or five times per week. The following tables show a few ways a weekly setup could be used for working out four to five times per week, starting with program 1.

Table 12.7   Gym-Based Function and Performance Program 1: Four or Five Times per Week

Program 1A: lower-body load					
	Workout 1: reload*	Workouts 2 and 5	Workouts 3 and 6	Workouts 4 and 7	Page
1. Load: barbell hybrid deadlift	2× 8-10 with 2-3 minutes rest between sets	4× 6-7 with 3-5 minutes rest between sets	5× 4-5 with 3-5 minutes rest between sets	6× 2-3 with 3-5 minutes rest between sets	124
2a. Dumbbell step-up	2× 6-8 each side	4× 6-8 each side	3× 10-14 each side	2× 17-20 each side	132
2b. Stability ball plate crunch	2× 6-8 with 90 seconds rest between paired sets	4× 6-8 with 90 seconds rest between paired sets	3× 10-12 with 90 seconds rest between paired sets	2× 15-17 with 90 seconds rest between paired sets	170
3a. One-leg 45-degree cable Romanian deadlift	2× 6-8 each side	4× 6-8 each side	3× 10-14 each side	2× 17-20 each side	147
3b. Dumbbell plank row	2× 6-8 each side with 90 seconds rest between paired sets	4× 5-6 each side with 90 seconds rest between paired sets	3× 8-9 each side with 90 seconds rest between paired sets	2× 11-12 each side with 90 seconds rest between paired sets	182
4. Hip adduction variations (exercises noted)	Machine hip adduction 2× 8-10 with 2-3 minutes rest between sets	Machine hip adduction 4× 6-8 with 2-3 minutes rest between sets	One-leg cable hip adduction 3× 10-14 each side with 2-3 minutes rest between sets	Side-lying hip adduction 2× 17-20 each side with 2-3 minutes rest between sets	152, 152, 148, and 153
Conditioning			High-resistance upright bike sprints: 10 sec on and 50 sec off × 4-8 rounds	Weight plate push: 40-50 yd (37-46 m) total distance × 3-5 sets. Rest 90 sec-3 min between sets	191 and 192

		Workout 1: reload*	Workouts 2 and 5	Workouts 3 and 6	Workouts 4 and 7	Page
	Program 1B: upper-body load					
1.	Load: chin-up (with machine or resistance band loop assistance if needed)	2× 6-8 with 2-3 minutes rest between sets	4× 6-7 with 3-5 minutes rest between sets	5× 4-5 with 3-5 minutes rest between sets	6× 2-3 with 3-5 minutes rest between sets	117
2a.	Dumbbell rotational shoulder press	2× 6-8 each side	4× 6-8 each side	3× 10-14 each side	2× 17-20 each side	83
2b.	One-arm cable row	2× 6-8 each side with 90 seconds rest between paired sets	4× 6-8 each side with 90 seconds rest between paired sets	3× 10-14 each side with 90 seconds rest between paired sets	2× 17-20 each side with 90 seconds rest between paired sets	93
3a.	Push-up variations (exercises noted)	Push-up 2× 8-10	Resistance band loop push-up 4× 6-8	Push-up or feet-elevated push-up (depending on your strength level) 3× 10-14	Stability ball push-up 2× 17-20	62, 105, 62 or 114, and 114
3b.	Supine resistance band shoulder L	2× 10-12 with 90 seconds rest between paired sets	4× 8-10 with 90 seconds rest between paired sets	3× 12-14 with 90 seconds rest between paired sets	2× 16-18 with 90 seconds rest between paired sets	110
4a.	E-Z bar preacher biceps curl	2× 6-8	4× 6-8	3× 10-14	2× 17-20	87
4b.	One-arm dumbbell overhead triceps extension	2× 6-8 each side with 90 seconds rest between paired sets	4× 6-8 each side with 90 seconds rest between paired sets	3× 10-14 each side with 90 seconds rest between paired sets	2× 17-20 each side with 90 seconds rest between paired sets	86
	Conditioning			Unilateral farmer's walk complex: 2-3 sets with 2-3 min rest between sets	Weight plate complex: 1× 3-4 rounds with 2-3 min rest between rounds	196 and 203
	Program 1C: lower-body explode					
1.	Explode: squat jump with arm drive	2× 3-4 with 2-3 minutes rest between sets	6× 3-4 with 3-5 minutes rest between sets	5× 5-6 with 3-5 minutes rest between sets	4× 7-8 with 3-5 minutes rest between sets	136
2a.	Traveling dumbbell Romanian deadlift lunge	2× 6-8 each side	2× 17-20 each side	3× 10-14 each side	4× 6-8 each side	144
2b.	Stability ball abdominal [illegible] (exercises noted)	Stability ball knee tuck 2× 8-10 with 90 seconds rest between paired sets	Stability ball knee tuck 2× 17-20 with 90 seconds rest between paired sets	Stability ball pike 3× 10-14 with 90 seconds rest between paired sets	Stability ball pike rollout 4× 6-8 with 90 seconds rest between paired sets	181, 181, 177, and 178

Table 12.7   *> continued*

		Workout 1: reload*	Workouts 2 and 5	Workouts 3 and 6	Workouts 4 and 7	Page
Program 1C: lower-body explode						
3a.	One-leg dumbbell bench hip thrust	2× 6-8 each side	2× 17-20 each side	3× 10-14 each side	4× 6-8 each side	145
3b.	Low-to-high cable chop	2× 8-10 with 90 seconds rest between paired sets	2× 5-17 with 90 seconds rest between paired sets	3× 10-12 with 90 seconds rest between paired sets	4× 6-8 with 90 seconds rest between paired sets	165
4.	Hamstring variations (exercises noted)	Machine lying hamstring curl 2× 8-10 with 2-3 minutes rest between sets	Machine seated hamstring curl 2× 17-20 with 2-3 minutes rest between sets	One-leg stability ball leg curl 3× 10-14 each side with 2-3 minutes rest between sets	Machine lying hamstring curl 4× 6-8 with 2-3 minutes rest between sets	151, 150, 154, and 151
	Conditioning		300-yd (274 m) shuttle run: 1-3 sets with 2-4 min rest between sets	One-mile (1.6 km) run (outside or on treadmill) for time		188 and 191
Program 1D: upper-body explode						
		Workout 1: reload*	Workouts 2 and 5	Workouts 3 and 6	Workouts 4 and 7	Page
1.	Explode: barbell high pull	2× 3-4 with 2-3 minutes rest between sets	6× 3-4 with 3-5 minutes rest between sets	5× 5-6 with 3-5 minutes rest between sets	4× 7-8 with 3-5 minutes rest between sets	76
2a.	Standing cable chest press	2× 8-10 each side	2× 17-20 each side	3× 10-14 each side	4× 6-8 each side	93
2b.	One-arm compound cable row	2× 8-10 each side with 90 seconds rest between paired sets	2× 17-20 each side with 90 seconds rest between paired sets	3× 10-14 each side with 90 seconds rest between paired sets	4× 6-8 each side with 90 seconds rest between paired sets	94
3a.	Lat pull-down (underhand grip)	2× 6-8	2× 17-20	3× 10-14	4× 6-8	58
3b.	Dumbbell triceps kickback	2× 6-8 with 90 seconds rest between paired sets	2× 17-20 with 90 seconds rest between paired sets	3× 10-14 with 90 seconds rest between paired sets	4× 6-8 with 90 seconds rest between paired sets	86
4a.	Dumbbell incline bench biceps curl	2× 6-8	2× 17-20	3× 10-14	4× 6-8	88
4b.	Dumbbell shoulder T	2× 8-10 with 90 seconds rest between paired sets	2× 18-20 with 90 seconds rest between paired sets	3× 14-15 with 90 seconds rest between paired sets	4× 10-12 with 90 seconds rest between paired sets	90
	Conditioning		Dumbbell farmer's walk complex: 3-5 sets with 2-3 min rest between sets	Weight plate complex: 3-4 rounds with 2-3 min rest between rounds		193 and 203

*Reload: Perform all exercises at a low intensity. On a scale of 1 to 10, you should be working at about a 3 or 4. Work at 7 to 9 on all other workouts.

Table 12.8 Gym-Based Function and Performance Program 2: Four or Five Times per Week

		Program 2A: lower-body load			
		Workout 1: reload*	Workouts 2 and 5	Workouts 3 and 6	Workouts 4 and 7	Page
1.	Load: trap bar squat or barbell front squat	2× 8-10 with 2-3 minutes rest between sets	4× 6-7 with 3-5 minutes rest between sets	5× 4-5 with 3-5 minutes rest between sets	6× 2-3 with 3-5 minutes rest between sets	139 or 122
2a.	Barbell Romanian deadlift	2× 6-8	4× 6-8	3× 10-14	2× 17-20	139
2b.	Reverse crunch	2× 18-10 with 90 seconds rest between paired sets	4× 6-8 (add medicine ball between knees) with 90 seconds rest between paired sets	3× 10-14 with 90 seconds rest between paired sets	2× 17-20 with 90 seconds rest between paired sets	160
3a.	Elevated dumbbell leaning reverse lunge	2× 4-5 each side	4× 6-8 each side	3× 10-12 each side	2× 14-15 each side	125
3b.	Cross-body plank	2× 5-6 each side with 90 seconds rest between paired sets	4× 6-8 each side with 90 seconds rest between paired sets	3× 10-12 each side with 90 seconds rest between paired sets	2× 14-15 each side with 90 seconds rest between paired sets	185
4.	Hamstring variations (exercises noted)	Machine seated hamstring curl 2× 8-10 with 2-3 minutes rest in between sets	Machine lying hamstring curl 4× 6-8 with 2-3 minutes rest in between sets	One-leg stability ball leg curl 3× 10-14 each side with 2-3 minutes rest in between sets	Machine seated hamstring curl 2× 17-20 with 2-3 minutes rest in between sets	150, 151, 154, and 150
	Conditioning			High-resistance upright bike sprints: 10 sec on and 50 sec off × 4-8 rounds	Weight plate push: 40-50 yd (37-46 m) total distance × 3-5 sets. Rest 90 sec-3 min between sets	191 and 192

		Program 2B: upper-body load			
		Workout 1: reload*	Workouts 2 and 5	Workouts 3 and 6	Workouts 4 and 7	Page
1.	Load: one-arm dumbbell row	2× 8-10 each side with 2-3 minutes rest between sets	4× 6-7 each side with 3-5 minutes rest between sets	5× 4-5 each side with 3-5 minutes rest between sets	6× 2-3 each side with 3-5 minutes rest between sets	64
2a.	One-arm angled barbell press	2× 6-8 each side	4× 6-8 each side	3× 10-14 each side	2× 17-20 each side	77
2b.	Lat pull-down	2× 8-10 with 90 seconds rest between paired sets	4× 6-8 with 90 seconds rest between paired sets	3× 10-14 with 90 seconds rest between paired sets	2× 17-20 with 90 seconds rest between paired sets	58

Table 12.8 *> continued*

	Program 2B: upper-body load				
	Workout 1: reload*	**Workouts 2 and 5**	**Workouts 3 and 6**	**Workouts 4 and 7**	**Page**
3a. Barbell bench press	2× 8-10	4× 6-8	3× 10-14	2× 17-20	79
3b. Dumbbell shoulder L	2× 8-10 each side with 90 seconds rest between paired sets	4× 6-8 each side with 90 seconds rest between paired sets	3× 10-14 each side with 90 seconds rest between paired sets	2× 17-20 each side with 90 seconds rest between paired sets	90
4a. Dumbbell triceps kickback	2× 8-10	4× 6-8	3× 10-14	2× 17-20	86
4b. Dumbbell biceps curl	2× 8-10 with 90 seconds rest between paired sets	4× 6-8 with 90 seconds rest between paired sets	3× 10-14 with 90 seconds rest between paired sets	2× 17-20 with 90 seconds rest between paired sets	68
Conditioning			Unilateral farmer's walk complex: 2-3 sets with 2-3 min rest between sets	Weight plate complex: 3-4 rounds with 2-3 min rest between rounds	196 and 203

	Program 2C: lower-body explode				
	Workout 1: reload*	**Workouts 2 and 5**	**Workouts 3 and 6**	**Workouts 4 and 7**	**Page**
1. Explode: lateral bound or lateral bench scissor jump	2× 3-4 with 2-3 minutes rest between sets	6× 3-4 each side with 3-5 minutes rest between sets	5× 5-6 each side with 3-5 minutes rest between sets	4× 7-8 each side with 3-5 minutes rest between sets	138
2a. One-leg squat	2× 6-8	2× 17-20	3× 10-14	4× 6-8	130
2b. Stability ball arc	2× 5-6 each side with 90 seconds rest between paired sets	2× 14-15 each side with 90 seconds rest between paired sets	3× 10-12 each side with 90 seconds rest between paired sets	4× 6-8 each side with 90 seconds rest between paired sets	172
3a. 45-degree hip extension	2× 6-8	2× 17-20	3× 10-14	4× 6-8	131
3b. High-to-low cable chop	2× 8-10 each side with 90 seconds rest between paired sets	2× 5-17 each side with 90 seconds rest between paired sets	3× 10-12 each side with 90 seconds rest between paired sets	4× 6-8 each side with 90 seconds rest between paired sets	168
4. Hip adduction variations (exercises noted)	One-leg cable hip adduction 2× 8-10 each side with 2-3 minutes rest between sets	Side-lying hip adduction 2× 17-20 each side with 2-3 minutes rest between sets	One-leg cable hip adduction 3× 10-14 each side with 2-3 minutes rest between sets	Machine hip adduction 4× 6-8 with 2-3 minutes rest between sets	148, 153, 148, and 152
Conditioning		300-yd (274 m) shuttle run: 1-3 sets with 2-4 min rest between sets	One-mile (1.6 km) run (outside or on treadmill) for time: ×1 set		188 and 191

Program 2D: upper-body explode					
	Workout 1: reload*	Workouts 2 and 5	Workouts 3 and 6	Workouts 4 and 7	Page
1. Explode: explosive box crossover push-up	2× 3-4 each side with 2-3 minutes rest between sets	6× 3-4 each side with 3-5 minutes rest between sets	5× 5-6 each side with 3-5 minutes rest between sets	4× 7-8 each side with 3-5 minutes rest between sets	113
2a. Fighter's cable lat pull-down	2× 6-8 each side	2× 17-20 each side	3× 10-14 each side	4× 6-8 each side	96
2b. Dumbbell rotational shoulder press	2× 6-8 each side with 90 seconds rest between paired sets	2× 17-20 each side with 90 seconds rest between paired sets	3× 10-14 each side with 90 seconds rest between paired sets	4× 6-8 each side with 90 seconds rest between paired sets	83
3a. Wide-elbow Smith bar row	2× 8-10	2× 17-20	3× 10-14	4× 6-8	116
3b. Smith bar triceps skull crusher	2× 8-10 with 90 seconds rest between paired sets	2× 17-20 with 90 seconds rest between paired sets	3× 10-14 with 90 seconds rest between paired sets	4× 6-8 with 90 seconds rest between paired sets	115
4a. Cable rope face pull	2× 8-10	2× 17-20	3× 10-14	4× 6-8	74
4b. Cable biceps curl	2× 8-10 with 90 seconds rest between paired sets	2× 17-20 with 90 seconds rest between paired sets	3× 10-14 with 90 seconds rest between paired sets	4× 6-8 with 90 seconds rest between paired sets	101
Conditioning		Dumbbell farmer's walk complex: 3-5 sets with 2-3 min rest between sets	Weight plate complex: 3-4 rounds with 2-3 min rest between rounds		193 and 203

*Reload: Perform all exercises at a low intensity. On a scale of 1 to 10, you should be working at about a 3 or 4. Work at 7 to 9 on all other workouts.

Table 12.9   Gym-Based Function and Performance Program 3: Four or Five Times per Week

Program 3A: lower-body load					
	Workout 1: reload*	Workouts 2 and 5	Workouts 3 and 6	Workouts 4 and 7	Page
1. Load: barbell rack pull	2× 8-10 with 2-3 minutes rest between sets	4× 6-7 with 3-5 minutes rest between sets	5× 4-5 with 3-5 minutes rest between sets	6× 2-3 with 3-5 minutes rest between sets	140
2a. Traveling dumbbell lunge	2× 6-8 each side	4× 6-8 each side	3× 10-14 each side	2× 17-20 each side	143
2b. Stability ball abdominal variations (exercises noted)	Stability ball knee tuck 2× 8-10 with 90 seconds rest between paired sets	Stability ball pike rollout 4× 6-8 with 90 seconds rest between paired sets	Stability ball pike 3× 10-14 with 90 seconds rest between paired sets	Stability ball knee tuck 2× 17-20 with 90 seconds rest between paired sets	181, 178, 177, and 181

> continued

Table 12.9   *> continued*

Program 3A: lower-body load					
	Workout 1: reload*	Workouts 2 and 5	Workouts 3 and 6	Workouts 4 and 7	Page
3a. One-leg hip lift with weight plate	2× 6-8 each side	4× 6-8 each side	3× 10-14 each side	2× 17-20 each side	146
3b. Low-to-high cable chop	2× 8-10 each side with 90 seconds rest between paired sets	4× 6-8 each side with 90 seconds rest between paired sets	3× 10-12 each side with 90 seconds rest between paired sets	2× 5-17 each side with 90 seconds rest between paired sets	165
4. Hip adduction variations (exercises noted)	Machine hip adduction 2× 8-10 with 2-3 minute rest between sets	Machine hip adduction 4× 6-8 with 2-3 minute rest between sets	One-leg cable hip adduction 3× 10-14 each side with 2-3 minute rest between sets	Side-lying hip adduction 2× 17-20 each side with 2-3 minute rest between sets	152, 152, 148, and 153
Conditioning			High-resistance upright bike sprints: 10 sec on and 50 sec off x 4-8 rounds	Weight plate push: 40-50 yd (37-46 m) total distance × 3-5 sets. Rest 90 sec-3 min between sets	191 and 192

Program 3B: upper-body load					
	Workout 1: reload*	Workouts 2 and 5	Workouts 3 and 6	Workouts 4 and 7	Page
1. Load: lat pull-down with neutral grip	2× 8-10 with 2-3 minutes rest between sets	4× 6-7 with 3-5 minutes rest between sets	5× 4-5 with 3-5 minutes rest between sets	6× 2-3 with 3-5 minutes rest between sets	91
2a. Dumbbell incline bench press	2× 8-10	4× 6-8	3× 10-14	2× 17-20	82
2b. Two-arm dumbbell bent-over row	2× 8-10 with 90 seconds rest between paired sets	4× 6-8 with 90 seconds rest between paired sets	3× 10-14 with 90 seconds rest between paired sets	2× 17-20 with 90 seconds rest between paired sets	66
3a. One-arm cable press	2× 8-10 each side	4× 6-8 each side	3× 10-14 each side	2× 17-20 each side	92
3b. Dumbbell shoulder T	2× 8-10 with 90 seconds rest between paired sets	4× 10-12 with 90 seconds rest between paired sets	3× 14-15 with 90 seconds rest between paired sets	2× 18-20 with 90 seconds rest between paired sets	90
4a. Cable biceps curl	2× 8-10	4× 6-8	3× 10-14	2× 17-20	101
4b. Cable triceps rope extension	2× 8-10 with 90 seconds rest between paired sets	4× 6-8 with 90 seconds rest between paired sets	3× 10-14 with 90 seconds rest between paired sets	2× 17-20 with 90 seconds rest between paired sets	98
Conditioning			Unilateral farmer's walk complex: 2-3 sets with 2-3 min rest between sets	Weight plate complex: 3-4 rounds with 2-3 min rest between rounds	196 and 203

	Program 3C: lower-body explode				
	Workout 1: reload*	Workouts 2 and 5	Workouts 3 and 6	Workouts 4 and 7	Page
1. Explode: broad jump	2× 3-4 with 2-3 minutes rest between sets	6× 3-4 with 3-5 minutes rest between sets	5× 5-6 with 3-5 minutes rest between sets	4× 7-8 with 3-5 minutes rest between sets	137
2a. Dumbbell step-up	2× 6-8 each side	2× 17-20 each side	3× 10-14 each side	4× 6-8 each side	132
2b. Stability ball plate crunch	2× 18-10 with 90 seconds rest between paired sets	2× 17-20 with 90 seconds rest between paired sets	3× 10-14 with 90 seconds rest between paired sets	4× 6-8 with 90 seconds rest between paired sets	170
3a. Dumbbell lateral Romanian deadlift lunge	2× 6-8 each side	2× 15-17 each side	3× 10-12 each side	4× 6-8 each side	142
3b. Dumbbell plank row	2× 6-8 each side with 90 seconds rest between paired sets	2× 11-12 each side with 90 seconds rest between paired sets	3× 8-9 each side with 90 seconds rest between paired sets	4× 5-6 each side with 90 seconds rest between paired sets	182
4. Hamstring variations (exercises noted)	Machine lying hamstring curl 2× 8-10 with 2-3 minutes rest between sets	Machine seated hamstring curl 2× 17-20 with 2-3 minutes rest between sets	One-leg stability ball leg curl 3× 10-14 each side with 2-3 minutes rest between sets	Machine lying hamstring curl 4× 6-8 with 2-3 minutes rest between sets	151, 150, 154, and 151
Conditioning		300-yd (274 m) shuttle run: 1-3 sets with 2-4 min rest between sets	One-mile (1.6 km) run (outside or on treadmill) for time: x1 set		188 and 191

	Program 3D: upper-body explode				
	Workout 1: reload*	Workouts 2 and 5	Workouts 3 and 6	Workouts 4 and 7	Page
1. Explode: angled barbell press and catch	2× 3-4 each side with 2-3 minutes rest between sets	6× 3-4 each side with 3-5 minutes rest between sets	5× 5-6 each side with 3-5 minutes rest between sets	4× 7-8 each side with 3-5 minutes rest between sets	76
2a. Barbell bent-over row	2× 6-8	2× 17-20	3× 10-14	4× 6-8	63
2b. Push-up variations (exercises noted)	Push-up 2× 8-10 with 90 seconds rest between paired sets	Stability ball push-up 2× 17-20 with 90 seconds rest between paired sets	Push-up or feet-elevated push-up (depending on your strength level) 3× 10-14 with 90 seconds rest between paired sets	Resistance band loop push-up 4× 6-8 with 90 seconds rest between paired sets	62, 114, 62 or 114, and 105

> continued

Table 12.9 > continued

Program 3D: upper-body explode					
	Workout 1: reload*	Workouts 2 and 5	Workouts 3 and 6	Workouts 4 and 7	Page
3a. Pull-up (with machine or resistance band loop assistance if needed)	2× 6-8	2× 17-20	3× 10-14	4× 6-8	118
3b. One-arm dumbbell overhead triceps extension	2× 8-10 each side with 90 seconds rest between paired sets	2× 17-20 each side with 90 seconds rest between paired sets	3× 10-14 each side with 90 seconds rest between paired sets	4× 6-8 each side with 90 seconds rest between paired sets	86
4a. E-Z bar preacher biceps curl	2× 6-8	2× 17-20	3× 10-14	4× 6-8	87
4b. Dumbbell shoulder A	2× 8-10 with 90 seconds rest between paired sets	2× 17-20 with 90 seconds rest between paired sets	3× 10-14 with 90 seconds rest between paired sets	4× 6-8 with 90 seconds rest between paired sets	88
Conditioning		Dumbbell farmer's walk complex: 3-5 sets with 2-3 min rest between sets	Weight plate complex: 3-4 rounds with 2-3 min rest between rounds		193 and 203

*Reload: Perform all exercises at a low intensity. On a scale of 1 to 10, you should be working at about a 3 or 4. Work at 7 to 9 on all other workouts.

Table 12.10 Gym-Based Function and Performance Program 4: Four or Five Times per Week

Workout 4A: lower-body load					
	Workout 1: reload*	Workouts 2 and 5	Workouts 3 and 6	Workouts 4 and 7	Page
1. Load: one-leg squat or dumbbell leaning Bulgarian split squat	2× 6-8 each side with 2-3 minutes rest between sets	4× 7-8 each side with 3-5 minutes rest between sets	5× 5-6 each side with 3-5 minutes rest between sets	6× 3-4 each side with 3-5 minutes rest between sets	130 or 128
2a. One-leg one-arm dumbbell Romanian deadlift	2× 6-8 each side	4× 6-8 each side	3× 10-14 each side	2× 17-20 each side	144
2b. Stability ball arc	2× 5-6 each side with 90 seconds rest between paired sets	4× 6-8 each side with 90 seconds rest between paired sets	3× 10-12 each side with 90 seconds rest between paired sets	2× 14-15 each side with 90 seconds rest between paired sets	172
3a. 45-degree hip extension	2× 6-8 each side	4× 6-8 each side	3× 10-14 each side	2× 17-20 each side	131
3b. High-to-low cable chop	2× 8-10 each side with 90 seconds rest between paired sets	4× 6-8 each side with 90 seconds rest between paired sets	3× 10-12 each side with 90 seconds rest between paired sets	2× 15-17 each side with 90 seconds rest between paired sets	168
4. Hamstring variations (exercises noted)	Machine seated hamstring curl 2× 8-10 with 2-3 minutes rest between sets	Machine lying hamstring curl 4× 6-8 with 2-3 minutes rest between sets	One-leg stability ball leg curl 3× 10-14 each side with 2-3 minutes rest between sets	Machine seated hamstring curl 2× 17-20 with 2-3 minutes rest between sets	150, 151, 154, and 150

Workout 4A: lower-body load

	Workout 1: reload*	Workouts 2 and 5	Workouts 3 and 6	Workouts 4 and 7	Page
Conditioning			High-resistance upright bike sprints: 10 sec on and 50 sec off × 4-8 rounds	Weight plate push: 40-50 yd (37-46 m) total distance × 3-5 sets. Rest 90 sec-3 min between sets	191 and 192

Workout 4B: upper-body load

		Workout 1: reload*	Workouts 2 and 5	Workouts 3 and 6	Workouts 4 and 7	Page
1.	Load: machine back row	2× 8-10 with 2-3 minutes rest between sets	4× 6-7 with 3-5 minutes rest between sets	5× 4-5 with 3-5 minutes rest between sets	6× 2-3 with 3-5 minutes rest between sets	102
2a.	One-arm dumbbell overhead press	2× 6-8 each side	4× 6-8 each side	3× 10-14 each side	2× 17-20 each side	82
2b.	Fighter's cable lat pull-down	2× 6-8 each side with 90 seconds rest between paired sets	4× 6-8 each side with 90 seconds rest between paired sets	3× 10-14 each side with 90 seconds rest between paired sets	2× 17-20 each side with 90 seconds rest between paired sets	96
3a.	Dumbbell bench press	2× 6-8	4× 6-8	3× 10-14	2× 17-20	81
3b.	Dumbbell shoulder L	2× 8-10 with 90 seconds rest between paired sets	4× 8-10 with 90 seconds rest between paired sets	3× 12-14 with 90 seconds rest between paired sets	2× 15-17 with 90 seconds rest between paired sets	90
4a.	Low-cable one-arm face-way biceps curl	2× 8-10 each side	4× 6-8 each side	3× 10-14 each side	2× 17-20 each side	101
4b.	Overhead cable triceps rope extension	2× 8-10 with 90 seconds rest between paired sets	4× 6-8 with 90 seconds rest between paired sets	3× 10-14 with 90 seconds rest between paired sets	2× 17-20 with 90 seconds rest between paired sets	97
Conditioning				Unilateral farmer's walk complex: 2-3 sets with 2-3 min rest between sets	Weight plate complex: 3-4 rounds with 2-3 min rest between rounds	196 and 203

Workout 4C: lower-body explode

		Workout 1: reload*	Workouts 2 and 5	Workouts 3 and 6	Workouts 4 and 7	Page
1.	Explode: deadlift jump	2× 3-4 with 2-3 minutes rest between sets	6× 3-4 with 3-5 minutes rest between sets	5× 5-6 with 3-5 minutes rest between sets	4× 7-8 with 3-5 minutes rest between sets	136
2a.	Barbell squat	2× 6-8	2× 17-20	3× 10-14	4× 6-8	121
2b.	Reverse crunch	2× 18-10 with 90 seconds rest between paired sets	2× 17-20 with 90 seconds rest between paired sets	3× 10-14 with 90 seconds rest between paired sets	4× 6-8 (Add medicine ball between knees) with 90 seconds rest between paired sets	160

257

> continued

Table 12.10 *> continued*

		Workout 1: reload*	Workouts 2 and 5	Workouts 3 and 6	Workouts 4 and 7	Page
	Workout 4C: lower-body explode					
3a.	Elevated dumbbell leaning reverse lunge	2× 6-8 each side	2× 17-20 each side	3× 10-14 each side	4× 6-8 each side	125
3b.	Cross-body plank	2× 5-6 each side with 90 seconds rest between paired sets	2× 14-15 each side with 90 seconds rest between paired sets	3× 10-12 each side with 90 seconds rest between paired sets	4× 6-8 each side with 90 seconds rest between paired sets	185
4.	Hip adduction variations (exercises noted)	One-leg cable hip adduction 2× 8-10 each side with 2-3 minutes rest between sets	Side-lying hip adduction 2× 17-20 each side with 2-3 minutes rest between sets	One-leg cable hip adduction 3× 10-14 each side with 2-3 minutes rest between sets	Machine hip adduction 4× 6-8 with 2-3 minutes rest between sets	148, 153, 148, and 152
	Conditioning		300-yd (274 m) shuttle run: 1-3 sets with 2-4 min rest between sets	One-mile (1.6 km) run (outside or on treadmill) for time: x1 set		188 and 191
	Workout 4D: upper-body explode					
1.	Explode: explosive push-up	2× 3-4 with 2-3 minutes rest between sets	6× 3-4 with 3-5 minutes rest between sets	5× 5-6 with 3-5 minutes rest between sets	4× 7-8 with 3-5 minutes rest between sets	112
2a.	Leaning lat pull-down	2× 8-10	2× 17-20	3× 10-14	4× 6-8	60
2b.	Angled barbell shoulder to shoulder press	2× 6-8 each side with 90 seconds rest between paired sets	2× 17-20 each side with 90 seconds rest between paired sets	3× 10-14 each side with 90 seconds rest between paired sets	4× 6-8 each side with 90 seconds rest between paired sets	77
3a.	One-arm dumbbell off-bench row	2× 8-10 each side	2× 17-20 each side	3× 10-14 each side	4× 6-8 each side	83
3b.	Dumbbell triceps skull crusher	2× 6-8 with 90 seconds rest between paired sets	2× 17-20 with 90 seconds rest between paired sets	3× 10-14 with 90 seconds rest between paired sets	4× 6-8 with 90 seconds rest between paired sets	73
4a.	Machine rear delt fly	2× 6-8	2× 17-20	3× 10-14	4× 6-8	103
4b.	Dumbbell biceps curl	2× 6-8 with 90 seconds rest between paired sets	2× 17-20 with 90 seconds rest between paired sets	3× 10-14 with 90 seconds rest between paired sets	4× 6-8 with 90 seconds rest between paired sets	68
	Conditioning		Dumbbell farmer's walk complex: 3-5 sets with 2-3 min rest between sets	Weight plate complex: 3-4 rounds with 2-3 min rest between rounds		193 and 203

*Reload: Perform all exercises at a low intensity. On a scale of 1 to 10, you should be working at about a 3 or 4. Work at a 7 to 9 on all other workouts.

Table 12.11 Sample Gym-Based Function and Performance Training Setup: Four Times per Week

Option 1	
Week 1	**Week 2***
Monday: Program 1A, Lower Body Load, workout 1	*Monday:* Program 1A, Lower Body Load, workout 2
Tuesday: Program 1B, Upper Body, Load, workout 1	*Tuesday:* Program 1B, Upper Body Load, workout 2
Wednesday: Rest	*Wednesday:* Rest
Thursday: Program 1C, Lower Body Explode, workout 1	*Thursday:* Program 1C, Lower Body Explode, workout 2
Friday: Program 1D, Upper Body Explode, workout 1	*Friday:* Program 1D, Upper Body Explode, workout 2
Saturday: Rest	*Saturday:* Rest
Sunday: Rest	*Sunday:* Rest

Option 2
Week 1*
Monday: Program 1A, Lower Body Load, workout 1
Tuesday: Program 1B, Upper Body Load, workout 1
Wednesday: Rest
Thursday: Program 1C, Lower Body Explode, workout 1
Friday: Rest
Saturday: Program 1D, Upper Body Explode, workout 1
Sunday: Rest

*Repeat this sequence four to seven times. You can change the days you perform the workouts from what is listed as long as you do the workouts on no more than two to three consecutive days before taking a rest day to maximize your recovery. Once you've completed program 1 four to seven times, you can move on to another program for four to seven times, and so on.

Table 12.12 Sample Gym-Based Function and Performance Training Setup: Four Times per Week

Week 1	Week 2
Monday: Program 1A, Lower Body Load, workout 1	*Monday:* Program 1B, Upper Body Load, workout 2
Tuesday: Program 1B, Upper Body Load, workout 1	*Tuesday:* Program 1C, Lower Body Explode, workout 2
Wednesday: Rest	*Wednesday:* Rest
Thursday: Program 1C, Lower Body Explode, workout 1	*Thursday:* Program 1D, Upper Body Explode, workout 2
Friday: Program 1D, Upper Body Explode, workout 1	*Friday:* Program 1A, Lower Body Load, workout 3
Saturday: Program 1B, Lower Body Load, workout 2	*Saturday:* Program 1B, Upper Body Load, workout 3
Sunday: Rest	*Sunday:* Rest

Week 3*
Monday: Program 1C, Lower Body Explode, workout 3
Tuesday: Program 1D, Upper Body Explode, workout 3
Wednesday: Rest
Thursday: Program 1A, Lower Body Load, workout 4
Friday: Program 1B, Upper Body Load, workout 4
Saturday: Program 1C, Lower Body Explode, workout 4
Sunday: Rest

Repeat this sequence the following week, and so on. You can change the days you perform the workouts from what is listed, as long as you perform the workouts on no more than two to three consecutive days before taking a rest day to maximize your recovery. Once you've completed program 1 four to seven times, you can move on to another program for four to seven times, and so on.

Function and Performance Home or Hotel Gym Workouts

On days that you're traveling, can't make it to the gym, or don't have access to a gym, you can use these home or hotel gym workouts or the band and bodyweight workouts. The two workouts in tables 12.13 and 12.14 use equipment that's either recommended for your home gym or that's commonly found in most hotel gyms. That equipment is as follows:

- A set of dumbbells (up to 50 lb or 20 kg)
- An adjustable weight bench that can be made flat or set at an incline
- A high-quality stability ball that's 55 to 65 centimeters
- A chin-up bar (many are designed to be easily placed inside the top of a doorway)
- A set of resistance bands with handles of varying strengths from light to very heavy
- Resistance band loops of varying strength from light to medium
- Resistance band mini loops of varying strength from light to medium

Resistance bands, resistance band loops, and resistance band mini loops are affordable and available at most sporting goods stores or online, but they are not often found at hotel gyms. I recommend traveling with at least one set of each type of band. They're portable and easy to pack in your luggage. It's also important to note that since the following workouts are designed to be done with limited equipment, some of the exercises included will require small modifications from how they're featured in the exercise descriptions. For example, for a cable-based exercise such as the One-Arm Cable Row, you'd perform it with a resistance band instead of cable if your training environment doesn't feature a cable column. Or, for a dumbbell exercise such as the Dumbbell Shoulder W, you'd simply perform the same movement as shown in the exercise description without holding dumbbells. These modifications are indicated within each of the following workouts.

Also, these workouts are intended to be used *only* as an addition to your regular weekly gym-based workouts on days when you're traveling, can't make it to the gym, or don't have access to a gym. These workouts are *not* intended to replace your gym-based workouts; your primary training should revolve around using the gym-based programs in the previous section. Before you begin any of the following workouts, be sure to perform one of the dynamic warm-up sequences in chapter 5.

The two workouts in tables 12.15 and 12.16 have bodyweight exercises and resistance band exercises utilizing three types of bands: resistance bands with handles (these can be attached to any doorway or stable object in matter of seconds), resistance band loops, and resistance mini band loops. A set of high-quality resistance bands with handles and both types of resistance band loops—they come in multiple resistances from light to very heavy—for home use and to take with you when you travel are a must. They are portable and add a number of effective exercise options to your bodyweight training workouts, delivering a value that far exceeds their cost.

Again, the following workouts are *not* intended to be done exclusively and are not designed to replace the gym-based programs earlier in this chapter. They are intended to be used only as an addition to your regular weekly gym based workouts on days when you don't have access to any kind of gym.

Table 12.13 Function and Performance Home or Hotel Gym Workout 1

Exercise	Sets and reps	Page
1. Load: one-leg squat	4× 5-7 each side with 3-5 minutes rest between sets	130
2. Explode: explosive push-up	6× 4-6 with 2-3 minutes rest between sets	112
3a. Dumbbell step-up	4× 6-8 each side	132
3b. Cable tight torso rotation with hip shift (with resistance band)*	4× 8-12 each side with 90 seconds rest between paired sets	166
4a. Resistance band step and chest press	3× 18-24 total	104
4b. One-arm compound cable row (with resistance band)*	4× 8-12 each side with 90 seconds rest between paired sets	94
5a. Dumbbell shoulder T	3× 10-15	90
5b. One-arm dumbbell overhead triceps extension	3× 10-15 each side with 90 seconds rest between paired sets	86
Conditioning	300-yd (274 m) shuttle run: 1-3 sets with 3-5 min rest between sets —or— Bodyweight leg complex: 2-3 sets with 2-4 min between sets	188 or 205

*Use a resistance band instead of a cable to perform this exercise in the manner provided in the exercise description.

Table 12.14 Function and Performance Home or Hotel Gym Workout 2

Exercise	Sets and reps	Page
1. Load: chin-up (with resistance band loop assistance if needed)	4× 6-7 with 3-5 minutes rest between sets	117
2. Explode: squat jump with arm drive	6× 3-4 with 2-3 minutes rest between sets	136
3a. Dumbbell rotational shoulder press	3× 10-14 each side	83
3b. Two-arm dumbbell bent-over row	3× 10-14 each side with 90 seconds rest between paired sets	66
4a. One-leg dumbbell bench hip thrust	3× 10-14 each side	145
4b. Dumbbell plank row	3× 8-10 each side with 90 seconds rest between paired sets	182
5a. Stability ball leg curl	3× 15-20	154
5b. Dumbbell biceps curl	3× 10-15 with 90 seconds rest between paired sets	68
Conditioning	Bodyweight and resistance band complex: 3-4 sets with 2-4 min rest between sets	209

Table 12.15 Function and Performance Bodyweight and Band Workout 1

Exercise	Sets and reps	Page
1. Load: one-leg squat	4× 5-7 each side with 3-5 minutes rest between sets	130
2. Explode: explosive push-up	6× 4-6 with 2-3 minutes rest between sets	112
3a. Resistance band loop hybrid deadlift	3× 10-15 as fast as possible without loss of technique	148
3b. Reverse crunch	3× 10-14 with 90 seconds rest between paired sets	160
4a. One-arm motorcycle cable row (with resistance band)*	3× 12-16 each side	94
4b. One-arm cable press (with resistance band)*	3× 12-16 each side with 90 seconds rest between paired sets	92
5a. Resistance band overhead triceps extension	3× 12-15	106
5b. Low-to-high cable chop (with resistance band)*	3× 12-15 each side with 90 seconds rest between paired sets	165
Conditioning	300-yard (274 m) shuttle run: 1-3 sets with 3-5 minutes rest between sets —or— Bodyweight leg complex: 2-3 sets with 2-4 min between sets	188 or 205

*Use a resistance band instead of a cable to perform this exercise in the manner provided in the exercise description.

Table 12.16 Function and Performance Bodyweight and Band Workout 2

Exercise	Sets and reps	Page
1. Load: one-arm push-up	4× 3-8 each side with 3-5 minutes rest between sets	111
2. Explode: lateral bound	6× 3-4 each side with 2-3 minutes rest between sets	138
3a. One-arm compound cable row (with resistance band)*	3× 10-14 each side	94
3b. Resistance band step and chest press	3× 20-24 total per stance with 90 seconds rest between paired sets	104
4a. One-leg 45-degree cable Romanian deadlift (with resistance band)*	3× 10-14 each side	147
4b. Cross-body plank	3× 10-12 each side with 90 seconds rest between paired sets	185
5a. Resistance band mini loop low lateral shuffle	3× 15-20 each side	149
5b. Resistance band biceps curl	3× 12-20 (to 45 degrees)	109
Conditioning	Bodyweight and resistance band complex: 3-4 sets with 2-4 min rest between sets	209

*Use a resistance band instead of a cable to perform this exercise in the manner provided in the exercise description.

13 } Fat Loss Programs

This chapter is for those who want to lose extra body fat while minimizing muscle loss. If you gauge success mainly by how you fit into your clothes, how you look in the mirror, reductions in your weight, or your body fat measurements, then the workout programs in this chapter are for you!

The Basics of Fat Loss Programs

The programs in this chapter are mainly total body circuits (i.e., trisets and quadsets), each consisting of three, four, or five resistance training exercises performed back-to-back. This maximizes the metabolic demand of the workouts by requiring you to use your whole body for an extended time—longer than you would to complete a paired set in the other workout chapters. These workout programs also include conditioning because they challenge your work capacity.

The only thing that separates these workouts from simply improving your conditioning is your diet. In other words, if your eating behaviors are *not* putting you in a consistent caloric deficit, these workout programs will help improve your workout capacity (i.e., your overall fitness and conditioning), but they aren't going to be very effective at helping you to lose fat.

As explained in chapter 3, you've got to be in a caloric deficit to consistently lose fat. The programs in this chapter are considered fat loss-specific. They help you accelerate fat loss by using resistance training to maximize metabolic demand instead of focusing on maximizing muscle size gains (like the physique programs featured in chapter 14) to improve the shape of your body while you watch your diet to reveal your shape.

If you're not as interested in changing your diet, the programs in this chapter can also be used as weight management to help offset the foods you love to eat while also improving your overall conditioning level.

There are some guidelines for using these programs. Some of these guidelines will be the same for all the program chapters in this book, but others differ depending on which type of program you're doing. Let's look at the key points to remember for your fat loss program.

- Perform the exercises designated with *a* or *b* as paired sets; the exercises with *a*, *b*, and *c* as trisets; and the exercises with *a*, *b*, *c* and *d* as quadsets. Perform all reps in each set before moving to the next set. Once all exercises within a set are complete, you can rest a bit longer than indicated between sets (if necessary) to complete the designated number of reps with good control. Completing one round of the exercises in a paired or triset is considered one set.

- The rep range (i.e., 10-15 reps) is next to each exercise in the workout programs in the next two sections. If you're using the same weight for each set, you may be able to do 15 reps on the first set, 12 reps on the next set, and 10 reps on the third set due to accumulated fatigue. Or, you can reduce the weight you're using with each consecutive set to achieve the higher end or given rep range on each consecutive set. Both methods will help you progress.

- When a program indicates to take a break before beginning a new cycle, this doesn't mean you have to do nothing. During your days off, you can do some low-impact activities, such as going for long walks, hikes, bike rides, or swims. Also, yoga can be a great option for your active rest periods. If you're already doing yoga each week, as recommended earlier, you can simply increase your yoga practice in your (active) rest week from the gym. Taking 4 to 7 days to "deload" before repeating a workout cycle can minimize the risk of overtraining and helps you continue to make gains. It also makes you hungry to get back into the gym, which can help you avoid getting in the habit of simply going through the motions.

- Maintain strict form, without cheating by using additional movements or momentum. Do the concentric (lifting) portion of each rep at a normal tempo and maintain control during the eccentric (lowering) portion.

- Use a weight load that leaves you close to being unable to perform any more reps than indicated while maintaining proper control and technique.

- Do not rest between exercises within a given set unless absolutely needed to finish each sequence without rushing through any exercise. In other words, minimize the transition time between exercises within a given sequence of exercises. Take as little rest as you need between exercises within given set or paired set to complete the reps indicated with good control and technique.

- If an exercise causes pain or discomfort beyond the sensation associated with muscle fatigue, utilize an alternative exercise that doesn't hurt. There are plenty of movements in the exercise chapters of this book to choose from.

- Remember, before you begin a workout in the following programs, be sure to perform one of the dynamic warm-up sequences in chapter 5.

Fat Loss Programs

I recommend that you first complete the beginner programs in chapter 10 if you're just starting out or haven't worked out in a while before you start any of these programs. If you have been regularly working out or you've completed the beginner programs, it's also recommended that you complete at least 6 to 8 weeks of the fitness programs in chapter 11.

Gym-based programs are the main focus of this chapter, but since you can't always make it to the gym and while your primary training should be done

Your Gym Bag

There are a couple pieces of portable equipment that I recommend you always have in your gym bag—resistance bands with handles and resistance band loops. These bands allow you to group exercises requiring immobile equipment (e.g., squat rack or machine) with bands, which are mobile equipment. This enables you to use band exercises within a paired set or triset while you remain at the immobile equipment and don't have to walk all over the gym, thus potentially losing your equipment to another member.

There are two places online that I recommend you go to purchase high-quality resistance bands: Power-Systems.com and Sorinex.com. At Power Systems, the resistance bands with handles to get are the *Double Cords*; the resistance band loops are called *strength bands*, and resistance band mini loops are called *Versa Loops*. At Sorinex Exercise Equipment, resistance band loops are called *strength bands*, and resistance band mini loops are called *short bands*.

using equipment, this chapter also provides two home and hotel gym workouts along with two workouts using only bodyweight and resistance band exercises that you can use on the days you're traveling or don't have access to any kind of gym equipment.

Gym-Based Fat Loss Programs

These programs alternate between eight different total body workouts and are to be used if you're training two, three, four, or five times per week. Doing these workouts five times per week is a challenge, but it's a challenge people who regularly enjoy pushing themselves with exercise are up for! Train no more than three days in a row to maximize recovery and minimize the risk of overtraining. The resistance exercise portion of the workouts has two different set/rep schemes to make your workouts more diverse and well-rounded. Each workout is designed with a constant theme to create the right stimulus for accelerating fat loss, and cycling through different workouts gives you the variety you crave!

If you're training four or five times per week, after finishing a cycle through all 16 workouts, take five days to a week off before repeating the sequence. Taking a break from the workouts doesn't mean you have to do nothing. As noted earlier, during your days off from training, you can do some low-impact activities, such as going for long walks, hikes, bike rides, or swims. Also, yoga can be a great option for your active rest periods between using the following programs.

There are two different versions of each program—A and B—for a total of 16 different routines to cycle through and repeat on an ongoing basis (see tables 13.1-13.8). A workout finishes with a conditioning component on the days you're performing fewer overall sets of the resistance exercises in the mixed set/rep scheme utilized.

The total body workout programs are designed to be used at least twice per week, but three to five times per week is recommended for best results. The following tables show a few ways a weekly setup could be used for working out two, three, four, and five times per week (see tables 13.9 to 13.12).

Table 13.1 Gym-Based Fat Loss Program 1

		Workout A	Workout B	Page
1a.	Barbell bent-over row	3× 12-16	4× 6-10	63
1b.	Elevated dumbbell reverse lunge	3× 10-12 each side	4× 6-8 each side	126
1c.	Push-up variations (exercises noted)	Push-up 3× max reps	Box crossover push-up 4× max reps	62 and 112
1d.	Weight plate around the world	3× 9-10 each side with 2-3 minutes rest between quadsets	4× 6-8 each side with 2-3 minutes rest between quadsets	182
2a.	Barbell hybrid deadlift	3× 12-16	4× 6-10	124
2b.	Dumbbell rotational shoulder press	3× 12-16 each side	4× 6-10 each side	83
2c.	Stability ball plate crunch	3× 12-16 with 2-3 minutes rest between trisets	4× 8-10 with 2-3 minutes rest between trisets	170
3a.	Chin-up (with machine or resistance band assistance if needed)	3× 12-16	4× 6-10	117
3b.	Weight plate speed chop	3× 12-16	4× 6-10	175
3c.	One-leg hip lift with weight plate	3× 25-30 each side with 2-3 minutes rest between trisets	4× 16-20 each side with 2-3 minutes rest between trisets	146
Conditioning		High-resistance upright bike sprints: 10 sec on and 50 sec off for 4-8 rounds		191

Table 13.2 Gym-Based Fat Loss Program 2

		Workout A	Workout B	Page
1a.	Dumbbell incline bench press	4× 6-8	3× 12-16	82
1b.	One-arm dumbbell row	4× 6-8 each side	3× 10-12 each side	64
1c.	Dumbbell lateral Romanian deadlift lunge	4× 6-8 each side	3× 10-12 each side	142
1d.	Reverse crunch	4× 6-9 with 2-3 minutes rest between quadsets	3× 12-15 with 2-3 minutes rest between quadsets	160
2a.	Leaning lat pull-down	4× 6-10	3× 12-16	60
2b.	Dumbbell leaning Bulgarian split squat (with back foot on top of lat pull-down seat)	4× 6-10 each side	3× 12-16 each side	128
2c.	Close-grip push-up	4× max reps with 2-3 minutes rest between trisets	3× max reps (hands elevated on seat) with 2-3 minutes rest between trisets	113
3a.	Machine lying hamstring curl	4× 6-10	3× 12-16	151
3b.	Dumbbell plank row	4× 6-7 each side	3× 9-10 each side	182
3c.	Dumbbell biceps curl	4× 6-10	3× 12-16	68
3d.	One-arm dumbbell overhead triceps extension	4× 6-10 each side with 2-3 minutes rest between quadsets	3× 12-16 each side with 2-3 minutes rest between quadsets	86
Conditioning			Dumbbell farmer's walk complex 2-3 sets with 2-3 min rest between sets	193

Table 13.3 Gym-Based Fat Loss Program 3

		Workout A	Workout B	Page
1a.	Fighter's cable lat pull-down	3× 12-16 each side	4× 6-10 each side	96
1b.	One-arm dumbbell overhead push press	3× 12-16 each side	4× 6-10 each side	81
1c.	Elevated dumbbell leaning reverse lunge	3× 12-16 each side with 2-3 minutes rest between trisets	4× 6-10 each side with 2-3 minutes rest between trisets	125
2a.	Barbell Romanian deadlift	3× 12-16	4× 6-10	139
2b.	Push-up variations (exercises noted)	Stability ball push-up 3× max reps	Close-grip push-up 4× max reps	114 and 113
2c.	Stability ball abdominal variations (exercises noted)	Stability ball knee tuck 3× 15-20	Stability ball pike 4× 6-12	181 and 177
2d.	Dumbbell side shoulder raise	3× 12-16 with 2-3 minutes rest between quadsets	4× 8-10 with 2-3 minutes rest between quadsets	71
3a.	One-arm dumbbell row	3× 12-16 each side	4× 6-10 each side	64
3b.	Dumbbell triceps skull crusher	3× 12-16	4× 6-10	73
3c.	One-leg stability ball leg curl	3× 12-16 each side	4× 6-10 each side	154
3d.	Abdominal rollout variations (exercises noted)	Stability ball rollout 3×15-20 with 2-3 minutes rest between quadsets	Arm walkout 4× 6-8 with 2-3 minutes rest between quadsets	176 and 183
Conditioning		Weight plate push: 40-50 yd (37-46 m) total distance for 3-5 sets. Rest 90 sec-3 min between sets		192

Table 13.4 Gym-Based Fat Loss Program 4

		Workout A	Workout B	Page
1a.	Lat pull-down with neutral grip	4× 6-8	3× 12-16	91
1b.	Angled barbell shoulder to shoulder press	4× 6-8 each side	3× 10-12 each side	77
1c.	One-leg angled barbell Romanian deadlift	4× 6-8 each side with 2-3 minutes rest between trisets	3× 10-12 each side with 2-3 minutes rest between trisets	140
2a.	Dumbbell bench press	4× 6-8	3× 12-16	81
2b.	One-arm dumbbell freestanding row	4× 6-8 each side	3× 10-12 each side	84
2c.	Dumbbell step-up	4× 6-8 each side	3× 10-12 each side	132
2d.	Reverse crunch	4× 6-9 with 2-3 minutes rest between quadsets	3× 12-15 with 2-3 minutes rest between quadsets	160
3a.	Low-to-high cable chop	4× 8-10 each side	3× 12-16 each side	165
3b.	Cable triceps rope extension	4× 8-12	3× 14-16	98
3c.	Cable rope face pull	4× 8-12	3× 14-16	74
3d.	Cross-body plank	4× 7-9 each side with 2-3 minutes rest between quadsets	3× 12-15 each side with 2-3 minutes rest between quadsets	105
Conditioning			Weight plate complex: 3-4 rounds with 2-3 min rest between rounds	203

Table 13.5 Gym-Based Fat Loss Program 5

		Workout A	Workout B	Page
1a.	Barbell bench press	3×12-16	4× 6-10	79
1b.	Two-arm dumbbell bent-over row	3× 12-16	4× 6-10	66
1c.	One-leg dumbbell bench hip thrust	3× 20-25 each side	4× 12-15 each side	145
1d.	Off-bench side lean hold	3× 20-25 seconds each side with 2-3 minutes rest between quadsets	4× 12-18 seconds each side with 2-3 minutes rest between quadsets	184
2a.	Trap bar squat or barbell squat	3× 12-16	4× 6-10	139 or 121
2b.	Dumbbell rotational shoulder press	3× 12-16 each side	4× 6-10 each side	83
2c.	Stability ball plate crunch	3× 12-16 with 2-3 minutes rest between trisets	4× 8-10 with 2-3 minutes rest between trisets	170
3a.	Leaning lat pull-down	3× 12-16	4× 6-10	60
3b.	One-leg one-arm dumbbell Romanian deadlift	3× 12-16 each side	4× 6-10 each side	144
3c.	One-arm dumbbell overhead triceps extension	3× 12-16 each side	4× 6-10 each side	86
3d.	One-arm plank	3× 20-25 seconds each side with 2-3 minutes rest between quadsets	4× 12-18 seconds each side with 2-3 minutes rest between quadsets	183
Conditioning		High-resistance upright bike sprints: 10 sec on and 50 sec off × 4-8 rounds		191

Table 13.6 Gym-Based Fat Loss Program 6

		Workout A	Workout B	Page
1a.	Lat pull-down (underhand grip)	4× 6-8	3× 12-16	58
1b.	Low foot Bulgarian split squat	4× 6-8 each side	3× 10-12 each side	129
1c.	Dumbbell overhead press	4× 6-8 each side with 2-3 minutes rest between trisets	3× 10-12 each side with 2-3 minutes rest between trisets	72
2a.	Underhand grip Smith bar row	4× 8-10	3× 14-16	115
2b.	Push-up variations (exercises noted)	Resistance band loop push-up 4× max reps	Push-up 3× max reps	105 and 62
2c.	Resistance band loop hybrid deadlift	4× 6-8 each side	3× 10-12 each side	148
2d.	Weight plate around the world	4× 6-8 each side with 2-3 minutes rest between quadsets	3× 9-10 each side with 2-3 minutes rest between quadsets	182
3a.	Machine lying hamstring curl	4× 8-12	3× 14-16	151
3b.	Stability ball abdominal variations (exercises noted)	Stability ball pike 4× 6-12	Stability ball knee tuck 3× 15-20	177 and 181

	Workout A	Workout B	Page
3c. Abdominal rollout variations (exercises noted)	Arm walkout 4× 6-8	Stability ball rollout 3× 15-20	183 and 176
3d. Dumbbell rear delt fly	4× 8-12 with 2-3 minutes rest between quadsets	3× 14-16 with 2-3 minutes rest between quadsets	67
Conditioning		Unilateral farmer's walk complex: 2-3 sets with 2-3 min rest between sets	196

Table 13.7   Gym-Based Fat Loss Program 7

	Workout A	Workout B	Page
1a. One-arm dumbbell freestanding row	3× 12-16 each side	4× 6-10 each side	84
1b. Dumbbell rotational shoulder press	3× 12-16	4× 6-10	83
1c. Stability ball wall squat	3× 20-25	4× 12-16	141
1d. Stability ball arc	3× 10-12 with 2-3 minutes rest between quadsets	4× 7-8 with 2-3 minutes rest between quadsets	172
2a. One-arm half-kneeling angled cable row	3× 12-16 each side	4× 6-10 each side	95
2b. High-to-low cable chop	3× 12-16 each side	4× 6-10 each side	168
2c. Traveling dumbbell Romanian deadlift lunge	3× 12-16 each side with 2-3 minutes rest between trisets	4× 6-10 each side with 2-3 minutes rest between trisets	144
3a. Machine chest press	3× 12-16	4× 6-10	102
3b. Stability ball leg curl variations (exercises noted)	Stability ball leg curl 3× 15-20	One-leg stability ball leg curl 4× 6-12	154 and 154
3c. Dumbbell biceps curl	3× 14-16	4× 8-12	68
3d. Dumbbell shoulder A	3× 14-16 with 2-3 minutes rest between quadsets	4× 8-12 with 2-3 minutes rest between quadsets	88
Conditioning	Weight plate push: 40-50 yd (37-46 m) total distance × 3-5 sets. Rest 90 sec-3min between sets		192

Table 13.8   Gym-Based Fat Loss Program 8

	Workout A	Workout B	Page
1a. One-arm cable press	4× 10-12	3× 14-16	92
1b. One-arm compound cable row	4× 10-12 each side	3× 14-16 each side	94
1c. One-leg one-arm dumbbell Romanian deadlift	4× 8-10 each side with 2-3 minutes rest between trisets	3× 12-15 each side with 2-3 minutes rest between trisets	144
2a. Pull-up (with machine or resistance band loop assistance if needed)	4× 6-8	3× 12-16	118

> continued

Table 13.8 > *continued*

	Workout A	Workout B	Page
2b. One-arm angled barbell press	4× 6-8 each side	3× 10-12 each side	77
2c. Elevated dumbbell reverse lunge	4× 6-8 each side with 2-3 minutes rest between trisets	3× 10-12 each side with 2-3 minutes rest between trisets	126
3a. Machine seated hamstring curl	4× 6-9	3× 12-15	150
3b. Shoulder tap plank	4× 15-20 seconds	3× 24-30 seconds	186
3c. Dumbbell shoulder T	4× 8-12	3× 14-16	90
3d. Dumbbell triceps kickback	4× 8-12 with 2-3 minutes rest between quadsets	3× 14-16 with 2-3 minutes rest between quadsets	86
Conditioning		Weight plate complex: 3-4 rounds with 2-3 min rest between rounds	203

Table 13.9   Sample Gym-Based Fat Loss Training Setup: Two Times per Week

Week 1	Week 2*
Monday: Fat loss program 1, workout A	*Monday:* Fat loss program 3, workout A
Tuesday: Rest	*Tuesday:* Rest
Wednesday: Rest	*Wednesday:* Rest
Thursday: Fat loss program 2, workout A	*Thursday:* Fat loss program 4, workout A
Friday: Rest	*Friday:* Rest
Saturday: Rest	*Saturday:* Rest
Sunday: Rest	*Sunday:* Rest

*On week three, you'd perform fat loss programs 5 and 6, workout A. On week four, you'd perform fat loss programs 7 and 8, workout A. Then, on week five, you'd repeat the sequence over again, starting again with program 1, workout B; and so on.

Table 13.10   Sample Gym-Based Fat Loss Training Setup: Three Times per Week

Week 1	Week 2*
Monday: Fat loss program 1, workout A	*Monday:* Fat loss program 4, workout A
Tuesday: Rest	*Tuesday:* Rest
Wednesday: Fat loss program 2, workout A	*Wednesday:* Fat loss program 5, workout A
Thursday: Rest	*Thursday:* Rest
Friday: Fat loss program 3, workout A	*Friday:* Fat loss program 6, workout A
Saturday: Rest	*Saturday:* Rest
Sunday: Rest	*Sunday:* Rest

*Once you go through the entire sequence of the "A" workouts for all eight programs, you'll repeat the cycle, starting over with the B workouts (e.g., program 1, workout B; program 2, workout B).

Table 13.11 Sample Gym-Based Fat Loss Training Setup: Four Times per Week

Week 1	Week 2*
Monday: Fat loss program 1, workout A	*Monday:* Fat loss program 5, workout A
Tuesday: Fat loss program 2, workout A	*Tuesday:* Fat loss program 6, workout A
Wednesday: Rest	*Wednesday:* Rest
Thursday: Fat loss program 3, workout A	*Thursday:* Fat loss program 7, workout A
Friday: Rest	*Friday:* Rest
Saturday: Fat loss program 4, workout A	*Saturday:* Fat loss program 8, workout A
Sunday: Rest	*Sunday:* Rest

*If you prefer to leave the weekend open and train on Monday, Tuesday, Thursday, and Friday, that's okay! On week three, you'll repeat the cycle, this time starting with program 1, workout B; program 2, workout B; and so on.

Table 13.12 Sample Gym-Based Fat Loss Training Setup: Five Times per Week

Week 1	Week 2*
Monday: Fat loss program 1, workout A	*Monday:* Fat loss program 6, workout A
Tuesday: Fat loss program 2, workout A	*Tuesday:* Fat loss program 7, workout A
Wednesday: Fat loss program 3, workout A	*Wednesday:* Fat loss program 8, workout A
Thursday: Rest	*Thursday:* Rest
Friday: Fat loss program 4, workout A	*Friday:* Fat loss program 1, workout B
Saturday: Fat loss program 5, workout A	*Saturday:* Fat loss program 2, workout B
Sunday: Rest	*Sunday:* Rest

*On week three, you'd perform program 3, workout B; program 4, workout B; program 5, workout B; and so on. Once you've completed fat loss program 8, workout B, you'll repeat the sequence over again, starting again with program 1, workout A; program 2, workout A; program 3, workout A; and so on.

Fat Loss Home or Hotel Gym Workouts

On days that you're traveling, can't make it to the gym, or don't have access to a gym, you can use these home or hotel gym workouts or the band and bodyweight workouts. The two workouts in tables 13.13 and 13.14 use equipment that's either recommended for your home gym or that's commonly found in most hotel gyms. That equipment is as follows:

- A set of dumbbells (up to 50 lb or 20 kg)
- An adjustable weight bench that can be made flat or set at an incline
- A high-quality stability ball that's 55 to 65 centimeters
- A chin-up bar (many are designed to be easily placed inside the top of a doorway)
- A set of resistance bands with handles of varying strengths from light to very heavy
- Resistance band loops of varying strength from light to medium
- Resistance band mini loops of varying strength from light to medium

Resistance bands, resistance band loops, and resistance band mini loops are affordable and available at most sporting goods stores or online, but they are not often found at hotel gyms. I recommend traveling with at least one set of each type of band. They're portable and easy to pack in your luggage. It's also important to note that since the following workouts are designed to be done with limited equipment, some of the exercises included will require small modifications from how they're featured in the exercise descriptions. For example, for a cable-based exercise such as the One-Arm Cable Row, you'd perform it with a resistance band instead of cable if your training environment doesn't feature a cable column. Or, for a dumbbell exercise such as the Dumbbell Shoulder W, you'd simply perform the same movement as shown in the exercise description without holding dumbbells. These modifications are indicated within each of the following workouts.

Also, these workouts are intended to be used *only* as an addition to your regular weekly gym-based workouts on days when you're traveling, can't make it to the gym, or don't have access to a gym. These workouts are *not* intended to replace your gym-based workouts; your primary training should revolve around using the gym-based programs in the previous section. Before you begin any of the following workouts, be sure to perform one of the dynamic warm-up sequences in chapter 5.

The two workouts in tables 13.15 and 13.16 are bodyweight exercises and resistance band exercises utilizing three types of bands: resistance bands with handles (these can be attached to any doorway or stable object in matter of seconds), resistance band loops, and resistance mini band loops. A set of high-quality resistance bands with handles and both types of resistance band loops—they come in multiple resistances from light to very heavy—for home use and to take with you when you travel are a must. They are portable and add a number of effective exercise options to your bodyweight training workouts, delivering a value that far exceeds their cost.

The following workouts are *not* intended to be done exclusively and are not designed to replace the gym-based programs earlier in this chapter. They are intended to be used only as an addition to your regular weekly gym-based workouts on days when you don't have access to any kind of gym. Remember, before you begin each of the following workouts, be sure to perform one of the dynamic warm-up sequences in chapter 5.

Table 13.13 Fat Loss Home or Hotel Gym Workout 1

Exercise	Sets and reps	Page
1a. Two-arm dumbbell bent-over row	3× 12-16	66
1b. Elevated dumbbell reverse lunge	3× 10-12 each side	126
1c. Push-up	3× max reps	62
1d. Weight plate around the world**	3× 9-10 each side with 2-3 minutes rest between quadsets	182
2a. Resistance band loop hybrid deadlift	3× 15-25	148
2b. Dumbbell rotational shoulder press	3× 12-16 each side	83
2c. Stability ball plate crunch**	3× 12-16 with 2-3 minutes rest between trisets	170
3a. Chin-up (with resistance band loop band assistance if needed)	3× 12-16	117
3b. Low-to-high cable chop (with resistance band)*	3× 12-15 each side	165
3c. One-leg dumbbell bench hip thrust	3× 12-20 each side with 2-3 minutes rest between trisets	145
Conditioning	Bodyweight and resistance band complex: 3 rounds of 15-20 reps of each exercise with 2-3 min rest between sets	209

*Use a resistance band instead of a cable to perform this exercise in the manner provided in the exercise description.

**If you don't have a weight plate, you can hold each side of a dumbbell instead.

Table 13.14 Fat Loss Home or Hotel Gym Workout 2

Exercise	Sets and reps	Page
1a. Dumbbell incline bench press	3× 14-20	82
1b. One-arm dumbbell row	3× 10-12 each side	64
1c. Dumbbell lateral Romanian deadlift lunge	3× 10-12 each side	142
1d. Reverse crunch	3× 12-15 with 2-3 minutes rest between quadsets	160
2a. One-arm motorcycle cable row (with resistance band)*	3× 14-20 each side	94
2b. Dumbbell leaning Bulgarian split squat	3× 12-16 each side	128
2c. Close-grip push-up	3× max reps with 2-3 minutes rest between trisets	113
3a. Stability ball leg curl	3× 12-20	154
3b. Dumbbell plank row	3× 9-10 each side	182
3c. Dumbbell biceps curl	3× 12-16	68
3d. One-arm dumbbell overhead triceps extension	3× 12-16 each side with 2-3 minutes rest between quadsets	86
Conditioning	Two-minute bodyweight complex: 2-3 rounds with 2-3 min rest between rounds	207

*Use a resistance band instead of a cable to perform this exercise in the manner provided in the exercise description.

Table 13.15 Fat Loss Bodyweight and Band Workout 1

Exercise		Sets and reps	Page
1a.	One-arm motorcycle cable row (with resistance band)*	3× 14-20 each side	94
1b.	One-arm cable press (with resistance band)*	3× 20-30 total each stance	92
1c.	Zombie squat	3× 20-30 (perform reps as fast as possible while maintaining form) with 2-3 minutes rest between trisets	152
2a.	Resistance band loop hybrid deadlift	3× 15-25	148
2b.	Push-up	3× max reps	62
2c.	One-arm plank	3× 15-20 seconds each side	183
2d.	Dumbbell shoulder T (without dumbbells)**	3× 15-25 with 2-3 minutes rest between quadsets	90
3a.	One-arm cable row (with resistance band)*	3× 14-20 each side	93
3b.	Resistance band overhead triceps extension	3× 14-20	106
3c.	One-leg hip lift***	3× 14-20 each side	147
3d.	Arm walkout	3× 4-7 with 2-3 minutes rest between quadsets	183
Conditioning		Bodyweight and resistance band complex: 3 rounds of 15-20 reps each exercise with 2-3 min rest between sets	209

*Use a resistance band instead of a cable to perform this exercise in the manner provided in the exercise description.

** Perform this movement without using dumbbells in the manner provided in the exercise description.

***If you don't have a weight bench, you can perform this exercise with your foot resting on the seat of a padded chair.

Table 13.16 Fat Loss Bodyweight and Band Workout 2

Exercise		Sets and reps	Page
1a.	Resistance band one-arm incline press	3× 12-20 each side	106
1b.	Resistance band one-arm bent-over row	3× 12-16 each side	108
1c.	One-leg 45-degree cable Romanian deadlift (with resistance band)*	3× 12-16 each side with 2-3 minutes rest between trisets	147
2a.	Resistance band step and chest press	3× 18-24	104
2b.	One-arm compound cable row (with resistance band)*	3× 12-15 each side	94
2c.	Dumbbell leaning Bulgarian split squat (without dumbbells)**	3× 10-12 each side	128
2d.	Reverse crunch	3× 8-15 with 2-3 minutes rest between quadsets	160
3a.	Low-to-high cable chop (with resistance band)*	3× 12-15 each side	165
3b.	Resistance band biceps curl	3× 14-16	109
3c.	Cross-body plank	3× 12-15 each side	185
3d.	Resistance band mini loop low lateral shuffle	3× 20-25 each side with 2-3 minutes rest between quadsets	149
Conditioning		Two-minute bodyweight complex: × 2-3 rounds with 2-3 min rest between rounds	207

*Use a resistance band instead of a cable to perform this exercise in the manner provided in the exercise description.

**Perform this movement without using dumbbells in the manner provided in the exercise description. You can also perform this movement without the front foot elevated.

14 } Physique Programs

This chapter is for those who are focused on aesthetics and are exercising to maximize muscular development (i.e., muscle size). If you tend to enjoy bodybuilding workouts and like to gauge success by how you look in the mirror (flexing) and by muscle circumference measurements, then the workout programs in this chapter are for you!

The Basics of Physique Programs

How frequently you work out each week often depends on the reason you're exercising to begin with. It is certainly possible to build muscle while training less often, but people who are focused on muscle building commonly train more frequently than those who are exercising for other goals. This chapter has two types of workout programs. The first series is for those who are training four times per week. The second series is for those who prefer to train five or six times per week. The details for each program are in the following two sections.

These programs differ from the programs found in the previous chapters because they create more overall training volume (i.e., amount of exercises, total sets and reps) per muscle group per week. Research shows that there's a dose-response to gains in muscle size. To accomplish this for those who are training four times per week, the first series of workouts alternates workouts for the upper and lower body. For those who are training five to six times per week, the second series of programs is rotating through a split involving a back/shoulders/biceps workout, a lower body/core workout, and a chest/shoulders/triceps workout. These workouts are designed to performed for three days, with one day off.

There are guidelines for the programs in this chapter. Some of these guidelines will be the same for all the program chapters featured in this book, but others differ depending on which type of program you're doing. Let's look at the key points to remember for your physique programs:

- Perform the exercises designated with *a* or *b* as paired sets, and perform exercises with *a*, *b*, and *c* as trisets. Perform all reps in a given set before moving to the next set. Once all exercises within a set are complete, you can rest a bit longer than indicated between sets (if necessary) to complete the designated number of reps with good control. Completing one round of the exercises in a paired or triset is considered one set.

- The rep range (i.e., 10-15 reps) is next to each exercise in the workout programs in the next two sections. If you're using the same weight for each set, you may be able to do 15 reps on the first set, 12 reps on the next set, and 10 reps on the third set due to accumulated fatigue. Or, you can reduce the weight you're using with each consecutive set to achieve the higher end or given rep range on each consecutive set. Both methods are effective at helping you to progress.

- When a program indicates to take a break before beginning a new cycle, this doesn't mean you have to do nothing. During your days off, you can do some low-impact activities, such as going for long walks, hikes, bike rides, or swims. Also, yoga can be a great option for your active rest periods. If you're already doing yoga each week, as recommended earlier, you can simply increase your yoga practice in your (active) rest week from the gym. Taking 4-7 days to deload before repeating a workout cycle can minimize the risk of overtraining and helps you continue to make gains. It also makes you hungry to get back into the gym, which can help you avoid getting in the habit of simply going through the motions.

- Maintain strict form, without cheating by using additional movements or momentum.

- Do the concentric (lifting) portion of each rep at a normal tempo while mentally focusing on the working muscles in each exercise. Maintain control during the eccentric (lowering) portion, taking 3-4 seconds to lower the weight on each rep.

- Use a weight load that leaves you unable to perform any more reps than indicated while maintaining proper control and technique.

- If an exercise causes pain or discomfort beyond the sensation associated with muscle fatigue, utilize an alternative exercise that doesn't hurt. There are plenty of movements in the exercise chapters of this book to choose from.

- Remember, before you begin a workout in the following programs, be sure to perform one of the dynamic warm-up sequences in chapter 5.

Physique Programs

Before you perform these programs, I recommend that you first complete the beginner programs in chapter 10 if you're just starting out or haven't worked out in a while. If you have been regularly working out or you've completed the beginner programs, it's also recommended that you complete at least six to eight weeks of the fitness programs in chapter 11 before using the following programs.

In addition, although the focus of the programs featured in this chapter are the gym-based programs, since you can't always make it to the gym, this chapter also provides two home and hotel gym workouts along with two workouts using only bodyweight and resistance band exercises that you can use on the days you're traveling or don't have access to any kind of gym equipment.

Your Gym Bag

There are a couple pieces of portable equipment that I recommend you always have in your gym bag—resistance bands with handles and resistance band loops. These bands allow you to group exercises requiring immobile equipment (e.g., squat rack or machine) with bands, which are mobile equipment. This enables you to use band exercises within a paired set or triset while you remain at the immobile equipment and don't have to walk all over the gym, thus potentially losing your equipment to another member.

There are two places online that I recommend you go to purchase high-quality resistance bands: Power-Systems.com and Sorinex.com. At Power Systems, the resistance bands with handles to get are the *Double Cords*; the resistance band loops are called *strength bands*, and resistance band mini loops are called *Versa Loops*. At Sorinex Exercise Equipment, resistance band loops are called *strength bands*, and resistance band mini loops are called *short bands*.

Gym-Based Physique Program: Four Times per Week

This program alternates between upper body and lower body and core workouts if you're training four times per week. There are two versions—A and B—of five upper-body workouts and lower-body and core workouts, for a total of ten different workouts (see tables 14.1-14.6). The B version of each workout has the same exercises performed in the A version, but they're done in the reverse order.

A good ongoing training program should be consistent enough to allow you to see progress but have enough variety to prevent staleness and boredom. This means using the same basic exercises but in different ways, which is exactly what you're doing when performing the exercises in the opposite order. It varies the workouts because it distributes fatigue to your body differently, without changing the workouts.

The programs featured here alternate between upper body and lower body and core workouts and are to be used if you're training four times per week, with no more than two consecutive days at a time for recovery. The following tables show how a weekly setup could be used for working out four times per week.

Gym-Based Physique Program: Five or Six Times per Week

This program starting in table 14.7 rotates through a split involving workouts focused on back, shoulders, and biceps; lower body and core; and chest, shoulders, and triceps. These workouts are to be used if you're training five to six times per week, but no more than three days in a row to maximize recovery and minimize the risk of overtraining.

There are five programs with workouts focused on back, shoulders, and biceps; lower body and core workouts, and workouts that focus on chest, shoulders, and triceps—each with an A and B version—for a total of 10 workouts (see tables 14.7-14.11). The B version of each workout has the same exercises performed in the A version, but they're done in the reverse order to distribute fatigue to your body differently, providing enough consistency to allow you to see progress while having enough variety to prevent staleness and boredom.

Table 14.1 Gym-Based Physique Program 1: Four Times per Week

Lower body/core			
Workout A	Page	Workout B	Page
1. Barbell squat 4× 8-12 with 3 minutes rest between sets	121	1. Copenhagen hip adduction 3× 12-16 each side with 90 seconds rest between sets	134
2. One-leg one-arm dumbbell Romanian deadlift 3× 10-12 each side with 2 minutes rest between sets	144	2a. Reverse crunch 3× 8-12	160
3. One-leg dumbbell bench hip thrust 3× 14-16 with 2 minutes rest between sets	145	2b. Machine lying hamstring curl 3× 8-10 with 90 seconds rest between paired sets	151
4a. Machine leg extension 3× 10-12	151	3a. Cable tight torso rotation with hip shift (with resistance band)* 3× 14-16 each side	166
4b. Cable tight torso rotation with hip shift (with resistance band)* 3× 14-16 each side with 90 seconds rest between paired sets	166	3b. Machine leg extension 3× 8-12 with 90 seconds rest between paired sets	151
5a. Machine lying hamstring curl 3× 10-12	151	4. One-leg dumbbell bench hip thrust 3× 14-16 with 2 minutes rest between sets	145
5b. Reverse crunch 3× 8-12 with 90 seconds rest between paired sets	160	5. One-leg one-arm dumbbell Romanian deadlift 3× 10-12 each side with 2 minutes rest between sets	144
6. Copenhagen hip adduction 3× 12-16 each side with 90 seconds rest between sets	134	6. Barbell squat 3× 12-15 with 3 minutes rest between sets	121

Upper body			
Workout A	Page	Workout B	Page
1a. Barbell bent-over row 4× 8-10	63	1a. Dumbbell side shoulder raise 3× 8-10	71
1b. Lockoff push-up 4× 6-8 each side with 2 minutes rest between paired sets	111	1b. E-Z bar preacher biceps curl 3× 8-10 with 90 seconds rest between paired sets	87
2a. Lat pull-down (underhand grip) 4× 8-10	58	2a. Cable biceps curl 3× 8-10	101
2b. Dumbbell overhead press 4× 8-10 with 2 minutes rest between paired sets	72	2b. Cable compound straight-arm pull-down 3× 8-10 with 90 seconds rest between paired sets	99
3a. Cable rope face pull 3× 12-15	74	3a. Cable rope triceps extension 3× 8-10	98
3b. Cable triceps rope extension 3× 10-15 with 90 seconds rest between paired sets	98	3b. Cable rope face pull 3× 12-15 with 90 seconds rest between paired sets	74
4a. Cable compound straight-arm pull-down 3× 10-15	99	4a. Dumbbell shoulder press 3× 12-15	72
4b. Cable biceps curl 3× 12-15 with 90 seconds rest between paired sets	101	4b. Lat pull-down (underhand grip) 3× 12-15 with 2 minutes rest between paired sets	58
5a. E-Z bar preacher biceps curl 3× 12-15	87	5a. Lockoff push-up 3× 6-10 each side	111
5b. Dumbbell side shoulder raise 3× 12-10 with 90 seconds rest between paired sets	71	5b. Barbell bent-over row 3× 8-12 each side with 2 minutes rest between paired sets	63

*Use a resistance band instead of a cable to perform this exercise in the manner provided in the exercise description.

278

Table 14.2 Gym-Based Physique Program 2: Four Times per Week

Lower body/core					
Workout A		Page	Workout B		Page
1.	Dumbbell leaning Bulgarian split squat 3× 8-12 each side with 2 minutes rest between sets	128	1a.	Weight plate speed chop 3× 8-10 each side	175
2.	Barbell Romanian deadlift 3× 12-15 with 2 minutes rest between sets	139	1b.	Machine hip adduction 3× 8-12 with 90 seconds rest between paired sets	152
3.	One-leg hip lift with weight plate 3× 8-12 each side with 90 seconds rest between sets	146	2a.	Stability ball pike rollout 4× 8-14	178
4a.	Stability ball wall squat 3× 12-16	141	2b.	Nordic hamstring curl 3× 8-10 with 90 seconds rest between paired sets	153
4b.	Stability ball plate crunch 3× 10-15 with 90 seconds rest between paired sets	170	3a.	Stability ball plate crunch 3× 10-15	170
5a.	Nordic hamstring curl 4× 6-8	153	3b.	Stability ball wall squat 3× 12-16 with 90 seconds rest between paired sets	141
5b.	Stability ball pike rollout 3× 8-14 with 90 seconds rest between paired sets	178	4.	One-leg hip lift with weight plate 3× 8-12 each side with 90 seconds rest between sets	146
6a.	Machine hip adduction 3× 10-15	152	5.	Barbell Romanian deadlift 3× 12-15 with 2 minutes rest between sets	139
6b.	Weight plate speed chop 3× 8-12 each side with 90 seconds rest between paired sets	175	6.	Dumbbell leaning Bulgarian split squat 3× 12-15 each side with 2 minutes rest between sets	128

Upper body					
Workout A		Page	Workout B		Page
1a.	Pull-up (with machine or resistance band loop assistance if needed) 4× 6-8	118	1a.	Dumbbell triceps skull crusher 3× 8-10	73
1b.	One-arm angled barbell press 4× 8-10 each side with 2 minutes rest between paired sets	77	1b.	Dumbbell biceps curl 3× 8-10 with 90 seconds rest between paired sets	68
2a.	One-arm dumbbell row 4× 8-10	64	2a.	One-arm dumbbell overhead triceps extension 3× 8-10	86
2b.	Barbell bench press 4× 8-10 with 2 minutes rest between paired sets	79	2b.	Cable pec fly 3× 8-10 with 90 seconds rest between paired sets	97
3a.	Wide-grip seated row 3× 10-12	96	3a.	Seated row shrug 3× 10-12	95
3b.	Seated row shrug 3× 8-10 with 90 seconds rest between paired sets	95	3b.	Wide-grip seated row 3× 12-15 with 2 minutes rest between paired sets	96
4a.	Cable pec fly 3× 12-15	97	4a.	Barbell bench press 3× 12-15	79
4b.	One-arm dumbbell overhead triceps extension 3× 12-15 with 90 seconds rest between paired sets	86	4b.	One-arm dumbbell row 3× 12-15 with 2 minutes rest between paired sets	64
5a.	Dumbbell biceps curl 3× 12-15	68	5a.	One-arm angled barbell press 3× 12-15 each side	77
5b.	Dumbbell triceps skull crusher 3× 12-15 with 90 seconds rest between paired sets	73	5b.	Pull-up (with machine or resistance band loop assistance if needed) 3× 12-15 with 3 minutes rest between paired sets	118

Table 14.3　Gym-Based Physique Program 3: Four Times per Week

Lower body/core				
Workout A	**Page**	**Workout B**	**Page**	
1. Barbell hybrid deadlift 4× 8-10 with 3 minutes rest between sets	124	1a. High-to-low cable chop 3× 10-12 each side	168	
2. Elevated dumbbell reverse lunge 3× 8-10 each side with 2 minutes rest between sets	126	1b. One-leg cable hip adduction 3× 12-15 each side with 90 seconds rest between paired sets	148	
3. 45-degree hip extension 3× 8-12 with 2 minutes rest between sets	131	2a. Plank march with resistance band mini loop 3× 6-8 each side	185	
4a. Mid-platform machine leg press 3× 12-15	149	2b. Machine seated hamstring curl 3× 8-10 with 2 minutes rest between paired sets	150	
4b. Arm walkout 3× 4-6 with 2 minutes rest between paired sets	183	3a. Arm walkout 3× 4-6	183	
5a. Machine seated hamstring curl 3× 10-14	150	3b. Mid-platform machine leg press 3× 12-15 with 2 minutes rest between paired sets	149	
5b. Plank march with resistance band mini loop 3× 6-8 each side with 2 minutes rest between paired sets	185	4. 45-degree hip extension 3× 12-15 with 2 minutes rest between sets	131	
6a. One-leg cable hip adduction 3× 12-15 each side	148	5. Elevated dumbbell reverse lunge 3× 10-12 each side with 2 minutes rest between sets	126	
6b. High-to-low cable chop 3× 10-12 each side with 90 seconds rest between paired sets	168	6. Barbell hybrid deadlift 3× 12-15 with 3 minutes rest between sets	124	
Upper body				
Workout A	**Page**	**Workout B**	**Page**	
1a. Machine chest press 4× 8-10	102	1. E-Z bar biceps curl 3× 8-10 with 2 minutes rest between sets	87	
1b. Two-arm dumbbell bent-over row 4× 8-10 with 2 minutes rest between paired sets	66	2. Low-cable one-arm face-away biceps curl 3× 8-10 each side with 2 minutes rest between sets	101	
2. Dumbbell incline bench press 4× 8-10 with 2 minutes rest between sets	82	3a. Close-grip push-up 3× 8-10 each side	113	
3. Leaning lat pull-down 4× 8-10 with 2 minutes rest between sets	60	3b. One-arm compound cable row 3× 8-10 each side with 2 minutes rest between paired sets	94	
4a. Machine chest fly 3× 12-15	104	4a. Dumbbell triceps kickback 3× 8-10	86	
4b. Dumbbell triceps kickback 3× 12-15 with 90 seconds rest between paired sets	86	4b. Machine chest fly 3× 8-10 with 2 minutes rest between paired sets	104	
5a. One-arm compound cable row 3× 12-15 each side	94	5. Leaning lat pull-down 4× 12-15 with 2 minutes rest between sets	60	
5b. Close-grip push-up 3× 12-15 each side with 2 minutes rest between paired sets	113	6. Dumbbell incline bench press 3× 12-15 with 2 minutes rest between sets	82	
6. Low-cable one-arm face-away biceps curl 3× 12-15 each side with 2 minutes rest between sets	101	7a. Two-arm dumbbell bent-over row 3× 12-15	66	
7. E-Z bar biceps curl 3× 12-15 with 2 minutes rest between sets	87	7b. Machine chest press 3× 12-15 with 2 minutes rest between paired sets	102	

Table 14.4 Gym-Based Physique Program 4: Four Times per Week

Lower body/core				
Workout A	**Page**	**Workout B**		**Page**
1. Trap bar squat 4× 8-10 with 3 minutes rest between sets	139	1.	Copenhagen hip adduction 3× 12-16 each side with 90 seconds rest between sets	134
2. Traveling dumbbell Romanian deadlift lunge 3× 8-10 each side with 2 minutes rest between sets	144	2a.	Stability ball arc 3× 5-8	172
3. One-leg dumbbell bench hip thrust 3× 12-16 each side with 2 minutes rest between sets	145	2b.	Stability ball leg curl 3× 12-20 with 2 minutes rest between paired sets	154
4a. Machine leg extension 3× 10-12	151	3a.	Reverse crunch 3× 8-15	160
4b. Reverse crunch 3× 8-15 with 2 minutes rest between paired sets	160	3b.	Machine leg extension 3× 12-15 with 2 minutes rest between paired sets	151
5a. Stability ball leg curl 3× 12-20	154	4.	One-leg dumbbell bench hip thrust 3× 12-16 each side with 2 minutes rest between sets	145
5b. Stability ball arc 3× 5-8 with 2 minutes rest between paired sets	172	5.	Traveling dumbbell Romanian deadlift lunge 3× 10-12 each side with 2 minutes rest between sets	144
6. Copenhagen hip adduction 3× 12-16 each side with 90 seconds rest between sets	134	6.	Trap bar squat 3× 12-15 with 3 minutes rest between sets	139

Upper body				
Workout A	**Page**	**Workout B**		**Page**
1. Chin-up (with machine or resistance band loop assistance if needed) 4× 6-8 with 3 minutes rest between sets	117	1a.	E-Z bar preacher biceps curl 3× 8-10	87
2a. Machine back row 4× 8-10	102	1b.	Dumbbell shoulder T 3× 8-10 each side with 2 minutes rest between paired sets	90
2b. Resistance band loop push-up 4× max reps with 3 minutes rest between paired sets	105	2a.	Overhead cable triceps rope extension 3× 8-10	97
3a. Dumbbell pec fly 3× 10-12	84	2b.	Low-cable angled upright row 3× 15-20 with 2 minutes rest between paired sets	99
3b. Dumbbell triceps skull crusher 3×10-12	73	3a.	Dumbbell biceps curl 3× 8-10	68
3c. Dumbbell biceps curl 3× 12-15 with 2 minutes rest between trisets	68	3b.	Dumbbell triceps skull crusher 3× 8-10	73
4a. Low-cable angled upright row 3× 15-20	99	3c.	Dumbbell pec fly 3× 12-15 with 2 minutes rest between trisets	84
4b. Overhead cable triceps rope extension 3× 12-15 with 2 minutes rest between paired sets	97	4a.	Resistance band loop push-up 3× max reps	105
5a. Dumbbell shoulder T 3× 12-15 each side	90	4b.	Machine back row 3× 12-15 with 3 minutes rest between paired sets	102
5b. E-Z bar preacher biceps curl 3× 12-15 with 2 minutes rest between paired sets	87	5.	Chin-up (with machine or resistance band loop assistance if needed) 3× 12-15 with 3 minutes rest between sets	117

Table 14.5 Gym-Based Physique Program 5: Four Times per Week

Lower body/core			
Workout A	Page	Workout B	Page
1. Mid-platform machine leg press 4× 8-10 with 3 minutes rest between sets	149	1a. One-arm plank 3× 15-20 seconds each side	183
2. Traveling dumbbell leaning lunge 3× 8-10 each side with 2 minutes rest between sets	127	1b. Machine hip adduction 3× 10-14 with 2 minutes rest between paired sets	152
3. One-leg 45-degree cable Romanian deadlift 3× 10-14 each side with 2 minutes rest between sets	147	2a. Stability ball plate crunch 3×8-14	170
4a. Stability ball wall squat 3× 10-15	141	2b. Machine lying hamstring curl 3× 8-12 with 2 minutes rest between paired sets	151
4b. Angled barbell rainbow 3× 8-10 each side with 2 minutes rest between paired sets	174	3a. Angled barbell rainbow 3× 8-10 each side	174
5a. Machine lying hamstring curl 3× 10-12	151	3b. Stability ball wall squat 3× 12-16 with 2 minutes rest between paired sets	141
5b. Stability ball plate crunch 3× 8-15 with 2 minutes rest between paired sets	170	4. One-leg 45-degree cable Romanian deadlift 3× 10-15 each side with 2 minutes rest between sets	147
6a. Machine hip adduction 3× 10-15	152	5. Traveling dumbbell leaning lunge 3× 10-12 each side with 2 minutes rest between sets	127
6b. One-arm plank 3× 15-20 seconds each side with 2 minutes rest between paired sets	183	6. Mid-platform machine leg press 3×12-16 with 3 minutes rest between sets	149

Upper body			
Workout A	Page	Workout B	Page
1a. Underhand grip Smith bar row 4× 8-10	115	1a. Dumbbell shoulder A 4× 8-10	88
1b. Wide-elbow Smith bar shrug 4× 8-10	116	1b. Dumbbell biceps curl 3× 8-10	68
1c. Smith bar triceps skull crusher 4× 8-10 each side with 2 minutes rest between trisets	115	1c. Dumbbell triceps kickback 3× 8-10 with 2 minutes rest between trisets	86
2a. Dumbbell bench press 4× 8-10	81	2a. Machine rear delt fly 3× 8-10	103
2b. Dumbbell shoulder L 3× 10-12 each side with 2 minutes rest between paired sets	90	2b. Machine chest fly 3× 8-10 with 2 minutes rest between paired sets	104
3a. One-arm dumbbell overhead press 3× 10-12 each side	82	3a. Lat pull-down with neutral grip 3× 12-15	91
3b. Lat pull-down with neutral grip 3× 8-10 with 3 minutes rest between paired sets	91	3b. One-arm dumbbell overhead press 3× 12-15 each side with 2 minutes rest between paired sets	82
4a. Machine chest fly 3× 12-15	104	4a. Dumbbell bench press 3× 12-15	81
4b. Machine rear delt fly 3× 12-15 with 2 minutes rest between paired sets	103	4b. Dumbbell shoulder L 3× 10-12 each side with 2 minutes rest between paired sets	90
5a. Dumbbell triceps kickback 3× 12-15	86	5a. Smith bar triceps skull crusher 3× 12-15	115
5b. Dumbbell biceps curl 3× 12-15	68	5b. Underhand grip Smith bar row 3× 12-15	115
5c. Dumbbell shoulder A 3× 12-15 with 2 minutes rest between trisets	88	5c. Wide-elbow Smith bar shrug 3×12-15 with 2 minutes rest between trisets	116

Table 14.6 Sample Gym-Based Physique Training Setup: Four Times per Week

Option 1	
Week 1	**Week 2**
Monday: Program 1, lower body/core, workout A	*Monday:* Program 3, lower body/core, workout A
Tuesday: Program 1, upper body, workout A	*Tuesday:* Program 3, upper body, workout A
Wednesday: Rest	*Wednesday:* Rest
Thursday: Program 2, lower body/core, workout A	*Thursday:* Program 4, lower body/core, workout A
Friday: Program 2, upper body, workout A	*Friday:* Program 4, upper body, workout A
Saturday: Rest	*Saturday:* Rest
Sunday: Rest	*Sunday:* Rest
Week 3	**Week 4**
Monday: Program 5, lower-body/core, workout A	*Monday:* Program 2, lower-body/core, workout B
Tuesday: Program 5, upper body, workout A	*Tuesday:* Program 2, upper body, workout B
Wednesday: Rest	*Wednesday:* Rest
Thursday: Program 1, lower body/core, workout B	*Thursday:* Program 3, lower body/core, workout B
Friday: Program 1, upper body, workout B	*Friday:* Program 3, upper body, workout B
Saturday: Rest	*Saturday:* Rest
Sunday: Rest	*Sunday:* Rest

Week 5*
Monday: Program 4, lower body/core, workout B
Tuesday: Program 4, upper body, workout B
Wednesday: Rest
Thursday: Program 5, lower body/core, workout B
Friday: Program 5, upper body, workout B
Saturday: Rest
Sunday: Rest

Option 2	
Week 1	**Week 2**
Monday: Program 1, lower body/core, workout A	*Monday:* Program 3, lower body/core, workout A
Tuesday: Program 1, upper body, workout A	*Tuesday:* Program 3, upper body, workout A
Wednesday: Rest	*Wednesday:* Rest
Thursday: Program 2, lower body/core, workout A	*Thursday:* Program 4, lower body/core, workout A
Friday: Rest	*Friday:* Rest
Saturday: Program 2, upper body, workout A	*Saturday:* Program 4, upper body, workout A
Sunday: Rest	*Sunday:* Rest

> continued

Table 14.6 > *continued*

Option 2	
Week 3	**Week 4**
Monday: Program 5, lower body/core, workout A	*Monday:* Program 2, lower body/core, workout B
Tuesday: Program 5, upper body, workout A	*Tuesday:* Program 2, upper body, workout B
Wednesday: Rest	*Wednesday:* Rest
Thursday: Program 1, lower body/core, workout B	*Thursday:* Program 3, lower body/core, workout B
Friday: Rest	*Friday:* Rest
Saturday: Program 1, upper body, workout B	*Saturday:* Program 3, upper body, workout B
Sunday: Rest	*Sunday:* Rest
Week 5*	
Monday: Program 4, lower body/core, workout B	
Tuesday: Program 4, upper body, workout B	
Wednesday: Rest	
Thursday: Program 5, lower body/core, workout B	
Friday: Rest	
Saturday: Program 5, upper body, workout B	
Sunday: Rest	

*At the end of a full cycle, it's recommended that you take four to seven days off from your workouts to allow your body and mind to recover and refocus before you continue with a new cycle.

Table 14.7 Gym-Based Physique Program 1: Five or Six Times per Week

Upper body (back, shoulders, biceps)			
Workout A	**Page**	**Workout B**	**Page**
1. Two-arm dumbbell bent-over row 4× 8-10 with 2 minutes rest between sets	66	1. E-Z bar preacher curl 3× 8-10 with 2 minutes rest between sets	87
2. Lat pull-down with underhand grip 4× 8-10 with 2 minutes rest between sets	58	2. Dumbbell biceps curl 3× 8-10 with 2 minutes rest between sets	68
3. One-arm cable row 3× 12-15 with 2 minutes rest between sets	93	3a. Cable compound straight-arm pull-down 3× 10-12	99
4a. Cable rope face pull 3× 12-15	74	3b. Cable rope face pull 3× 10-12 with 2 minutes rest between paired sets	74
4b. Cable compound straight-arm pull-down 3× 10-15 with 2 minutes rest between paired sets	99	4. One-arm cable row 3× 12-15 with 2 minutes rest between sets	93
5. Dumbbell biceps curl 3× 10-12 with 2 minutes rest between sets	68	5. Lat pull-down with underhand grip 3× 12-15 with 2 minutes rest between sets	58
6. E-Z bar preacher biceps curl 3× 10-12 with 2 minutes rest between sets	87	6. Two-arm dumbbell bent-over row 4× 8-10 with 2 minutes rest between sets	66

Lower body/core				
Workout A	**Page**	**Workout B**		**Page**
1. Barbell squat 4× 8-12 with 3 minutes rest between sets	121	1. Copenhagen hip adduction 3× 12-16 each side with 90 seconds rest between sets		134
2. One-leg one-arm dumbbell Romanian deadlift 3× 10-12 each side with 2 minutes rest between sets	144	2a. Reverse crunch 3× 8-12		160
3. One-leg dumbbell bench hip thrust 3× 14-16 with 2 minutes rest between sets	145	2b. Machine lying hamstring curl 3× 8-10 with 2 minutes rest between paired sets		151
4a. Machine leg extension 3× 10-12	151	3a. Cable tight torso rotation with hip shift (with resistance band)* 3× 14-16 each side		166
4b. Cable tight torso rotation with hip shift (with resistance band)* 3× 14-16 each side with 2 minutes rest between paired sets	166	3b. Machine leg extension 3× 8-12 with 2 minutes rest between paired sets		151
5a. Machine lying hamstring curl 3×10-12	151	4. One-leg dumbbell bench hip thrust 3× 14-16 with 2 min. rest between sets		145
5b. Reverse crunch 3× 8-12 with 2 minutes rest between paired sets	160	5. One-leg one-arm dumbbell Romanian deadlift 3× 10-12 each side with 2 minutes rest between sets		144
6. Copenhagen hip adduction 3× 12-16 each side with 90 seconds rest between sets	134	6. Barbell squat 3× 12-15 with 3 minutes rest between sets		121

Upper body (chest, shoulders, triceps)				
Workout A	**Page**	**Workout B**		**Page**
1. Dumbbell bench press 4× 8-10 with 2 minutes rest between sets	81	1a. Dumbbell triceps skull crusher 3× 10-12		73
2. Machine shoulder press 4× 8-10 with 2 minutes rest between sets	103	1b. Dumbbell pullover 3× 10-12 with 2 minutes rest between paired sets		91
3. Lockoff push-up 3× 6-10 each side with 2 minutes rest between sets	111	2a. Dumbbell triceps kickback 3× 12-15		86
4a. Dumbbell side shoulder raise 3× 10-12	71	2b. Dumbbell side shoulder raise 3× 12-15 with 2 minutes rest between paired sets		71
4b. Dumbbell triceps kickback 3× 10-12 with 2 minutes rest between paired sets	86	3. Lockoff push-up 3× 6-10 each side with 2 minutes rest between sets		111
5a. Dumbbell pullover 3× 12-15	91	4. Machine shoulder press 3× 12-16 with 2 minutes rest between sets		103
5b. Dumbbell triceps skull crusher 3× 12-15 with 2 minutes rest between paired sets	73	5. Dumbbell bench press 3× 12-16 with 2 minutes rest between sets		81

*Use a resistance band instead of a cable to perform this exercise in the manner provided in the exercise description.

Table 14.8 Gym-Based Physique Program 2: Five or Six Times per Week

Upper body (back, shoulders, biceps)				
Workout A	**Page**	**Workout B**	**Page**	
1. Pull-up (with machine or resistance band loop assistance if needed) 4× 6-8 with 3 minutes rest between sets	118	1. Dumbbell incline bench biceps curl 3× 8-10 with 2 minutes rest between sets	88	
2. One-arm dumbbell row 4× 8-10 with 2 minutes rest between sets	64	2a. E-Z bar biceps curl 3× 8-10	87	
3a. Wide-grip seated row 3× 10-12	96	2b. Machine rear delt fly 3× 10-12 with 2 minutes rest between paired sets	103	
3b. Seated row shrug 3× 8-10 with 2 minutes rest between paired sets	95	3a. Wide-grip seated row 3× 8-10	96	
4a. Machine rear delt fly 3× 12-15	103	3b. Seated row shrug 3× 12-14 with 2 minutes rest between paired sets	95	
4b. E-Z bar biceps curl 3× 12-15 with 2 minutes rest between paired sets	87	4. One-arm dumbbell row 3× 10-12 each side with 2 minutes rest between sets	64	
5. Dumbbell incline bench biceps curl 3× 10-12 with 2 minutes rest between sets	88	5. Pull-up (with machine or resistance band loop assistance if needed) 3× 10-12 with 3 minutes rest between sets	118	

Lower body/core				
Workout A	**Page**	**Workout B**	**Page**	
1. Dumbbell leaning Bulgarian split squat 3× 8-12 each side with 2 minutes rest between sets	128	1a. Weight plate speed chop 3× 8-10 each side	175	
2. Barbell Romanian deadlift 3× 12-15 with 3 minutes rest between sets	139	1b. Machine hip adduction 3× 8-12 with 2 minutes rest between paired sets	152	
3. One-leg hip lift with weight plate 3× 8-12 each side with 2 minutes rest between sets	146	2a. Stability ball pike rollout 4× 8-14	178	
4a. Stability ball wall squat 3× 12-16	141	2b. Nordic hamstring curl 3× 8-10 with 2 minutes rest between paired sets	153	
4b. Stability ball plate crunch 3× 10-15 with 2 minutes rest between paired sets	170	3a. Stability ball plate crunch 3× 10-15	170	
5a. Nordic hamstring curl 4× 6-8	153	3b. Stability ball wall squat 3× 12-16 with 2 minutes rest between paired sets	141	
5b. Stability ball pike rollout 3× 8-14 with 2 minutes rest between paired sets	178	4. One-leg hip lift with weight plate 3× 8-12 each side	146	
6a. Machine hip adduction 3× 10-15	152	5. Barbell Romanian deadlift 3× 12-15 with 3 minutes rest between sets	139	
6b. Weight plate speed chop 3× 8-12 each side with 2 minutes rest between paired sets	175	6. Dumbbell leaning Bulgarian split squat 3× 12-15 each side with 2 minutes rest between sets	128	

Upper body (chest, shoulders, triceps)				
Workout A	**Page**	**Workout B**	**Page**	
1. One-arm angled barbell press 4× 8-10 each side with 2 minutes rest between sets	77	1a. Low-cable one-arm side shoulder raise 3× 12-16 each side	100	
		1b. Cable triceps rope extension 3× 8-12 with 2 minutes rest between paired sets	98	

Upper body (chest, shoulders, triceps)				
Workout A	Page		Workout B	Page
2a. Barbell bench press 4× 8-10	79		2a. One-arm dumbbell overhead triceps extension 3× 8-12 each side	86
2b. Dumbbell shoulder L 3× 10-12 each side with 2 minutes rest between paired sets	90			
3a. Cable pec fly 3× 12-15	97		2b. Cable pec fly 3× 10-12 with 2 minutes rest between paired sets	97
3b. One-arm dumbbell overhead triceps extension 3× 12-15 each side with 2 minutes rest between paired sets	86		3a. Barbell bench press 3× 12-15	79
4a. Cable triceps rope extension 3× 12-15	98		3b. Dumbbell shoulder L 3× 10-12 each side with 2 minutes rest between paired sets	90
4b. Low-cable one-arm side shoulder raise 3× 10-15 each side with 2 minutes rest between paired sets	100		4. One-arm angled barbell press 3× 12-15 each side with 2 minutes rest between sets	77

Table 14.9 Gym-Based Physique Program 3: Five or Six Times per Week

Upper body (back, shoulders, biceps)				
Workout A	Page		Workout B	Page
1. Barbell bent-over row 4× 8-10 with 2 minutes rest between sets	63		1. Low cable one-arm face-away biceps curl 3× 8-10 each side with 2 minutes rest between sets	101
2. Leaning lat pull-down 4× 8-10 with 2 minutes rest between sets	60		2a. Dumbbell biceps curl 3× 8-10	68
3. One-arm compound cable row 3× 10-12 each side with 2 minutes rest between sets	94		2b. Wide-elbow Smith bar row 3× 6-8	116
4a. Wide-elbow Smith bar row 3× 12-15	116		2c. Wide-elbow Smith bar row shrug 3× 8-10 with 2 minutes rest between trisets	116
4b. Wide-elbow Smith bar row shrug 3× 10-12	116		3. One-arm compound cable row 3× 12-15 each side with 2 minutes rest between sets	94
4c. Dumbbell biceps curl 3× 12-15 with 2 minutes rest between trisets	68		4. Leaning lat pull-down 3× 12-15 with 2 minutes rest between sets	60
5. Low cable one-arm face-away biceps curl 3× 12-15 each side with 2 minutes rest between sets	101		5. Barbell bent-over row 3× 12-15 with 2 minutes rest between sets	63

Lower body/core				
Workout A	Page		Workout B	Page
1. Barbell hybrid deadlift 4× 8-10 with 3 minutes rest between sets	124		1a. High-to-low cable chop 3× 10-12 each side	168
2. Elevated dumbbell reverse lunge 3× 8-10 each side with 2 minutes rest between sets	126		1b. One-leg cable hip adduction 3× 12-15 each side with 2 minutes rest between paired sets	148
3. 45-degree hip extension 3× 8-12 with 2 minutes rest between sets	131		2a. Plank march with resistance band mini loop 3× 6-8 each side	185
4a. Mid-platform machine leg press 3× 12-15	140		2b. Machine seated hamstring curl 3× 8-10 with 2 minutes rest between paired sets	160

> continued

Table 14.9   > continued

Lower body/core					
Workout A		**Page**	**Workout B**		**Page**
4b.	Arm walkout 3× 4-6 with 2 minutes rest between paired sets	183	3a.	Arm walkout 3× 4-6	183
5a.	Machine seated hamstring curl 3× 10-14	150	3b.	Mid-platform machine leg press 3× 12-15 with 2 minutes rest between paired sets	149
5b.	Plank march with resistance band mini loop 3× 6-8 each side with 2 minutes rest between paired sets	185	4.	45-degree hip extension 3× 12-15 with 2 minutes rest between sets	131
6a.	One-leg cable hip adduction 3× 12-15 each side	148	5.	Elevated dumbbell reverse lunge 3× 10-12 each side with 2 minutes rest between sets	126
6b.	High-to-low cable chop 3× 10-12 each side with 2 minutes rest between paired sets	168	6.	Barbell hybrid deadlift 3× 12-15 with 3 minutes rest between sets	124

Upper body (chest, shoulders, triceps)					
Workout A		**Page**	**Workout B**		**Page**
1a.	Machine chest press 4× 8-10 with 2 minutes rest between sets	102	1a.	Overhead cable triceps rope extension 3× 8-12	97
1b.	Dumbbell shoulder L (from a standing position) 3× 10-12 each side with 2 minutes rest between paired sets	90	1b.	Dumbbell overhead press 3× 8-12 with 2 minutes rest between paired sets	72
2.	Dumbbell incline bench press 4× 8-10 with 2 minutes rest between sets	82	2a.	Dumbbell triceps kickback 3× 8-12	86
3a.	Machine chest fly 3× 12-15	104	2b.	Machine chest fly 3× 12-15 with 2 minutes rest between paired sets	104
3b.	Dumbbell triceps kickback 3× 12-15 with 2 minutes rest between paired sets	86	3.	Dumbbell incline bench press 3× 12-16 with 2 minutes rest between sets	82
4a.	Dumbbell overhead press 3× 12-15	72	4a.	Machine chest press 3× 12-16	102
4b.	Overhead cable triceps rope extension 3× 12-15 with 2 minutes rest between paired sets	97	4b.	Dumbbell shoulder L (from a standing position) 3× 10-12 each side with 2 minutes rest between paired sets	90

Table 14.10   Gym-Based Physique Program 4: Five or Six Times per Week

Upper body (back, shoulders, biceps)					
Workout A		**Page**	**Workout B**		**Page**
1.	Chin-up (with machine or resistance band loop assistance if needed) 4× 6-8 with 3 minutes rest between sets	117	1.	Cable biceps curl 3× 8-10 with 2 minutes rest between sets	101
2.	Machine back row 4× 8-10 with 2 minutes rest between sets	102	2.	E-Z bar preacher biceps curl 3× 8-10 with 2 minutes rest between sets	87
3.	Underhand grip Smith bar row 3× 8-12 with 2 minutes rest between sets	115	3a.	Low-cable angled upright row 3× 15-20	99
4a.	Cable compound straight-arm pull-down 3× 10-12	99	3b.	Cable compound straight-arm pull-down 3× 8-12 with 2 minutes rest between paired sets	99
4b.	Low-cable angled upright row 3× 15-20 with 2 minutes rest between paired sets	99	4.	Underhand grip Smith bar row 3× 15-20 with 2 minutes rest between sets	115

Upper body (back, shoulders, biceps)

Workout A	Page	Workout B	Page
5. E-Z bar preacher biceps curl 3× 12-15 with 2 minutes rest between sets	87	5. Machine back row 3× 12-15 with 2 minutes rest between sets	102
6. Cable biceps curl 3× 12-15 with 2 minutes rest between sets	101	6. Chin-up (with machine or resistance band loop assistance if needed) 3× 12-15 with 3 minutes rest between sets	117

Lower body/core

Workout A	Page	Workout B	Page
1. Trap bar squat or barbell front squat 4× 8-10 with 3 minutes rest between sets	139 or 122	1. Copenhagen hip adduction 3× 12-16 each side with 90 seconds rest between sets	134
2. Traveling dumbbell Romanian deadlift lunge 3× 8-10 each side with 2 minutes rest between sets	144	2a. Stability ball arc 3× 5-8	172
3. One-leg dumbbell bench hip thrust 3× 12-16 each side with 2 minutes rest between sets	145	2b. Stability ball leg curl 3× 12-20 with 2 minutes rest between paired sets	154
4a. Machine leg extension 3× 10-12	151	3a. Reverse crunch 3× 8-15	160
4b. Reverse crunch 3× 8-15 with 2 minutes rest between paired sets	160	3b. Machine leg extension 3× 12-15 with 2 minutes rest between paired sets	151
5a. Stability ball leg curl 3× 12-20	154	4. One-leg dumbbell bench hip thrust 3× 12-16 each side with 2 minutes rest between sets	145
5b. Stability ball arc 3× 5-8 with 2 minutes rest between paired sets	172	5. Traveling dumbbell Romanian deadlift lunge 3× 10-12 each side with 2 minutes rest between sets	144
6. Copenhagen hip adduction 3× 12-16 each side with 90 seconds rest between sets	134	6. Trap bar squat or barbell front squat 3× 12-15 with 3 minutes rest between sets	139 or 122

Upper body (chest, shoulders, triceps)

Workout A	Page	Workout B	Page
1. One-arm dumbbell overhead press 4× 7-8 each side with 2 minutes rest between sets	82	1. Dumbbell shoulder Y 3× 10-15 with 2 minutes rest between sets	89
2a. Resistance band loop push-up 4× max	105	2a. Overhead cable triceps rope extension 3× 8-12	97
2b. Supine resistance band shoulder L 3× 10-12 with 2 minutes rest between paired sets	110	2b. Low-cable one-arm side shoulder raise 3× 8-12 each side with 2 minutes rest between paired sets	100
3a. Dumbbell chest squeeze press 3× 10-12	85	3a. Dumbbell triceps skull crusher 3× 8-12	73
3b. Dumbbell triceps skull crusher 3× 10-12 with 2 minutes rest between paired sets	73	3b. Dumbbell chest squeeze press 3× 12-15 with 2 minutes rest between paired sets	85
4a. Low-cable one-arm side shoulder raise 3× 12-15 each side	100	4a. Resistance band loop push-up 3× max	105
4b. Overhead cable triceps rope extension 3× 12-15 with 2 minutes rest between paired sets	97	4b. Supine resistance band shoulder L 3× 10-12 with 2 minutes rest between paired sets	110
5. Dumbbell shoulder Y 2× 20-25 with 2 minutes rest between sets	89	5. One-arm dumbbell overhead press 3× 8-10 each side with 2 minutes rest between sets	82

Table 14.11 Gym-Based Physique Program 5: Five or Six Times per Week

Upper body (back, shoulders, biceps)			
Workout A	**Page**	**Workout B**	**Page**
1. Lat pull-down with neutral grip 4× 8-10 with 2 minutes rest between sets	91	1a. E-Z bar biceps curl 3× 8-10	87
2. Machine back row 4× 8-10 with 2 minutes rest between sets	102	1b. Fighter's cable lat pull-down 3× 8-12 each side with 2 minutes rest between paired sets	96
3. One-arm compound cable row 3× 10-12 each side with 2 minutes rest between sets	94	2a. Low-cable one-arm face-away biceps curl 3× 8-12 each side	101
4a. Low-cable one-arm rear delt fly 3× 8-12	98	2b. Low-cable one-arm rear delt fly 3× 12-15 each side with 2 minutes rest between paired sets	98
4b. Low-cable one-arm face-away biceps curl 3× 8-12 each side with 2 minutes rest between paired sets	101	3. One-arm compound cable row 3× 12-15 each side with 2 minutes rest between sets	94
5a. Fighter's cable lat pull-down 3× 10-15 each side	96	4. Machine back row 3× 12-16 with 2 minutes rest between sets	102
5b. E-Z bar biceps curl 3× 10-15 with 2 minutes rest between paired sets	87	5. Lat pull-down with neutral grip 3× 12-16 with 2 minutes rest between sets	91
Lower body/core			
Workout A	**Page**	**Workout B**	**Page**
1. High-platform machine leg press 4× 8-10 with 2 minutes rest between sets	150	1a. One-arm plank 3× 15-20 seconds each side	183
2. Traveling dumbbell leaning lunge 3× 8-10 each side with 2 minutes rest between sets	127	1b. Machine hip adduction 3× 10-14 with 2 minutes rest between paired sets	152
3. One-leg 45-degree cable Romanian deadlift 3× 10-14 each side with 2 minutes rest between sets	147	2a. Stability ball plate crunch 3× 8-14	170
4a. Stability ball wall squat 3× 10-15	141	2b. Machine lying hamstring curl 3× 8-12 with 2 minutes rest between paired sets	151
4b. Angled barbell rainbow 3× 8-10 each side with 2 minutes rest between paired sets	174	3a. Angled barbell rainbow 3× 8-10 each side	174
5a. Machine lying hamstring curl 3× 10-12	151	3b. Stability ball wall squat 3× 12-16 with 2 minutes rest between paired sets	141
5b. Stability ball plate crunch 3× 8-15 with 2 minutes rest between paired sets	170	4. One-leg 45-degree cable Romanian deadlift 3× 10-15 each side with 2 minutes rest between sets	147
6a. Machine hip adduction 3× 10-15	152	5. Traveling dumbbell leaning lunge 3× 10-12 each side with 2 minutes rest between sets	127
6b. One-arm plank 3× 15-20 seconds each side with 2 minutes rest between paired sets	183	6. High-platform machine leg press 3× 12-16 with 2 minutes rest between sets	150

Upper body (chest, shoulders, triceps)			
Workout A	**Page**	**Workout B**	**Page**
1a. Dumbbell bench press 4× 6-8 each side with 3 minutes rest between sets	81	1. Close-grip push-up 2× max reps with 3 minutes rest between sets	113
1b. Dumbbell shoulder L 3× 10-12 each side with 2 minutes rest between paired sets	90	2. Resistance band side shoulder raise 3× 8-10 with 2 minutes rest between sets	107
2a. Standing cable chest press 3× 10-12 each side	93	3. One-arm angled barbell press 3× 8-10 each side with 2 minutes rest between sets	77
2b. One-arm dumbbell overhead triceps extension 3× 10-12 each side with 2 minutes rest between paired sets	86	4a. One-arm dumbbell overhead triceps extension 3× 8-10 each side	86
3. One-arm angled barbell press 3× 10-12 each side with 2 minutes rest between sets	77	4b. Standing cable chest press 3× 12-15 with 2 minutes rest between paired sets	93
4. Resistance band side shoulder raise 3× 10-12 with 2 minutes rest between sets	107	5a. Dumbbell bench press 3× 8-10 each side	81
5. Close-grip push-up 2× max reps with 3 minutes rest between sets	113	5b. Dumbbell shoulder L 3× 10-12 each side with 2 minutes rest between paired sets	90

These programs are designed to be used if you're training five to six times per week, but no more than 3 days in a row in order to maximize recovery and minimize the risk of overtraining. Table 14.12 shows how a weekly setup could be used for the five to six times per week workout program.

Table 14.12 Sample Gym-Based Physique Training Setup: Five or Six Times per Week

Week 1	Week 2
Monday: Program 1, back/shoulders/biceps, workout A	*Monday:* Rest
Tuesday: Program 1, lower body/core, workout A	*Tuesday:* Program 3, back/shoulders/biceps, workout A
Wednesday: Program 1, chest/shoulders/triceps, workout A	*Wednesday:* Program 3, lower body/core, workout A
Thursday: Rest	*Thursday:* Program 3, chest/shoulders/triceps, workout A
Friday: Program 2, back/shoulders/biceps, workout A	*Friday:* Rest
Saturday: Program 2, lower body/core, workout A	*Saturday:* Program 4, back/shoulders/biceps, workout A
Sunday: Program 2, chest/shoulders/triceps, workout A	*Sunday:* Program 4, lower body/core, workout A
Week 3	**Week 4**
Monday: Program 4, chest/shoulders/triceps, workout A	*Monday:* Program 1, lower body/core, workout B
Tuesday: Rest	*Tuesday:* Program 1, chest/shoulders/triceps, workout B

> continued

Table 14.12   *> continued*

Week 3	Week 4
Wednesday: Program 5, back/shoulders/biceps, workout A	*Wednesday:* Rest
Thursday: Program 5, lower body/core, workout A	*Thursday:* Program 2, back/shoulders/biceps, workout B
Friday: Program 5, chest/shoulders/triceps, workout A	*Friday:* Program 2, lower body/core, workout B
Saturday: Rest	*Saturday:* Program 2, chest/shoulders/triceps, workout B
Sunday: Program 1, back/shoulders/biceps, workout B	*Sunday:* Rest
Week 5	**Week 6***
Monday: Program 3, back/shoulders/biceps, workout B	*Monday:* Rest
Tuesday: Program 3, lower body/core, workout B	*Tuesday:* Program 5, back/shoulders/biceps, workout B
Wednesday: Program 3, chest/shoulders/triceps, workout B	*Wednesday:* Program 5, lower body/core, workout B
Thursday: Rest	*Thursday:* Program 5, chest/shoulders/triceps, workout B
Friday: Program 4, back/shoulders/biceps, workout B	*Friday:* Rest
Saturday: Program 4, lower body/core, workout B	*Saturday:* Rest
Sunday: Program 4, chest/shoulders/triceps, workout B	*Sunday:* Rest

*At the end of a full cycle, it's recommended that you take four to seven days off from your workouts to allow your body and mind to recover and refocus before you continue with a new cycle.

Physique Home or Hotel Gym Workouts

On days that you're traveling, can't make it to the gym, or don't have access to a gym, you can use these home or hotel gym workouts or the band and bodyweight workouts. The two workouts in tables 14.13 and 14.14 use equipment that's either recommended for your home gym or that's commonly found in most hotel gyms. That equipment is as follows:

- A set of dumbbells (up to 50 lb or 20 kg)
- An adjustable weight bench that can be made flat or set at an incline
- A high-quality stability ball that's 55 to 65 centimeters
- A chin-up bar (many are designed to be easily placed inside the top of a doorway)
- A set of resistance bands with handles of varying strengths from light to very heavy
- Resistance band loops of varying strength from light to medium
- Resistance band mini loops of varying strength from light to medium

Resistance bands, resistance band loops, and resistance band mini loops are affordable and available at most sporting goods stores or online, but they are not often found at hotel gyms. I recommend traveling with at least one set of each type of band. They're portable and easy to pack in your luggage. It's also important to note that since the following workouts are designed to be done with limited equipment, some of the exercises included will require small modifications from how they're featured in the exercise descriptions. For example, for a cable-based exercise such as the One-Arm Cable Row, you'd perform it with a resistance band instead of cable if your training environment doesn't feature a cable column. Or, for a dumbbell exercise such as the Dumbbell Shoulder W, you'd simply perform the same movement as shown in the exercise description without holding dumbbells. These modifications are indicated within each of the following programs.

Note that these workouts are intended to be used *only* as an addition to your regular weekly gym-based workouts on days when you're traveling, can't make it to the gym, or don't have access to a gym. These workouts are *not* intended to replace your gym-based workouts; your primary training should revolve around using the gym-based programs in the previous section. Before you begin any of the following workouts, be sure to perform one of the dynamic warm-up sequences in chapter 5.

The two workouts in tables 14.13 and 14.14 have bodyweight exercises and resistance band exercises utilizing three types of bands: resistance bands with handles (these can be attached to any doorway or stable object in matter of seconds), resistance band loops, and resistance mini band loops. A set of high-quality resistance bands with handles and both types of resistance band loops—they come in multiple resistances from light to very heavy—for home use and to take with you when you travel are a must. They are portable and add a number of effective exercise options to your bodyweight training workouts, delivering a value that far exceeds their cost.

Again, the following workouts are *not* intended to be done exclusively and are not designed to replace the gym-based programs earlier in this chapter. They are only an addition to your regular weekly gym-based workouts on days when you don't have access to any kind of gym.

Table 14.13 Physique Home or Hotel Gym Workout

Exercise	Sets and reps	Page
Lower body/core		
1. Dumbbell leaning Bulgarian split squat	3× 10-15 each side	128
2. One-leg one-arm dumbbell Romanian deadlift	3× 12-15 each side	144
3. One-leg hip lift	3× 15-20 each side	147
4a. Stability ball wall squat	3× 14-20	141
4b. Stability ball plate crunch**	3× 10-15	170
5a. Stability ball leg curl	3× 15-25	154
5b. Stability ball pike rollout	3× 12-20	178
6a. Side-lying hip adduction	3× 15-20 each side	153
6b. Low to high cable chop (with resistance band)*	3× 8-12 each side	183

(continued)

Table 14.13   *> continued*

Upper body		
1a. Pull-up (with resistance band loop assistance if needed)	4× 6-10	118
1b. Dumbbell overhead press	4× 8-10	72
2a. One-arm dumbbell freestanding row	4× 8-10 each side	84
2b. Dumbbell bench press	4× 8-10	81
3a. Dumbbell shoulder Y	3× 10-15	89
3b. Two-arm dumbbell bent-over row	3× 12-15	66
4a. Close-grip push-up	3× max reps	113
4b. Cable compound straight-arm pull-down (with resistance band)*	3× 12-20	99
5a. Dumbbell biceps curl	3× 12-15	68
5b. One-arm dumbbell overhead triceps extension	3× 12-15	86

Rest 2 minutes between all straight sets. Rest 90 seconds between all paired sets.

*Use a resistance band instead of a cable to perform this exercise in the manner provided in the exercise description.

**If you don't have a weight plate, you can hold each side of a dumbbell instead.

Table 14.14   Physique Bodyweight and Band Workout

Exercise	Sets and reps	Page
Lower body/core		
1. Resistance band loop hybrid deadlift	4× 15-20	148
2. Dumbbell leaning Bulgarian split squat (without dumbbells)**	3× 15-20 each side	128
3. One-leg 45-degree cable Romanian deadlift (with resistance band)*	3× 15-20 each side	147
4a. Zombie squat	3× 20-30	152
4b. Arm walkout	3× 4-7	183
5a. Stability ball leg curl	3× 15-20	154
5b. Side-lying hip adduction	3× 15-20 each side	153
6a. Plank march with resistance band mini loop	3× 20-25 each side	185
6b. Low-to-high cable chop (with resistance band)*	3× 8-12 each side	165
Upper body		
1a. Push-up	3× max reps	62
1b. One-arm motorcycle cable row (with resistance band)*	3× 14-20 each side	94
2. Resistance band one-arm incline press	3× 15-20 each side	106
3. Resistance band one-arm bent-over row	3× 15-20 each side	108
4a. Resistance band chest fly	3× 15-20	108
4b. Resistance band overhead triceps extension	3× 15-20	106
5a. Cable compound straight-arm pull-down (with resistance band)*	3× 15-20	99
5b. Resistance band triceps extension	3× 15-20	105
6. Resistance band biceps curl	3× 15-20	109
7. Resistance band loop pull-apart	3× 15-20	109

Rest 2 minutes between all straight sets. Rest 90 seconds between all paired sets.

*Use a resistance band instead of a cable to perform this exercise in the manner provided in the exercise description.

** Perform this movement without using dumbbells in the manner provided in the exercise description.

15 { Strategies for Minimizing Injury

Whether your goal is related to general fitness, function and performance, fat loss, or physique, the best *ability* in exercise is the *availability* to do it in the first place. You don't just want to exercise toward your goal; you also want to do so in a way that allows you to keep training, which means taking steps to reduce the risk of an exercise-related injury. That's what this chapter is all about!

Injury risk factors and concerns often vary by sport (factors for swimmers aren't the same as those for soccer players, for example) and body region or joint (factors for ACL rupture are different than for low-back pain). Jason Silvernail, DPT, coauthored this chapter with me. We have reviewed the literature and used professional experience to bring you this list of factors that are generalized for exercise and strength training. We believe everyone should be aware of these high-value areas and address them in their programs.

Exercise training is generally a low-risk activity, but it's not a no-risk activity (1). You can use the following practical strategies, regardless of your training goal, to successfully use exercise as medicine while minimizing the risk of having to take medicine because you exercise.

When it comes to minimizing a training-related injury, almost everyone is familiar with the old advice of "don't overdo it" and to avoid exercises that tend to put the body into an awkward position, such as end-range spine movements (e.g., performing deadlifts with your back fully rounded forward). Although that advice is fine, far more can be added to the conversation.

The following are a variety of general, practical exercise programming strategies you can immediately use, along with the rationale behind why they can help you reduce the risk of suffering a training-related injury.

Exercise Around Pain, Not Through It!

You're not helping the situation by exercising through pain that's aggravated by exercise. Although this should be obvious, many athletes and hardcore exercisers are stubborn and use exercises that cause pain—a practice that is often the product of letting your ego get the best of you. Continuing to perform exercises that cause pain could very well make things worse and lead to further damage, which could change a painful area from something one can easily train around to something that's more debilitating.

Don't exercise through pain; exercise *around* it. This recommendation isn't referring to the sensation associated with muscle fatigue. This refers to any aches and pains that exist outside the gym or that flare up when you perform certain exercise movements. Such problem areas may simply need time to heal through rest, or they may be injuries—compromised areas of the body that can no longer tolerate the same level of load and do not improve without appropriate care.

If an exercise hurts you—for whatever reason—find a modification or an alternative that doesn't hurt. There are plenty of exercise options in this book that can allow you to do just that.

Avoid Forcing End Ranges of Motion When Lifting

Generally, avoiding attempts to force end-range joint and spine actions is the way to go when lifting heavy loads or using medium loads for high repetitions. It has been demonstrated that as the spine reaches full flexion (i.e., being fully bent forward), such as can happen when performing deadlifts with an excessively rounded back, the support responsibilities of the spine are shifted from the muscles to the disks and ligamentous tissues (2). These shifts in shear loading associated with a fully flexed spine posture are quite dramatic and can easily cause excessive shear load (3). In spinal full flexion, not only is anterior shear loading higher, but the ligaments are also at risk of injury (4). Repetitive compressive loading in the spine can exceed tissue tolerance and cause injury (5). Therefore, maintaining a relatively neutral spine posture when lifting heavy loads, as directed in the exercise descriptions in this book, is sound training advice.

When joints are moved to their end range as you are lifting weights, the load is shifted from the contracting muscle to the noncontractile connective tissue (ligaments, joint capsules, etc.). This isn't good for two reasons: you're no longer providing as good a training load for the muscles, and you may injure or damage the other connective tissues. Now, weight training helps build those connective tissues as well, and tissue responds positively to load—they get stronger over time. You shouldn't be afraid to load your body by lifting challenging weights. But loading up your joints at the end ranges of motion while exercising doesn't have a good risk–benefit ratio.

Joints function very well in their middle ranges of motion, but they also need some full range of motion activity to stay healthy and maintain their current range of movement. To support that, doing some yoga or mobility drills, such as the exercises in chapter 5, Warm-Up and Mobility Exercises, can serve as a nice complement to comprehensive resistance training workouts. Because of its low-load, slow-paced nature, many yoga moves and mobility exercises require the joints and spine to move into their end range of motion, something that one usually doesn't get from weight training. They provide more activity variety and help give you a more well-rounded body that's not just stronger and leaner but also mobile.

Use Care with Previous Injuries

Injury risk is usually increased in those with a previous injury (6, 7, 8, 9). Most strength and conditioning professionals already know this, and clients and athletes will often tell trainers or coaches about previous injuries and return to training after rehabilitation. In addition to the advice about not forcing end-range joint motion and working around pain, here are other points to consider:

- Progress (i.e., increase) the load you lift and the amount you do (i.e., how many total sets and reps you perform) very carefully around injured areas.
- Be especially careful with movements and positions that were part of the previous injury (for example, a person who injured a knee coming down from a jump in basketball should be extra careful on single-leg jumping exercises).
- Don't neglect injured areas. Building strength around an injured joint is important. Specific training of injured areas has been shown to help prevent future injuries (10).

Single-leg exercises have been shown to potentially help reduce injury risk and are discussed in the following section.

Do Single-Leg Strength Exercises

The variety of research discussed in chapter 2, Function and Performance, comparing unilateral versus bilateral leg training demonstrated that both single-leg and double-leg exercises for the lower body optimize performance.

In addition to that, a study suggested using single-leg performance to detect deficits in unilateral force development (i.e., strength) (11), while another study demonstrated that a 15 percent or greater variance in closed kinetic chain strength (i.e., strength when your foot is on the ground) or movement control ability in single limb performance between the right and left leg (limb symmetry index) is a good indicator of increased injury risk (12).

With this in mind, it's important to regularly incorporate some single-leg training exercise variations into your training, regardless of the main exercise goal, to work on improving your single-leg control, strength, and strength endurance.

Improve Conditioning Levels

Fatigue is a risk factor in musculoskeletal injuries. Those with low levels of conditioning have been found to be at risk for injury in several studies (9,13,14,15,16). Therefore, improving your conditioning level can help you to become more resistant to fatigue and recover more quickly between fatiguing efforts and potentially reduce your risk of suffering an injury due to fatigue.

In addition to conditioning levels, total training load is emerging as a risk factor for injury (17). This is where the fine art of progressive overload comes in and was discussed in chapter 2. All exercise training is an applied stress to the body. This stress causes the body to adapt by becoming stronger, bigger, and fitter to accommodate the stress with more efficiency and to better tolerate it and reduce the chance of injury. Smart exercise training is about applying enough stress to the body—based on your current ability—to make it adapt without applying too much stress and overloading the tissues to the point where they become damaged. Be patient and smart when you're exercising. Don't try to do too much, too fast.

Don't Smoke

It's no secret that smoking is generally bad for human health, but some studies have demonstrated that it is also can be a risk factor for injury (9, 18, 19, 20). Smoking is a consistent risk factor for poor recovery after injury and poor healing, so there is good reason to avoid smoking, both to reduce injury risk and to improve recovery after an injury or surgery.

Get Enough Sleep

There has been an increasing interest in the science of sleep and its effect on health, illness, fat loss, and athletic performance. A major modifiable risk factor for training injury risk might be right in front of everyone—in one's bedroom.

Adolescents and adults not getting 7 to 10 hours of sleep per night may be at increased risk of injury (21,22,23,24). Reviewing appropriate sleep guidelines (21,22,25) for performance enhancement and injury reduction is a solid, evidence-based practice for everyone.

This chapter identified several potential risk factors for injury and then provided generalized, simple, and practical exercise recommendations you can immediately use—strategies that have been used to design the workout programs in this book—to reduce the risk of suffering an exercise- or sports-related injury.

Remember that risk factors aren't guarantees. Having one of these factors present doesn't doom you to injury, and having none of them does not guarantee an injury-free future. These factors vary in predictive ability and relevance across different groups of individuals, and the recommendations here are considered a practical interpretation for you to apply.

It's important to note that many people confuse identifying risk factors for making promises. A good example of this confusion is tobacco use. For example, health organizations don't say that science has shown that tobacco use causes cancer; they say that tobacco use greatly increases the risk of developing cancer (and dying from it). Just because someone does not have an injury from the risk factors identified doesn't mean the general training recommendations are wrong, any more than one's grandfather smoking until age 95 doesn't disprove the general health recommendations on tobacco use.

Take this opportunity to think about the next steps on your exercise journey. What is your main exercise goal: fat loss, muscle building, improved performance, or general fitness and health? You now have the programming path toward it and the knowledge to be well on your way to success. There's a saying to "plan your work, then work your plan." This book has the right game plan, regardless of your goal. Now it's time for you to work the plan!

The great thing about exercise is that it works if you work it! As with most worthwhile things in life, the main building block you need for continued success in exercise is consistent effort. Be patient, be realistic, and be consistent in your effort. When you continue to lay a foundation of effort, you can build just about anything on it.

References

Chapter 1   Fitness

1. Malik S, Wong ND, Franklin SS, et al. Impact of the metabolic syndrome on mortality from coronary heart disease, cardiovascular disease, and all causes in United States adults. *Circulation*. 2004;110(10):1245-50.

2. Hunter GR, Brock DW, Byrne NM, Chandler-Laney PC, Del Corral P, Gower BA. Exercise training prevents regain of visceral fat for 1 year following weight loss. *Obesity* (Silver Spring). 2010;18(4):690-5.

3. FitzGerald SJBC, Kampert JB, Morrow Jr JR, Jackson AW, Blair SN. Muscular fitness and all-cause mortality: a prospective study. *J Phys Act Health*. 2004;1:7-18.

4. Tanasescu M, Leitzmann MF, Rimm EB, Willett WC, Stampfer MJ, Hu FB. Exercise type and intensity in relation to coronary heart disease in men. *JAMA*. 2002;288(16):1994-2000.

5. Brill PA, Macera CA, Davis DR, Blair SN, Gordon N. Muscular strength and physical function. *Med Sci Sports Exerc*. 2000;32(2):412-6.

6. Puetz TW. Physical activity and feelings of energy and fatigue: epidemiological evidence. *Sports Med*. 2006;36(9):767-80.

7. Maimoun L, Sultan C. Effects of physical activity on bone remodeling. *Metabolism*. [Epub ahead of print]. 2010 [cited 2010 Mar 30].

8. Slemenda C, Heilman DK, Brandt KD, et al. Reduced quadriceps strength relative to body weight: a risk factor for knee osteoarthritis in women? *Arthritis Rheum*. 1998;41(11):1951-9.

9. Suominen H. Muscle training for bone strength. *Aging Clin Exp Res*. 2006;18(2):85-93.

10. Miller MC. Understanding depression. Boston: Harvard Medical School. 2011 Mar 1. Available from: http://hrccatalog.hrrh.on.ca/InmagicGenie/DocumentFolder/understanding%20 depression.pdf

11. Schoenfeld TJ, Rada P, et al. Physical exercise prevents stress-induced activation of granule neurons and enhances local inhibitory mechanisms in the dentate gyrus. *J Neurosci*. 2013 May 1;33(18):7770-7.

12. Laurin D, et al. Physical activity and risk of cognitive impairment and dementia in elderly persons. *Arch Neurol*. 2001 Mar;58(3):498-504.

13. Friedland, RP, et al. Patients with Alzheimer's disease have reduced activities in midlife compared with healthy control-group members. Proceeding of the National Academy of Sciences of USA. 2001 Mar 13;98(6):3440-5.

14. Driver HS, Taylor SR. Exercise and sleep. *Sleep Med Rev*. 2000 Aug;4(4):387-402.

15. Lee D, Pate RR, Lavie CJ, Sui X, Church TS, Blair SN. Leisure-time running reduces all-cause and cardiovascular mortality risk. *J Am Coll Cardiol*. 2014;64(5):472-81. doi:10.1016/j.jacc.2014.04.058

16. Zuhl M, Kravitz L. HITT vs. continuous endurance training: battle of the aerobic titans. *IDEA Fitness Journal*. 2012 Feb. www.ideafit.com/fitness-library/hiit-vs-continuous-endurance-training-battle-of-the-aerobic-titans

17. Mikkola J, Rusko H, et al. Neuromuscular and cardiovascular adaptations during concurrent strength and endurance training in untrained men. *Int J Sports Med*. 2012;33(9):702-10.

18. Harber MP, et al. Aerobic exercise training induces skeletal muscle hypertrophy and age-dependent adaptations in myofiber function in young and older men. *J Appl Physiol*. 2012;113(9):1495-504.

19. Konopka AR, Harber M. Skeletal muscle hypertrophy after aerobic exercise training. *Exerc Sport Sci Rev*. 2014;42(2):53-61.

20. Chtara M, Chamari K, Chaouachi M, Chaouachi A, Koubaa D, Feki Y, et al. Effects of intra-session concurrent endurance and strength training sequence on aerobic performance and capacity. *Br J Sports Med*. 2005;39(8):555-60.

21. Kang, J, Ratamess, N. Which comes first: resistance before aerobic exercise or vice versa? *ACSM Health Fit J*. 2014 Jan/Feb;18(1):9-14.

22. Kang J, Rashti SL, Tranchina CP, Ratamess NA, Faigenbaum AD, Hoffman JR. Effect of preceding resistance exercise on metabolism during subsequent aerobic session. *Eur J Appl Physiol.* 2009;107(1):43-50.

23. Dudley GA, Djamil R. Incompatibility of endurance- and strength-training modes of exercise. *J Appl Physiol.* 1985;59(5):1446-51.

24. Kraemer WJ, Patton JF, Gordon SE, Harman EA, Deschenes MR, Reynolds K, et al. Compatibility of high-intensity strength and endurance training on hormonal and skeletal muscle adaptations. *J Appl Physiol.* 1995;78(3):976-89.

25. Leveritt M, Abernethy PJ. Acute effects of high-intensity endurance exercise on subsequent resistance activity. *J Strength Cond Res.* 1999;13(1):47-51.

26. Goto K, Ishii N, Sugihara S, Yoshioka T, Takamatsu K. Effects of resistance exercise on lipolysis during subsequent submaximal exercise. *Med Sci Sports Exerc.* 2007;39(2):308-15.

Chapter 2   Function and Performance

1. Swinton PA, et al. Regression models of sprint, vertical jump, and change of direction performance. *J Strength Cond Res.* 2014 Jul;28(7):1839-48.

2. Sheppard JM, Triplett NT. Program design for resistance training. In: Haff GG, Triplett, NT, editors. *NSCA's Essentials of Strength Training and Conditioning.* (4th ed.) Champaign (IL): Human Kinetics; 2016. p. 439-69.

3. Mangine, GT, et al. Resistance training intensity and volume affect changes in rate of force development in resistance-trained men. *Eur J Appl Physiol.* 2016;116:2367. doi:10.1007/s00421-016-3488-6

4. Tumminello, N. Resistance exercise programming: a mixed training approach. *Personal Training Quarterly* 2015;2(3):8-11.

5. Haff, GH. Resistance training program design. In: Coburn JW, Malek MH, editors. *NSCA's Essentials of Personal Training.* 2nd ed. Champaign (IL): Human Kinetics; 2012. p. 347-388.

6. Santana JC. *Functional Training.* Champaign (IL): Human Kinetics; 2016. p.13-25.

7. Speirs D, et al. Unilateral vs. bilateral squat training for strength, sprints, and agility in Academy rugby players. *J. Strength Cond Res.* 2016 Feb;30(2):386-92.

8. Rube N, Secher NH. Effect of training on central factors in fatigue follows two- and one-leg static exercise in man. *Acta Physiol Scand.* 1991;141(1):87-95.

9. Hakkinen, K, Kallinen, M, Linnamo, V, Pastinen, UM, Newton, RU, and Kraemer, WJ. Neuromuscular adaptations during bilateral versus unilateral strength training in middle-aged and elderly men and women. *Acta Physiol Scand.* 1996:158(1): 77-88.

10. Schoenfeld BJ, et al. Differential effects of heavy versus moderate loads on measures of strength and hypertrophy in resistance-trained men. *J Sports Sci Med.* 2016 Dec;15(4):715-22.

11. Coyle EF, et al. Specificity of power improvements through slow and fast isokinetic training. *J Appl Physiol Respir Environ Exerc Physiol.* 1981 Dec;51(6):1437-42.

12. Mora-Custodio R, et al. Effect of low- vs moderate-load squat training on strength, jump and sprint performance in physically active women. *Int J Sports Med* 2016;37(06):476-82.

13. Schoenfeld BJ, et al. Effects of low- vs. high-load resistance training on muscle strength and hypertrophy in well-trained men. *J Strength Cond Res.* 2015 Oct;29(10):2954-63.

14. De Salles BF, et al. Rest interval between sets in strength training. *Sports Med.* 2009;39(9):765-77.

15. Lyons BD, Hoffman BJ, Michel JW, Williams KJ. On the predictive efficiency of past performance and physical ability: the case of the National Football League. *Hum Perform.* 2011;24(2):158-72.

16. Kuzmits FE, Adams AJ. The NFL combine: does it predict performance in the National Football League? *J Strength Cond Res.* 2008 Nov;22(6):1721-7.

17. Bazyler, CD, et al. The efficacy of incorporating partial squats in maximal strength training. *J Strength Cond Res.* 2014 Nov;28(11):3024-32.

18. Anderson KG, Behm DG. Maintenance of EMG activity and loss of force output with instability. *J Strength Cond Res.* 2004 Aug;18(3):637-40

19. Willardson, J. The effectiveness of resistance exercises performed on unstable equipment. *Strength Cond J.* 2004;26. doi:10.1519/00126548-200410000-00015

20. Whiting WC, Stuart R. *Dynatomy: dynamic human anatomy*. Human Kinetics 2006. Available from: www.humankinetics.com/excerpts/excerpts/Five-factors-determine-stability-and-mobility

21. Askling C, Karlsson J, Thorstensson A. (2003), Hamstring injury occurrence in elite soccer players after preseason strength training with eccentric overload. *Scand J Med Sci Sports*. 2003;13:244-250. doi:10.1034/j.1600-0838.2003.00312

22. Schoenfeld B, Contreras B, Tiryaki-Sonmez R, Wilson J, Kolber M, Peterson M. Regional differences in muscle activation during hamstrings exercise. *Journal Strength Cond Res*. 2014;29.

23. Whittaker JL, Small C, Maffey L, et al. Risk factors for groin injury in sport: an updated systematic review. *Br J Sports Med*. 2015;49:803-9.

24. Tyler TF, et al. The association of hip strength and flexibility with the incidence of adductor muscle strains in professional ice hockey players. *Am J Sports Med*. 2001 Mar-Apr;29(2):124-8.

25. Pereira GR, Leporace G, Chagas D, et al. Influence of hip external rotation on hip adductor and rectus femoris myoelectric activity during a dynamic parallel squat. *J Strength Cond Res* 2010;24:2749-54.

26. Clark DR, Lambert MI, Hunter AM. Muscle activation in the loaded free barbell squat: a brief review. *J Strength Cond Res* 2012;26:1169-78.

27. Dwyer MK, Boudreau SN, Mattacola CG, Uhl TL, Lattermann C. Comparison of lower extremity kinematics and hip muscle activation during rehabilitation tasks between sexes. *J Athl Train*. 2010;45(2):181-90. doi:10.4085/1062-6050-45.2.181

Chapter 3   Fat Loss

1. Aragon AA, Schoenfeld BJ, Wildman R, et al. International society of sports nutrition position stand: diets and body composition. *J Int Soc Sports Nutr*. 2017;14:16. doi:10.1186/s12970-017-0174-y

2. Poortmans JR, Dellalieux O. Do regular high-protein diets have potential health risks on kidney function in athletes? *Int J Sport Nutr Exerc Metab*. 2000;10(1):28-38.

3. Martin WF, Armstrong LE, Rodriguez NR. Dietary protein intake and renal function. *Nutr Metab*. 2005;2:25. doi:10.1186/1743-7075-2-25

4. Heaney RP. Effects of caffeine on bone and the calcium economy. *Food Chem Toxicol*. 2002;40(9):1263-70.

5. Kerstetter JE, et al. Low protein intake: the impact on calcium and bone homeostasis in humans. *J Nutr*. 2003;133(3):855S-61S.

6. Porter KH, Johnson MA. Dietary protein supplementation and recovery from femoral fracture. *Nutr Rev*. 1998 Nov;56(11):337-40.

7. Clark JE. Diet, exercise or diet with exercise: comparing the effectiveness of treatment options for weight-loss and changes in fitness for adults (18–65 years old) who are overfat, or obese; systematic review and meta-analysis. *J Diabetes Metabolic Disord*. 2015;14:31.

8. Tumminello, N. *Strength training for fat loss*. Champaign (IL): Human Kinetics; 2014. pp. 7-9.

9. Willis LH, et al. Effects of aerobic and/or resistance training on body mass and fat mass in overweight or obese adults. *J App Phys*. 2012;113(12):1831-7.

10. Wallace MB, et al. Effects of cross-training on markers of insulin resistance/hyperinsulinemia. *Med Sci Sports Exerc*. 1997 Sep;29(9):1170-5.

11. Iglay HB, et al. Resistance training and dietary protein: effects on glucose tolerance and contents of skeletal muscle insulin signaling proteins in older persons. *Am J Clin Nutr*. 2007 Apr;85(4):1005-13.

12. Dolezal B, Potteiger J. Concurrent resistance and endurance training influence basal metabolic rate in nondieting individuals. *Journal Appl Physiol* (1985). 1998;85:695-700. doi:10.1152/jappl.1998.85.2.695

13. Josse AR, et al. Body composition and strength changes in women with milk and resistance exercise. *Med Sci Sports Exerc*. 2010 Jun;42(6):1122-30.

14. Urbanchek MG, Picken EB, Kalliainen LK, Kuzon WM. Specific force deficit in skeletal muscles of old rats is partially explained by the existence of denervated muscle fibers. *J Gerontol A Biol Sci Med Sci*. 2001 May;56(5):B191-7.

15. Farvid MS, et al. Association of adiponectin and resistin with adipose tissue compartments, insulin resistance and dyslipidaemia. *Diabetes Obes Metab*. 2005 Jul;7(4):406-13

16. Stallknecht B, et al. Are blood flow and lipolysis in subcutaneous adipose tissue influenced by contractions in adjacent muscles in humans? *Am J Physiol Endocrinol Metab* 2007 Feb;292(2):E394-9.

17. Kostek MA, et al. Subcutaneous fat alterations resulting from an upper-body resistance training program. *Med Sci Sports Exerc*. 2007 Jul;39(7):1177-85.

18. Ramírez-Campillo R, et al. Regional fat changes induced by localized muscle endurance resistance training. *J Strength Cond Res*. 2013 Aug;27(8):2219-24.

19. Vispute SS, et al. The effect of abdominal exercise on abdominal fat. *J Strength Cond Res*. 2011 Sep;25(9):2559-64.

20. Katch FI, et al. Effects of sit-up exercise training on adipose cell size and adiposity. *Res Q Exerc Sport*. 1984;55(3):242-7.

Chapter 4   Physique

1. Schoenfeld BJ. The mechanisms of muscle hypertrophy and their application to resistance training. *J Strength Cond Res*. 2010 Oct;24(10):2857-72.

2. Mitchell CJ, Churchward-Venne TA, West DWD, et al. Resistance exercise load does not determine training-mediated hypertrophic gains in young men. *J Appl Physiol*. 2012;113(1):71-7.

3. Arandjelović O. Does cheating pay: the role of externally supplied momentum on muscular force in resistance exercise. *Eur J Appl Physiol*. 2013 Jan;113(1):135-45.

4. Pinto RS, et al. Effect of range of motion on muscle strength and thickness. *J Strength Cond Res*. 2012 Aug;26(8):2140-5.

5. Hartmann H, et al. Influence of squatting depth on jumping performance. *J Strength Cond Res*. 2012 Dec;26(12):3243-61.

6. McMahon GE, et al. Impact of range of motion during ecologically valid resistance training protocols on muscle size, subcutaneous fat, and strength. *J Strength Cond Res*. 2014 Jan;28(1):245-55.

7. Pereira PE, Motoyama Y, Esteves G, Carlos Quinelato W, Botter L, Tanaka K, Azevedo P. Resistance training with slow speed of movement is better for hypertrophy and muscle strength gains than fast speed of movement. *Int J Appl Exerc Physiol*. 2016;5:37-43.

Chapter 6   Upper-Body Exercises

1. Signorile JF, Zink AJ, Szwed SP. A comparative electromyographical investigation of muscle utilization patterns using various hand positions during the lat pull-down. *J Strength Cond Res*. 2002 Nov;16(4):539-46.

2. Andersen V, Fimland M, Wiik E, Skoglund A, Saeterbakken A. Effects of grip width on muscle strength and activation in the lat pull-down. *J Strength Cond Res*. 2014;28:1135-42.

3. Contreras B, et al. The biomechanics of the push-up: implications for resistance training programs. *Strength Cond J*. 2011 Oct;34(5):41-6.

4. Schoenfeld B, et al. Effect of hand position on EMG activity of the posterior shoulder musculature during a horizontal abduction exercise. *J Strength Cond Res*. 2013 Oct;27(10):2644-9.

5. Reinold MM, Wilk KE, et al. Electromyographic analysis of the rotator cuff and deltoid musculature during common shoulder external rotation exercises. *J Orthop Sports Phys Ther*. 2004 Jul;34(7):385-94.

6. McAllister MJ, et al. Effect of grip width on electromyographic activity during the upright row. *J Strength Cond Res*. 2013 Jan;27(1):181-7.

7. Schoenfeld B, et al. The upright row: implications for preventing subacromial impingement *Strength Cond J*. 2011 Oct;33(5):25-8.

8. Cools A, Borms D, Cottens S, Himpe M, Meersdom S, Barbara C. Rehabilitation exercises for athletes with biceps disorders and slap lesions a continuum of exercises with increasing loads on the biceps. *Am J Sports Med*. 2014;42:1315-22.

9. Johnston TB. Movements of the shoulder joint—a plea for use of "plane of the scapula" as a plane of reference for movements occurring in at humeroscapula joint. *Br J Surg*. 1937; 25:252.

10. Greenfield B. Special considerations in shoulder exercises: plane of the scapula. In: Andrews JR, Wilk KE. *The athlete's shoulder*. New York: Churchill Livingstone; 1994: 513-22.

11. Flatow EL, et al. Excursion of the rotator cuff under the acromion. Patterns of subacromial contact. *Am J Sports Med*. 1994 Nov-Dec;22(6):779-88.

Chapter 7   Lower-Body Exercises

1. Zalawadia A, et al. Study of femoral neck anteversion of adult dry femora in Gujarat region. *NJIRM*. 2010 Jul-Sep;1(3):7-11.

2. Kingsley PC, Olsmtead KL. A study to determine the angle of anteversion of the neck of femur. *Journ Bone Joint Surg* 1948;30-A:745-51.

3. D'lima DD, Urquhart AG, Buehler KO, Walker RH, Colwell CW. The effect of the orientation of the acetabular and femoral components on the range of motion of the hip at different head-neck ratios. *J Bone Joint Surg Am*. 2000;82:315-21.

4. Yi C, Ma C, Wang Q, Zhang G, Cao Y. Acetabular configuration and its impact on cup coverage of a subtype of Crowe type 4 DDH with bi-pseudoacetabulum. *Hip Int*. 2013;23:135-42.

5. Swinton PA, et al. A biomechanical analysis of straight and hexagonal barbell deadlifts using submaximal loads. *J Strength Cond Res* 2011;25(7):2000-2009.

6. Youdas JW, Hollman JH, Hitchcock JR, Hoyme GJ, Johnsen JJ. Comparison of hamstring and quadriceps femoris electromyographic activity between men and women during a single-limb squat on both a stable and labile surface. *J Strength Cond Res*. 2007 Feb;21(1):105-11.

7. Kannus P, Beynnon B. Peak torque occurrence in the range of motion during isokinetic extension and flexion of the knee. *Int J Sports Med*. 1993 Nov;14(8):422-26.

8. Anderson AF, Dome DC, Gautam S, Awh MH, Rennirt GW. Correlation of anthropometric measurements, strength, anterior cruciate ligament size, and intercondylar notch characteristics to sex differences in anterior cruciate ligament tear rates. *Am J Sports Med*. 2001 Jan-Feb;29(1):58-66.

9. Griffin LY, Agel J, Albohm MJ, et al. Noncontact anterior cruciate ligament injuries: risk factors and prevention strategies. *J Am Acad Orthop Surg*. 2000 May-Jun;8(3):141-150.

10. Tumminello, N, Vigotsky, A. Are the seated leg extension, leg curl, and adduction machine exercises non-functional or risky? *Personal Training Quarterly*. 2017:4(4).

Chapter 8   Core Exercises

1. Martuscello JM, et al. Systematic review of core muscle activity during physical fitness exercises. *J Strength Cond Res*. 2013 Jun;27(6):1684-98.

2. Prieske O, et al. The role of trunk muscle strength for physical fitness and athletic performance in trained individuals: a systematic review and meta-analysis. *Sports Med*. 2016 Mar;46(3):401-19.

3. Nuzzo JL, et al. Trunk muscle activity during stability ball and free weight exercises. *J Strength Cond Res*. 2008 Jan;22(1):95-102.

4. Wilk BR, Stenback JT, Gonzalez C, Jagessar C, Nau S, Muniz A. Core muscle activation during Swiss ball and traditional abdominal exercises. *J Orthop Sports Phys Ther*. 2010;40:538-9; author reply 539.

5. Gottschall JS, Mills J, Hastings B. Integration core exercises elicit greater muscle activation than isolation exercises. *J Strength Cond Res*. 2013 Mar;27(3):590-6.

6. Schoenfeld BJ, Morey J. Abdominal crunches are/are not a safe and effective exercise. *Stren Cond Jour*. 2016 Dec;38(6):61-4.

Chapter 15   Strategies for Minimizing Injury

1. Keogh JW, Winwood PW. The epidemiology of injuries across the weight-training sports. *Sports Med*. 2016 Jun;21.

2. McGill SM, Kippers V. Transfer of loads between lumbar tissues during the flexion-relaxation phenomenon. *Spine*. 1994;19:2190.

3. McGill SM. The biomechanics of low back injury: implications on current practice in industry and the clinic. *J Biomech*. 1997;30:465-75.

4. McGill SM. Low back exercises: evidence for improving exercise regimens. *Phys Ther*. 1998 Jul;78(7):754-65.

5. Gooyers CE et al. Characterizing the combined effects of force, repetition and posture on injury pathways and micro-structural damage in isolated functional spinal units from sub-acute-failure magnitudes of cyclic compressive loading. *Clin Biomech* (Bristol, Avon). 2015 Nov;30(9):953-9.

6. van der Worp MP, et al. Injuries in runners; a systematic review on risk factors and sex differences. *PLoS One*. 2015 Feb 23;10(2):e0114937.

7. McCall A, et al. Injury risk factors, screening tests and preventative strategies: a systematic review of the evidence that underpins the perceptions and practices of 44 football (soccer) teams from various premier leagues. *Br J Sports Med*. 2015 May;49(9):583-9.

8. Saragiotto BT, et al. What are the main risk factors for running-related injuries? *Sports Med*. 2014 Aug;44(8):1153-63.

9. Zambraski EJ, Yancosek KE. Prevention and rehabilitation of musculoskeletal injuries during military operations and training. *J Strength Cond Res*. 2012 Jul;26(Suppl 2):S101-6.

10. Leppänen M, et al. Interventions to prevent sports related injuries: a systematic review and meta-analysis of randomised controlled trials. *Sports Med*. 2014 Apr;44(4):473-86.

11. Myer GD, et al. No association of time from surgery with functional deficits in athletes after anterior cruciate ligament reconstruction: evidence for objective return-to-sport criteria. *Am J Sports Med*. 2012 Oct;40(10):2256-63.

12. Rohman E, et al. Changes in involved and uninvolved limb function during rehabilitation after anterior cruciate ligament reconstruction: implications for Limb Symmetry Index measures. *Am J Sports Med*. 2015 Jun;43(6):1391-8.

13. Bulchazelli MT, et al. Injury during U.S. Army basic combat training: a systematic review of risk factor studies. *Am J Prev Med*. 2014 Dec;47(6):813-22.

14. Malone S, et al. Aerobic fitness and playing experience protect against spikes in workload: the role of the acute:chronic workload ratio on injury risk in elite Gaelic football. *Int J Sports Physiol Perform*. 2016 Aug 24:1-25.

15. Watson A, et al. Preseason aerobic capacity is an independent predictor of in-season injury in collegiate soccer players. *Clin J Sport Med*. 2016 Jun 22.

16. Jones BH, Hauschild VD. Physical training, fitness, and injuries: lessons learned from military studies. *J Strength Cond Res*. 2015 Nov;29(Suppl 11):S57-64.

17. Jones CM, et al. Training load and fatigue marker associations with injury and illness: a systematic review of longitudinal studies. *Sports Med*. 2016 Sep 28.

18. Bulzacchelli MT, et al. Injury during U.S. Army basic combat training: a systematic review of risk factor studies. *Am J Prev Med*. 2014 Dec;47(6):813-22.

19. Kaufman KR, Brodine S, Shaffer R. Military training-related injuries: surveillance, research, and prevention. *Am J Prev Med*. 2000 Apr;18(3 Suppl):54-63.

20. Van Middelkoop M. Risk factors for lower extremity injuries among male marathon runners. *Scand J Med Sci Sports*. 2008 Dec;18(6):691-7.

21. Yarnell AM, Deuster P. Sleep as a strategy for optimizing performance. *J Spec Oper Med*. 2016 Spring;16(1):81-5.

22. Simpson NS, Gibbs EL, Matheson GO. Optimizing sleep to maximize performance: implications and recommendations for elite athletes. *Scand J Med Sci Sports*. 2016 Jul 1.

23. Milewski MD, et al. Chronic lack of sleep is associated with increased sports injuries in adolescent athletes. *J Pediatr Orthop*. 2014 Mar;34(2):129-33.

24. Uehli K, et al. Sleep problems and work injuries: a systematic review and meta-analysis. *Sleep Med Rev*. 2014 Feb;18(1):61-73.

25. American Sleep Association. What is sleep? Available from: www.sleepassociation.org/patients-general-public/what-is-sleep

About the Author

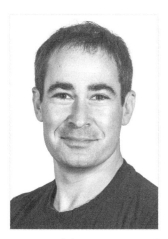

Nick Tumminello is the owner of Performance University International, which provides strength training and conditioning for athletes and educational programs for trainers and coaches all over the world.

As an educator, Tumminello has become known as the trainer of trainers. He has presented at international fitness conferences in Australia, Norway, Iceland, China, and Canada. He has been a featured presenter at conferences held by such organizations as the IDEA Health & Fitness Association and the National Strength and Conditioning Association (NSCA), along with conducting staff trainings at fitness clubs throughout the United States. Tumminello does workshops and mentorship programs in his hometown of Fort Lauderdale, Florida. He is the author of *Building Muscle and Performance* (Human Kinetics, 2016) and *Strength Training for Fat Loss* (Human Kinetics, 2014). He has produced more than 20 instructional DVDs and is the coauthor of the National Strength and Conditioning Association's *Program Design Essentials* and *Foundations of Fitness Programming*. Tumminello is also the editor in chief of the National Strength and Conditioning Association's *Personal Training Quarterly (PTQ)* journal.

Tumminello has been a fitness professional since 1998 and co-owned a private training center in Baltimore, Maryland, from 2001 to 2011. He has worked with a variety of exercise enthusiasts of all ages and fitness levels, including physique and performance athletes from the amateur level to the professional ranks. From 2002 to 2011, Tumminello was the strength and conditioning coach for the Ground Control MMA fight team. He has been a consultant and expert for clothing and equipment companies such as Sorinex, Dynamax, Hylete, Reebok, and Power Systems.

Tumminello's articles have appeared in more than 50 major health and fitness magazines, including *Men's Health, Men's Fitness, Muscle and Performance, Women's Health, Oxygen, Fitness Rx*, and *TRAIN*. He is also a featured contributor to several popular fitness training websites. He has been on the advisory board for Yahoo! Health and has been featured in two exercise books on the *New York Times*–best seller list, on the home page of Yahoo! and YouTube, and in the *ACE Personal Trainer Manual*. In 2015 Tumminello was inducted into the Personal Trainer Hall of Fame. In 2016 he won the NSCA Personal Trainer of the Year.

Tumminello writes a popular fitness training blog at NickTumminello.com.

You read the book—now complete an exam to earn continuing education credit.

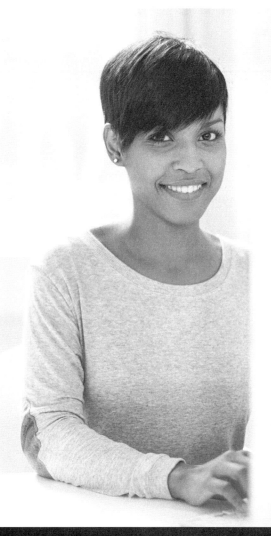

Congratulations on successfully preparing for this continuing education exam!

If you would like to earn CE credit, please visit

www.HumanKinetics.com/CE-Exam-Access

for complete instructions on how to access your exam.

Take advantage of a discounted rate by entering promo code **YWP2019** when prompted.

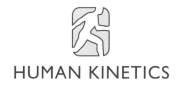

HUMAN KINETICS